ANNUAL PROGRESS IN CHILD PSYCHIATRY AND CHILD DEVELOPMENT 2002

Edited by
MARGARET E. HERTZIG, M.D.
Professor of Psychiatry
Cornell University Medical College

and

ELLEN A. FARBER, Ph.D.
Clinical Assistant Professor of Psychology
Cornell University Medical College

Routledge
Taylor & Francis Group
NEW YORK AND LONDON

This edition published 2012 by Routledge

Published in 2005 by
Routledge
Taylor & Francis Group
711 Third Avenue,
New York, NY 10017

Published in Great Britain by
Routledge
Taylor & Francis Group
27 Church Road
Hove, East Sussex BN3 2FA

Routledge is an imprint of Taylor & Francis Group
Formerly a Brunner-Routledge title.

First issued in paperback 2012

International Standard Book Number-13: 978-0-415-64587-4 (Paperback)
International Standard Book Number-13: 978-0-415-94917-0 (Hardcover)

Library of Congress Cataloging-in-Publication Data

Catalog record is available from the Library of Congress

T&F informa

Taylor & Francis Group
is the Academic Division of T&F Informa plc.

Visit the Taylor & Francis Web site at
http://www.taylorandfrancis.com

and the Routledge Web site at
http://www.routledgementalhealth.com

ANNUAL PROGRESS IN CHILD PSYCHIATRY AND CHILD DEVELOPMENT 2002

CONTENTS

INTRODUCTION

DEVELOPMENTAL TOPICS

The first section contains five papers on child development. The first two papers discuss attachment theory. Dozier and her colleagues present an intriguing study of foster parents' attachment organization and the resulting classification for the foster infants. Early placement, in the first 18 months of life, resulted in secure attachments when the foster parents were emotionally available. The authors contend that the concordance of the foster infant's attachment security with the foster parent's state of mind was similar to that among biologically intact families. This is an important finding relevant for both attachment researchers and for foster care practitioners. The Adult Attachment Instrument is cumbersome to score. Future work might address whether user-friendly measures of caregiver availability can be developed as useful screening methods for foster parents.

In the second paper, Schneider, Atkinson and Tardif present a meta-analytic study of close friendships. The attachment relationship that forms in infancy is considered important because it creates internal working models that children bring forward to new relationships. Schneider and colleagues summarize the data addressing the association of infant attachment with peer relationships. They found that overall sociability (likely a temperamental variable) is not that relevant. A low but consistent association between secure attachment and the ability to have close friends was found. This association provides support for the view that one comes away from infancy with models of how people will interact and notions that potential playmates might be receptive or rejecting. These internal working models play a part in shaping new relationships.

The third article describes relationships between parents and older children. Hock extends her research on separation anxiety with parents of infants to parents of adolescents. In this paper, Hock, Eberly, Bartle-Haring, Ellwanger and Widaman develop a measure of separation anxiety for parents of adolescents. After testing a number of items, they found a 35-item scale with two factors was useful. This paper briefly describes construct validity: a method for developing and assessing the utility of new measures. The paper cited by Cronbach and Meehl is a classic in the field of measurement and should be read by every professional to understand how to differentiate a well-established construct from a less well-established construct.

Hock's work with infants yielded three factors. In this study parents of older children were less concerned with routine absences than parents of infants. Hock and colleagues labeled the two factors from the new separation anxiety measure: anxiety about adolescent distancing and comfort with secure base role. The comfort with secure base role is a concept borrowed from the attachment literature. Parents who were comfortable being there when needed reported less conflictual communication with their adolescents. Parents of college seniors reported lower separation anxiety than parents of sixth through twelfth graders. Parents of adolescents have long known about parental separation anxiety but this is one of the few studies that attempted to define it and assess relationship correlates. This type of anxiety is within the realm of normal, functional anxiety.

The fourth paper in this section describes a study of fantasy play in young children. Dunn and Hughes found that the themes of children's fantasy play were significant. They chose a group of preschoolers who were described as "hard to manage" in the classroom and compared them to a group of "not difficult to manage" preschoolers. Each child was observed with a peer from their preschool class in a play setting. Both groups engaged in a variety of fantasy play themes. The "normal" group engaged in a greater percentage of benign play themes such as fantasy characters or doctors. The identified group had a greater percentage of violent themes and play episodes including killings and making arrests.

In addition to studying play themes, tests of social cognitive functioning were administered. The children with more violent fantasy themes had poorer performance on executive control tasks, more difficulty managing conflict with a peer, and somewhat more difficulty understanding others' thoughts. This intriguing study provides useful information that is relevant for clinical and developmental understanding.

The next paper is titled, "Ordinary Magic: Resilience Processes in Development." Once mental illness researchers realized that both genetic and environmental factors were important in developing disease, researchers began to delineate factors, such as life stress, that increased one's chance of developing mental illness. Initially, the focus was on why certain individuals developed mental illness. Eventually, researchers focused more on the group that did not develop mental health problems. What strengths or resources created this group of invulnerable or resilient individuals who despite having significant life stressors or a genetic predisposition for illness did not develop illness?

The field of resiliency research grew from the 1970s to include children with either the genetic predisposition or experiential stressors that put them at risk for psychopathology. The fifth paper in this section, by Ann Masten, is a cogent review of the topic of resilience. She adds an interesting spin as she reverses the direction of the resilience research questions. The typical question asked is what characteristics and environment enable children to do well in spite of adversity? Masten contends that resilience is the norm, that many children thrive. She reviews the current models and concepts in resilience research.

BIOLOGY AND BEHAVIOR

This section includes six papers that examine a range of topics, all of which expand our understanding of the biologic bases of behavior. The section opens with Moldavsky, Lev, and Lerman-Sagie's reference guide for psychiatrists of behavioral phenotypes of genetic syndromes. As these authors point out, it is only recently that geneticists have begun to recognize behavioral patterns specific to genetic syndromes, previously characterized only in terms of dysmorphology. A behavioral phenotype (Flint and Yule, 1994) is defined as the specific and characteristic behavioral repertoire exhibited by individuals with a genetic or chromosomal disorder. As such it includes cognitive, language, and social aspects of behavior as well as behavioral problems and psychopathology. As a causal relationship is implied between the genetic lesion and behavior, specific behavioral patterns must be consistently associated with the condition. However, just as in the case of physical phenotypes, not all individuals with the same syndrome will express the same abnormality to the same extent—variability of expression.

The authors review currently available information on the following 11 genetic/chromosomal conditions: Down Syndrome, Fragile X Syndrome, Rett Syndrome, Prader-Willi Syndrome, Angelman Syndrome, Smith-Magenis Syndrome, Isodicentric Chromosome 15, Williams Syndrome, Velocardiofacial Syndrome, Brunner Syndrome, and Turner Syndrome. Two useful tables summarize the cognitive features of genetic syndromes and commonly associated psychopathology. Updated knowledge of behavioral phenotypes of genetic syndromes is of considerable importance to clinicians who may be called upon to evaluate the behavior problems of affected children. The identification of presenting problems as part of a behavioral phenotype will pave the way for accurate genetic diagnosis, appropriate parental counseling regarding prognosis and risk in future pregnancies, as well as specific treatment recommendations.

In the second paper Asherson and Curran direct attention to the study of disorders that do not conform to Mendelian patterns of segregation, including autism, reading disability, and attention-deficit hyperactivity disorder (ADHD). In these conditions, the combined effects of several genes (oligogenic) or perhaps many genes (polygenic), each of which, on its own, has only a small effect, are thought to contribute to the emergence of an observable phenotype. Advances in molecular genetics enable the identification of genes involved in complex disorders and permit the study of molecular mechanisms and gene–environment interactions. Although mapping and identifying the genes responsible for such complex disorders is additionally complicated by the difficulties surrounding definition and the identification of heritable phenotypes, contemporary approaches to gene discovery are being applied to conditions arising during the developmental period.

In this paper, strategies employed in molecular genetic research including linkage analysis using multiply affected families, linkage analysis using affected sibling pairs, association strategies, quantitative trait loci mapping, genetic maps and high-throughput genotyping, and new approaches to very rapid genotyping are briefly but comprehensively reviewed. Progress toward the identification of susceptibility genes is illustrated by examples from autism, reading disability, and ADHD. Asherson and Curran predict that in the next 5 to 10 years susceptibility genes for these disorders will be established. However, as they go on to emphasize, the identification of susceptibility genes is only an initial step. Molecular genetic studies that aim to identify common genetic risk factors provide a starting point for expanding our understanding of gene–environment interactions. Further clarification of both genetic and environmental influences on child behavioral and neurodevelopmental disorders will require bridges between structure and function; between molecular mechanisms and behavior; and between social, genetic, and developmental psychiatry. This paper provides a thoughtful introduction to this challenging but potentially promising area of investigation.

In their report of the functional neuroanatomy of visuospatial working memory in fragile X syndrome, Kwon and colleagues examine relationships between genes and behavior from yet another perspective. These workers have used a working memory task to investigate deficits in higher-order cognition in subjects with fragile X syndrome. The syndrome arises from disruption in expression of the FMR1 gene, which is most commonly caused by expansion of a CGG repeat stretch in the gene, with resultant methylation and silencing of expression. The absence of the FMR1 gene product (FMRP) in neurons is associated with abnormal morphology of dendritic spines and a reduction in the length of synapses in the cortex. As neurophysiological studies have suggested that the prefrontal cortex plays a critical role in recent memory, and as subjects with fragile X syndrome show significant deficits in visuospatial cognition, as well as in executive functions, the authors hypothesized that individuals with fragile X will also exhibit significant impairment in visuospatial memory tasks.

This study examined brain activation in four regions of the cortex known to play a critical role in visuospatial working memory in 10 female subjects with fragile X and in 15 typically developing females as they performed both

1-back and 2-back visuospatial memory tasks. Relative to the comparison group, subjects with fragile X performed significantly more poorly on the 2-back task (which places a greater demand on working memory), but not on the 1-back task. The results of further region of interest and correlational analyses have led the authors to conclude that subjects with fragile X syndrome exhibit significant visuospatial working memory deficits that extend beyond the effects of differences in IQ that are correlated with abnormalities in activation in brain areas known to be involved in working memory. Moreover, FMRP expression was found to be correlated with brain activation, a finding that may reflect the involvement of this protein in the dynamic response to working memory load. The authors further suggest that as the gene defect in this disorder can be readily quantified, fragile X syndrome may serve as a model for bridging the gap between the molecular biology of neurogenetic disorders and their neuronal and behavioral manifestations.

As Siegel's review of the developmental, interpersonal and neurobiological aspects of memory clearly illustrates, working memory is but one of many aspects of this fundamental property of the human mind. Memory has been the focus of research of a wide range of academic disciplines including cognitive psychology, developmental psychology, neuropsychology, cognitive neuroscience, psychiatry, neurology, anthropology, and psycholinguistics. Siegel's review integrates clinically relevant concepts deriving from these various disciplines. Memory is broadly defined as the way past events affect future function. Information regarding the ways in which the brain processes and encodes information is briefly summarized as the process of memory is explicated. The types and characteristics of memory, most particularly implicit or nondeclarative memory and explicit or declarative memory, and their developmental course are described. Other topics considered include: the phases and timing of memory, the subjective experience of memory, childhood amnesia, trauma and memory, memory and the accuracy of recounting, and memory and narrative. The practicing clinician will find this review and the accompanying references an invaluable guide to the interpretation of clinical assessments of memory functioning as well as to current research on memory.

In the next paper in this section, Woodward, McManis, Kagan, Deldin, Snidman, Lewis, and Kahn examine possible associations between differences in temperamental organization and aspects of brain function. These authors begin their report by noting that the theoretical definition of human temperament lies at the interface of behavior and biology. However, most research on temperament has relied solely on behavioral variables derived from parental reports or direct observations. As the authors note, technical advances make it feasible to add biological measures to behavioral assessments. As the authors suggest, this strategy can be of importance because as children grow, the expected association between behavioral and biological correlates of infant temperament become attenuated in the laboratory setting, in part because the defining behaviors seen in very young children tend to become masked by the influences of socialization. Consequently, physiological measures might be of help in discriminating among older children who possess different temperaments early in life, but have become more behaviorally homogeneous with advancing age. In the reported study, 56 ten to twelve-year-old children, 32 if whom had been characterized as high reactives (15 boys and 17 girls) and 24 low reactives (16 boys and 8 girls) completed a 3-hour battery of physiological and behavioral tasks. The physiological task included the elicitation of brainstem auditory evoked response (BAER) while the behavioral variables included the determination of the number of smiles and number of spontaneous unprovoked remarks or elaborations made to the examiner.

The data revealed differences in the BAERs of preadolescent children that were in accord with their infant temperamental categories. Specifically, children who were high reactive infants had larger V-wave amplitudes than children who were low reactive infants, implying that the two temperamental groups differ in a significant property of brainstem function. However, as the authors note, the results of this study do not reveal the nature of that difference. Several alternative explanations requiring further experimentation to elucidate are offered. Moreover, no significant differences between high and low reactives for the mean number of smiles and spontaneous comments made to the examiner at the 10- to 12-year visit were found. Thus the data support the notion that behavioral distinctions between temperamental groups become increasingly subtle with development. Consequently, physiological variables become a critical addition to traditional behavioral batteries. Additionally, the authors suggest that because wave V magnitude appears to be a sensitive marker of a temperamental bias for infant reactivity, regardless of contemporary sociability, measurement of wave V as part of a larger test battery might help identify children and adolescents who are vulnerable to the development of anxious psychopathology.

The final paper in this section by Henderson, Fox, and Rubin examines yet another aspect of the interface between temperament and biology. As the authors point out, the majority of studies of relations between early temperament and later social and emotional development have followed a direct linkage model, in which early temperament is thought to be directly and linearly related to later adjustment. However, the degree of discontinuity in temperament-adjustment linkages is quite high, suggesting that other variables may well act to moderate social outcomes. In particular, frontal EEG asymmetry, which reflects the difference in the degree of activation between the left and right frontal regions, is a plausible candidate variable. A variety of data from adult clinical and normal populations, as well as from infant and child studies, suggests that the two sides of the frontal cortex may be differentially specialized for approach or withdrawal tendencies. Other bodies of data strongly suggest that gender may also potentially influence the relation between negative reactivity and social behavior.

This report summarizes the results of a longitudinal study of 97 children that explores these issues through an examination of the moderating roles of frontal electroencephalogram (EEG) asymmetry at 9 months and gender on relations between maternal reports of negative reactivity at 9 months of age and maternal ratings and laboratory observations of social wariness and sociability at 4 years of age. The data indicate that maternal report of negative reactivity during the first year of life, by itself, did not significantly predict either sociability or social wariness. However, negative emotionality was predictive of social wariness for infants who also displayed a pattern of right frontal EEG asymmetry at 9 months of age, but not for infants with a pattern of left frontal EEG asymmetry. Additionally, the influence of negative reactivity on social wariness was also moderated by gender with negative reactivity during infancy being positively related to social wariness for boys, but not for girls.

This report highlights the importance of temperamental differences in understanding the etiology of internalizing behaviors in young children. The authors suggest that clinicians should pay particular attention to patterns of temperamental negative reactivity in infants who may be predisposed to a pattern of right frontal EEG asymmetry (such as infants of depressed women) or a bias toward withdrawing from novelty. However, as the authors emphasize, simple fussiness or irritability does not predict risk for maladaptive social behavior. Rather it is the interaction of this particular temperamental bias with other biological and social factors that best accounts for variability in social outcome.

CLINICAL ISSUES

The five papers in this section focus on a range of issues of interest to clinicians. In the first paper, Chakrabarti and Fombonne report on the results of a study designed to estimate the prevalence of pervasive developmental disorders (PDDs) in a geographically defined population of preschool children residing in Staffordshire, England. Since the first epidemiological survey of autism was conducted in England in the mid-1960s more than 30 surveys have been performed worldwide. Rates of autism have typically been reported to range between 4 and 6 per 10,000 although to some extent these figures appear to have increased in the past 15 years. In addition the above quoted estimates do not account for a large group of children falling short of strict diagnostic criteria for autism but whose behavior is nonetheless characterized by disturbances in social relatedness, impairments in the ability to use language effectively for communicative purposes, and narrow and restricted interests (the other PDDs). In this survey, which was conducted between July 1998 and June 1999, 15,500 children aged 2.5 to 6.5 years were screened for developmental problems. Children with symptoms of PDD were intensively assessed by a multidisciplinary team, which conducted standardized diagnostic interviews and administered psychometric tests.

A total of 97 children (79.4% male) were confirmed to have a PDD. The prevalence of the PDDs was estimated to be 62.6%. Prevalences were 16.8 per 10,000 for autistic disorder and 45.8 for other PDDs. These results are consistent with the 57.9 and 67.4 per 10,000 reported in two other recent investigations, which also utilized intensive screening procedures, focused on children below the age of 10 years, and used modern standardized diagnostic measures such as the Autism Diagnostic Interview or the Autism Diagnostic Observation schedule. Whether the higher prevalence rates reported recently derive from a secular increase in the incidence of the disorder or merely reflect a broadening of the concept of PDD together with improved detection and recognition cannot be determined from these data. Nevertheless, a prevalence of approximately 60 per 10,000 children draws attention to the needs of a substantial minority of children. Additionally, the children with PDD identified during the course of the present survey as a group are less impaired than what has been classically described. Although the average rate of mental retardation was near 75% in previous autism surveys this rate has fallen to much lower figures of 40% to 50% in other recent surveys and was 26% in this survey. This shift has important implications for intervention as a considerable number of these children may well require education in mainstream schools with the provision of individual support. Moreover, as it is possible that very early intervention in autism and the other PDDs might be associated with improved cognitive outcome, it behooves clinicians to act promptly in the face of early identification of developmental delays and behavioral deviance in preschool children.

While it is clear that pharmacological treatments are only minimally effective on the core symptoms of autism and the other pervasive developmental disorders (PDDs): social withdrawal, lack of emotional reciprocity, and absent or stereotyped language, neuroleptic medications have been noted to be helpful in reducing hyperactivity, aggression, and temper tantrums in older children with PDD. Although clinicians often extrapolate information on older children, adolescents, or adults, downward to include the preschool age group, to date, little systematic information has been available regarding the safety and efficacy of neuroleptic treatment of very young children with PDD. In the second paper in this section, Masi, Cosenza, Mucci and Brovedani address this gap in their report of the results of an open trial of risperidone in 24 young children with PDDs and persistent uncontrollable behavior. The 24 subjects (21 boys and 3 girls) were clinically diagnosed with PDD (19 autistic, 5 PDD-NOS). In addition they had a Childhood Autism Rating Scale

(CARS) score greater than 30. Behavioral symptoms were assessed in each subject by two independent examiners at baseline and again at the end of the 16-week treatment. In addition to ratings of videotaped play sessions with a familiar adult, the following rating scales were completed on all patients at baseline and 16 weeks: Children's Psychiatric Rating Scale (CPRS), Clinical Global Impression-Improvement (CGI-I), and the CARS. All children were begun on a dose of 0.25 mg at bedtime. Subsequent titration was 0.25 mg with increments no more frequent than on weekly intervals, depending on a clinical response and occurrence of side effects to a maximum dose of 0.75 mg or 0.04 mg/kg.

Two children did not complete the trial because parents requested discontinuation because of side effects. One child experienced marked sedation and hyporexia after 2 weeks of treatment. The other child exhibited episodes of tachycardia after 7 days of treatment that did not recur after discontinuation. Other side effects were reported as follows: Subjects' mean weight increased from 20.18 kg to 21.31 kg. Three patients experienced a weight gain of more than 10%. In six children appetite increased and in three children it decreased. Three children exhibited modest agitation and/or enuresis. One child had transitory dystonic episodes involving the neck. No changes in blood count, liver enzymes, or ECG were noted. Modest improvements in behavior were reported. Items that improved more than 25% on the CPRS included hyperactivity, fidgetiness, rhythmic motions, lability of affect, angry affect, and withdrawal. Although controlled studies are required for confirmation, the results of this open trial are reassuring to clinicians in demonstrating that low-dose risperidone is well tolerated in preschool children and may well be effective in treating some aspects of autistic symptomatology.

Firesetting among children and adolescents is a prevalent and serious problem. In the fourth paper in this section, Kolk, Day, Bridge, and Kazdin provide a prospective evaluation of the course and predictors of children's involvement with fire over a 2-year period in a total of 268 (N =106 patients and N = 162 community non patient) children and adolescents. Cases with no history of treatment within the past 12 months were recruited through the Pittsburgh public school system, while outpatients were recruited after their assessment in an outpatient clinic serving children and youth and their families at Western Psychiatric Institute and Clinic. Children in both groups were predominantly male and ranged in age from 6 to 13 years. The child's firesetting status was assessed based on child and parent responses to the Firesetting History Screen (FHS). Screening questions evaluated the children's interest in fire, frequency of matchplay and firesetting, and if applicable the severity of firesetting. Three time periods were sampled on two separate occasions: at initial assessment the questionnaire was administered to reflect the child's firesetting history in two separate time periods, during the past 12 months and more than 12 months ago. At follow-up the questionnaire was readministered to obtain an interval history. Children were classified as firesetters if they were involved in burning some type of property or setting a fire as acknowledged by themselves or their parents. The definition included any act in which an object was burned or set on fire, including small objects, personal property, furniture, or a residence or structure. Children were classified as nonfiresetters if both sources agreed about the absence of firesetters. Nonfiresetters included children whose fireplay was limited to matchplay (e.g., playing with candles, striking matches). Across both periods, children were classified into one of four mutually exclusive firesetting history patterns. Among children with no initial history of firesetting, those who did vs. did not exhibit firesetting on follow-up were described as late-starters and controls, respectively. Among children with an initial history of firesetting, those who did vs. did not exhibit firesetting at follow-up were described as recidivists and desistors, respectively. A large number of other measures were utilized to measure the following constructs: fire-specific risk including curiosity and exposure to fire-related activities; child dysfunction and social competence; parental practices/dysfunction; and family functioning and stress.

Involvement with fire was high among both nonpatients and patients. During the current year, in the nonpatient sample there were 50 firesetters (31.3%), 15 matchplayers only (9.4%) and 95 nonfiresetters (59%). Similar percentages were found for the follow-up period. Among the patients, there were 44 firesetters (51.2%), 10 matchplayers only (11.6%) and 32 nonfiresetters (37.2%) initially, and similar percentages were also found at follow-up 2 years later. In terms of the course of firesetting in the two samples, 13% and 26% of the nonpatient and patient nonfiresetters at initial assessment became late-starters by 2-year follow-up respectively, whereas 50% and 59% of the firesetters in these two samples became recidivists. Overall, approximately half of a sample of firesetters will set at least one additional fire and a modest percentage of children will become firesetters for the first time within a 2-year period regardless of their patient status. The high frequency of occurrence of fire-related activities among patients not originally identified because of firesetting behavior underscores the importance of expanding routine assessment to include careful attention to obtaining a firesetting history.

In the fifth paper in this section, Cannon, Walsh, Hollis, Kargin, Taylor, Murray, and Jones utilize standard psychological data collected over many years from a large child psychiatric service to examine predictors of later schizophrenia and affective psychosis. Beginning in 1968, the Children's and Adolescent's Department of the Maudsley and Bethlem Royal Hospital has used a computer-based system of clinical data gathering, storage, and retrieval. The system uses an item sheet that employs Likert-type scales, which is completed in addition to the usual medical file. Each symptom or sign occurring over the past 12 months is rated by the assessing psychiatrist within 2 weeks of the child's initial evaluation as absent (0), minimal or dubious (1), or definitely present (2). The rated symptoms were grouped as follows: emotional symptoms; somatic symptoms; disturbances of relationships; speech and language; motor disturbances; antisocial behavior; and an assortment of socio-demographic and administrative variables. The cases that provided the data of the present report selected from among those discharges from the Maudsley Hospital Adult Psychiatric Service up to 1993 who had previously attended the Children's and Adolescent Department between 1968 and 1989. In total, 56 cases fulfilling ICD-10 criteria for schizophrenia and 24 fulfilling ICD-10 criteria for affective psychosis (bipolar affective disorder or severe depression with psychotic symptoms) were identified. The comparison group was selected as follows: The next four children, of the same age and gender, who were registered at the clinic after the index psychosis case were taken as the initial "raw" comparison group. Next, tracing, utilizing the resources of the National Health Service Central Register at the Office of Censuses and Surveys, the name of the relevant Family Health Service Authority (FHSA) was identified and provided the names of the general practitioner for each subject who then completed a questionnaire on the adult psychiatric history of each potential subject. The final sample available for analysis (7 data sheets were not able to be located) consisted of 59 childhood attendees with an adult diagnosis of schizophrenia, 27 childhood attendees with an adult diagnosis of affective psychosis (20 bipolar and 8 psychotic depression), and 86 childhood attendees who had not suffered mental illness during adulthood.

Data analysis proceeded in two stages: In the first stage, univariate analyses were conducted to separately identify items that were associated with later schizophrenia and later affective psychosis. In the second stage all variables that were associated significantly with schizophrenia or affective psychosis on univariate analyses were entered into multivariate analyses. After logistic regression, the final model for schizophrenia comprised two symptom variables ("abnormal suspiciousness or sensitivity" and "relationship difficulties") and two sociodemographic variables ("family psychiatric history" and "past psychiatric contact"). The positive predictive power of the model was 81.2% (26/32 cases correctly classified) and the model sensitivity was 65%. The final model for affective psychosis comprised three variables: "hysterical symptoms," "disturbance of eating," and "family psychiatric history." The positive predictive power of the model for affective cases was 63.6% (7/11 cases correctly classified) and the model sensitivity was 43.8%. The authors conclude that symptoms detected on routine psychological assessment can predict adult psychotic illness and that there appear to be separate childhood precursors for schizophrenia and affective psychosis. Strictly speaking the results apply only to children who attend a child psychiatry service. The predictive power of childhood symptoms is generally low in the general population owing to the high prevalence of childhood difficulties and the rarity of adult psychotic outcomes. This study underscores the value of systematically collected clinical data and the ability to reliably determine adult outcome in examining the childhood antecedents of serious psychiatric disorder in adults.

The final report in this section examines prediction from yet another vantage. Specifically, Ialongo, Edelsohn, and Kellam seek to determine the prognostic power of first graders' self-reports of depressed mood and feelings with respect to later psychopathology and adaptive functioning in a population of urban school children (N = 946). This study is rooted in an ongoing controversy over childhood depression. As the authors point out, after decades of debate there is a growing consensus that children as young as 8 or 9 years of age do experience depressive syndromes similar to those seen in adults in terms of social and cognitive impairment and symptom presentation. Additionally, there is general agreement that by the middle to late elementary school years children can provide reliable and valid reports of their symptoms. However, it is less clear whether or not children as young as 5 or 6 years can experience and report on depressive phenomena and feelings. This report is based on data gathered in the fall of the first grade and the spring of the fourth, sixth, and eighth grades. The data gathered in the first grade included children's self-reports responses to the Children's Depression Inventory (CDI) modified so as not to require reading skills as well as other demographic information and standardized achievement scores. Parent reports of child mental health service use were obtained in fourth and sixth grades. Teacher reports of the need for child mental health service use were obtained in the sixth grade. Grades and special education services use were also obtained in sixth grade from school records, along with grade retentions. Finally, child self-reports of depressive symptoms (including suicidal ideation and behavior) were obtained in eighth grade. After appropriate consolidation of the data and adjustments for missing data points, logistic regression analysis was used to examine the prognostic value of first graders' reports of depressed mood and feelings. All analyses were conducted separately by gender.

The principal findings of this series of meticulously conducted analyses are that first grade self-reports of depressed mood predicted later child academic functioning, the need for and use of mental health services, suicidal ideation, and a diagnosis of major depressive disorder by age 14. The authors interpret these results as providing support for the view that children as young as 5 or 6 years of age are capable of providing valid reports of depressed mood and feelings. Nevertheless, as they point out, these findings on prognostic power do not suggest a causal relation between a depressed mood in first grade and later mental health and academic outcomes. They offer several alternative explanations. The findings may simply reflect the fact that children who fail to meet the academic challenges of first grade are likely to experience emotional distress with early academic failures setting the stage for subsequent failures and increased punishment and reductions in reinforcement from parents, teachers, and peers. This chronic history of failure may result in sustained emotional distress and increased risk of major depressive disorder. Alternatively, it might be the case that a third variable—such as a chronically poor caregiving environment—may explain both social adaptational failures and decrements in psychological well being. Whatever may ultimately prove to be the mechanisms through which unhappy first graders develop later impairments with respect to academic and psychological functioning, the take-home message for clinicians as well as teachers is to seriously and systematically assess mood disturbances in young children with an eye to the development of appropriate intervention strategies.

CULTURE AND SOCIETY

The last section, titled "Culture and Society," has four papers dealing with societal or crosscultural issues. The first two papers are studies of children's adaptation after disasters. Studies of children's adaptation to disasters may be particularly informative to researchers and clinicians in the post–9/11 world. Studies of children's responses to other incidences of organized violence may inform us as to ways to proceed in the present.

Laor, Wolmer, and Cohen present data from a longitudinal study of children who experienced the 1991 Gulf War. The initial sample was 101 families who were exposed to SCUD missile attacks. Some of the families were displaced from their homes for up to 6 months and others remained in their homes. At the 5-year follow-up 81 families participated in the study. The initial sample of children were of preschool age. The children were first assessed 6 months after the missile attack and then again 2½ years and 5 years after the attack. The first two data points were summarized in other papers. Those papers summarized the symptoms of displaced preschool children and the association of parental reactions and children's reactions. Young children's reactions to trauma and displacement closely mirrored their mother's reactions.

This paper analyzed the reactions from the 5-year data. Children were assessed using the Child Behavior Checklist, the Preschool Children's Assessment of Stress Scale, and the Child Posttraumatic Stress Reaction Index. Mothers were assessed using the Bell Object Relations Inventory, the Defense Style Questionnaire, the SCL-90, the Impact of Event Scale, and the Gordon Test of Visual Imagery Control. At the 30-month assessment, mothers completed a measure of family cohesion, the FACES. Mothers were divided into three groups of functioning—poor, moderate, and good. Children's externalizing symptoms decreased over time irrespective of mother's functioning.

For some children, posttraumatic symptoms increased over time and for others they decreased. Family functioning and cohesiveness 30 months after the incident exerted a long-term effect on the children's symptoms. Also of significance was the finding that the caretaker was much more important for the younger child's processing of a traumatic event than for older children.

The next paper by Angel, Hjern, and Ingleby collected data on 99 children who relocated from Bosnia to Sweden following war in Bosnia in 1992. The authors emphasize that war trauma and PTSD are often studied as a unidimensional event. They highlighted that war trauma is multifaceted including exposure to violence, loss of home, loss of significant others, and other stressors. The authors' goals were to document the stressors that families are exposed to and the effect on children's mental health. They collected data 18 months after the families arrived in Sweden. Data collection involved interviews with parents alone and with parents and children together. The authors suggested that war-related stressors could be divided into five categories: violence, resistance, disruption, threat, and loss. The authors also created subscales for children's psychological symptoms based on the interview data. They named the subscales: behavior problems, generalized anxiety, and phobic and depressive symptoms.

In this study, about a third of the children were judged to suffer from post-traumatic stress symptoms. The authors describe the different types of stresses that children and families were exposed to before, during, and after displacement. Of particular interest was their finding that for children exposed to high levels of stress, parental encouragement of talking about the stress exacerbated their problems.

The notion that "working through" traumatic experiences is important to mental health was clearly seen following the September 11, 2001, terrorist attacks. Mental health professionals were asked to volunteer their time in crisis intervention centers set up by private businesses, hospitals, and the Red Cross. The paper by Angel, Hjern, and Ingleby did not support the notion that talking is uniformly therapeutic. Research now being conducted on children's reactions following the 9/11 incidents may inform us as to whether cross-cultural differences are partly accountable. Other factors are of course relevant including how the parent or therapist responds to the child's talking through.

The third paper by Doi, Roberts, Takeuchi, and Suzuki is a crosscultural study of Japanese and American adolescent depression. There have been epidemiological studies in the United States to identify rates of depression in nonidentified samples. However, little is known about the rate of adolescent depression in Japan. The authors wondered whether differences in emotional expression between Japanese and American cultures might lead to different rates of identification.

The paper describes why epidemiological research has not been undertaken previously in Japan including reluctance of school boards and parents to contact students, the lack of measures written in Japanese, and lack of knowledge about whether the standard diagnostic criteria developed for Western culture would be applicable to Japanese children.

As part of a large Teen Life Changes Survey study, questionnaires were administered to children in Houston, Texas, and in Japan. The Japanese children were in a public junior high school. The DISC, a standardized measure of depression, was used following three translations (translations and back-translation). Adolescents were designated as cases based on their self-reports on the questionnaires. Compared to youth living in Texas, the Japanese youth had lower rates of depression. The Texas sample was divided into three ethnic groups. African Americans and Mexican Americans had higher rates of depressions than Anglo Americans. The prevalence rates for the Japanese youth were 1.3% for major depression with impairment and 5.6% for major depression without impairment. In part, socioeconomic factors accounted for the differences in rates of depression. The authors concur that more research is needed to understand both incidence and meaning of depression in Japanese adolescents. They discuss the concept of etic and emic research and the need to include both orientations. Etic research refers to validity across cultures and emic research refers to concepts valid only within a culture.

The final paper deals with the cultural issues of emergency placement and child maltreatment. Ballou, Barry, Billingham, Boorstein, Butler and colleagues describe a procedure that can be used in emergency situations when judges need to make decisions without the benefit of an extended forensic evaluation. The important criteria that should be considered in forensic placement were cogently described in a series of books by Goldstein, Solnit, and Freud. The authors reference those authors as well as others who have written about standards for child placement. Family preservation and the best interests of the child are two concepts that are usually considered.

Using multidisciplinary focus and discussion groups, the authors identified six factors that should be considered in determining whether a child should be placed at home or out of the home. They present a six-factor psychological model to be used when there is not enough time for a standard forensic evaluation. The experts they consulted described six factors: (1) caretaker's history of behavior/relationship with the child, (2) caretaker's history of violent behavior, (3) caretaker's substance abuse, (4) caretaker's major mental illness, (5) caretaker's adaptive coping skills, and (6) other considerations. Each of these factors was defined as clearly as possible with an attempt to limit psychological jargon. This study presents an important first step in producing a measure useful for child placement that combines legal and psychological research on child maltreatment and placement. It is an interesting discussion of social policy research.

REFERENCES

Flint, J., & Yule, V. (1994). Behavioral phenotypes. In M. Rutter, E. Taylor, & L. Hersov (Eds.), *Child and Adolescent Psychiatry*. Oxford, England: Blackwell Scientific Publications.

Part I

DEVELOPMENTAL TOPICS

1

Attachment for Infants in Foster Care: The Role of Caregiver State of Mind

Mary Dozier, K. Chase Stovall, Kathleen E. Albus, and Brady Bates

The concordance between foster mothers' attachment state of mind and foster infants' attachment quality was examined for 50 foster mother–infant dyads. Babies had been placed into the care of their foster mothers between birth and 20 months of age. Attachment quality was assessed between 12 and 24 months of age, at least 3 months after the infants' placement into foster care. The two-way correspondence between maternal state of mind and infant attachment quality was 72%, $\kappa = .43$, similar to the level seen among biologically intact mother–infant dyads. Contrary to expectations, age at placement was not related to attachment quality. Rather, concordance between maternal state of mind and infant attachment was seen for relatively late-placed babies, as well as early-placed babies. These findings have two major implications. First, following a disruption in care during the first year and a half of life, babies appear capable of organizing their behavior around the availability of new caregivers. Second, these data argue for a nongenetic mechanism for the intergenerational transmission of attachment.

INTRODUCTION

Babies entering foster care are faced with the task of forming attachments to new primary caregivers. When placed later than birth, these infants have often experienced problematic rearing conditions as well as disruptions in their previous caregiving relationships. It is conceivable that these previous experiences diminish foster infants' chances of forming trusting relationships with new caregivers. It is possible, however, that these infants organize their attachment behavior around the availability of their new caregivers. In this study we examined the nature of the attachments formed by these foster infants with their new surrogate caregivers. Little research on foster infants' attachments to their caregivers has yet been reported in the literature. Nonetheless, the extensive literature regarding intact dyads, as well as the more limited literature regarding adopted infants, and infants with other-than-primary caregivers, is useful in suggesting hypotheses regarding foster infant attachments.

Attachment

Infants in biologically intact dyads organize their attachment behaviors around the availability of their caregivers. When infants find caregivers to be available in times of need, they develop expectations that caregivers will be available when needed in the future. Behaviorally, these infants then seek out the comfort they need (Sroufe, 1989) from caregivers, with the confident expectation that they will be soothed. Such infants are classified as having secure attachments to their caregivers (Ainsworth, Blehar, Waters, & Wall, 1978).

When caregivers are not responsive to infants' needs for reassurance, their babies do not develop confident expectations regarding parental availability. Instead, these babies develop alternative strategies for interacting with their parents when distressed. Some infants turn away from caregivers under conditions of moderate stress, giving the appearance of not needing nurturance. These infants are classified as having avoidant attachments. Other infants show a pattern of seeking out caregivers while simultaneously resisting contact and are classified as having resistant attachments. Finally, some infants show a breakdown in strategy when they are distressed and in their caregivers' presence, displaying behaviors that appear disoriented or disorganized (Main & Solomon, 1990). These infants are classified as having disorganized attachments. Because disorganized attachment is seen as a breakdown in strategy, infants who are classified as disorganized receive a secondary classification of secure, avoidant, or resistant.

Attachment quality is considered important by attachment researchers because it reflects the quality of the infant's relationship with the caregiver, and also because it is associated with the child's later interpersonal functioning. Children who develop secure attachments to caregivers show more competent problem-solving skills as toddlers (Matas, Arend, & Sroufe, 1978), more independent and confident behaviors with teachers as preschoolers (Sroufe, 1983), and more competent interactive behaviors with peers at school age (Elicker, Englund, & Sroufe, 1992) than do other children. Attachment strategies that are insecure but organized (i.e., avoidant and resistant attachments) may not place children at substantially increased risk for later disorder (e.g., Lewis, Feiring, McGuffog, & Jaskir, 1984; Lyons-Ruth, Alpern, & Repacholi, 1993). Those children with disorganized attachments, however, are at risk for a host of problematic outcomes, including aggressive behavior with peers (Lyons-Ruth et al. 1993; Lyons-Ruth, Easterbrooks,

& Cibelli, 1997) and dissociative symptomatology evidenced throughout childhood (Carlson, 1998). Identifying predictors of disorganized attachment is, therefore, of particular importance.

Maternal state of mind and infant attachment. Among biologically intact mother–infant dyads, the strongest predictor of infant attachment found thus far is the caregiver's state of mind with regard to attachment (van IJzendoorn, 1995). Attachment state of mind refers to the way in which adults process thoughts and feelings regarding their own attachment experiences. State of mind is assessed through a process of discourse analysis developed by Main and colleagues (Main & Goldwyn, 1998).

Adults who value attachment and are coherent in processing their own attachment experiences are classified as having autonomous states of mind. As parents, these adults are most likely to have infants who are securely attached to them (van IJzendoorn, 1995). Adults who are not coherent in their processing of attachment-related experiences are said to have nonautonomous states of mind. These adults violate rules of conversational discourse in their discussion of attachment experiences, with the violations taking one of several forms. Some adults idealize attachment experiences and attachment figures, showing a lack of coherence in terms of the consistency and completeness of their discourse regarding attachments (Main & Goldwyn, 1998). These adults are classified as having dismissing states of mind with regard to attachment. Parents with dismissing states of mind are most likely to have infants with avoidant attachments to them (van IJzendoorn, 1995). A second form of violation occurs among adults who show angry involvement with attachment figures, or ramble in their discourse, providing excessive, irrelevant detail in their discussion of attachment issues. These adults are classified as having preoccupied states of mind and are somewhat more likely than others to have infants with resistant attachments. Finally, a third form of violation occurs among adults who show a breakdown in reasoning or discourse when discussing a loss or trauma. These adults are classified as unresolved and are likely to have infants with disorganized attachments (van IJzendoorn, 1995). Parallel to infant disorganized attachment, unresolved state of mind is assumed to represent a breakdown in strategy; thus, a secondary (autonomous, dismissing, or preoccupied) classification is given to adults classified as unresolved.

Associations between parental state of mind and infant attachment quality have been assessed in a number of investigations. In a meta-analysis of 18 samples, van IJzendoorn (1995) found a concordance of 75%, $\kappa = .49$, between parental state of mind and infant attachment security when two categories (autonomous/nonautonomous and secure/insecure) were considered. When four categories of parental state of mind and infant attachment security were considered, there was a concordance of 63%, $\kappa = .42$.

It has generally been assumed that unresolved state of mind wields more influence on parenting than the secondary autonomous, dismissing, or preoccupied state of mind (Main & Hesse, 1990). Main and Hesse proposed that parents who are unresolved tend to behave in ways that are frightening to children. Their children are thus disorganized in the face of threat because they need comfort from caregivers, but caregivers are frightening to them. Recent findings of Schuengel, Bakersman-Kranenburg, and van IJzendoorn (1999), however, suggest the possibility that this link between unresolved maternal state of mind and infant disorganized attachment may be limited to those unresolved mothers with nonautonomous secondary classifications. Schuengel et al. found that unresolved mothers with secondary autonomous classifications displayed low levels of frightening behaviors toward their infants relative to other caregivers and were not at increased risk for having disorganized infants.

Questions regarding genetic factors. Some researchers have questioned whether the association between caregiver state of mind and child attachment is a function of biological relatedness or shared temperament (e.g., Fox, 1995), rather than the caregiving environment. Although temperament has not been strongly associated with infant attachment quality (e.g., Goldsmith & Alansky, 1987), the possibility of some form of genetic transmission is difficult to rule out. There are no studies reported in the literature that examined differential predictability from maternal state of mind to infant attachment quality for monozygotic and dizygotic twins. However, several studies have compared concordance of attachment quality for twins and for siblings (Goldsmith & Campos, 1990; Minde, Corter, Goldberg, & Jeffers, 1990; Vandell, Owen, Wilson, & Henderson, 1988; van IJzendoorn et al., 2000), and failed to provide strong support for the importance of genetic factors in attachment quality. In Ricciuti's 1992 reanalysis of three twin data sets (Goldsmith & Campos, 1990; Minde et al., 1990; Vandell et al., 1988), 78% of the dizygotic infant pairs were concordant for attachment quality and 66% of the monozygotic infant pairs were concordant. In a meta-analysis of 138 sibling pairs, van IJzendoorn (1995) found that the level of concordance between siblings was 62% using the two-way classification scheme, with discordance partially attributable to differences in maternal sensitivity for the two siblings.

If genetic transmission is the primary source of the covariation between maternal state of mind and infant attachment security, little association should be found among nonbiologically related mother–infant dyads. Although negative findings for infants in foster care could be attributable to a host of factors, including prenatal environment, early experiences of maltreatment, and the effects of relationship disruption, strong positive findings would provide compelling evidence that genetic factors are not the primary source of intergenerational transmission of attachment.

Children's Attachments to Nonbiologically Related Caregivers

Attachment quality of children with nonbiological caregivers has been investigated for children placed soon after birth with adoptive parents (Juffer & Rosenboom, 1997; Singer, Brodzinsky, Ramsay, Steir, & Waters, 1985), for children placed with adoptive parents after extended stays in orphanages (Chisholm, 1998; O'Connor, Bredenkamp, & Rutter, 1999), for children on kibbutzim with metapelet (Sagi et al., 1995), and for children with child-care providers (Howes & Hamilton, 1992). These various investigations are useful in suggesting the range of possible outcomes for foster children forming new attachments to surrogate caregivers.

Attachment of early adopted children. Several investigations of attachment security among children adopted from relatively benign conditions have been reported in the literature (Juffer & Rosenboom, 1997; Singer et al., 1985). Juffer and Rosenboom found that of Asian and South American children adopted before 6 months of age by parents in the Netherlands, 74% were classified as secure. Singer et al. reported a relatively lower percentage of secure infants (52%) among a sample of 56 babies between the ages of 3 days and 10 months who were adopted by parents in the United States. Because the coding of disorganized attachment is a relatively new addition to the coding scheme, neither of these groups reported disorganized attachments among their samples. Juffer, Stams, Bakermans-Kranenburg, and van IJzendoorn (1999), however, found a disproportionately high percentage of disorganized attachments in a subsequent investigation of a small subset of their sample.

These two studies suggest that attachment quality among some adopted children may be compromised, although the findings are not consistent and the underlying reasons are unclear. Findings reported to date do not make it possible to disentangle the effects of adoptive parent state of mind, timing of relationship disruption, and previous relationship experiences on the child's attachment quality.

Children adopted following extreme privation. Following extended stays in the extreme conditions of Romanian orphanages, children have been studied in their adoptive homes in the United Kingdom, Canada, and the United States. Chisholm (1998) found that 66% of children adopted by 4 months of age developed secure attachments to their adoptive parents. This figure is not significantly different from that found for a control group of nonadopted children, 58% of whom developed secure attachments. Of children who had been in the institutional setting for at least 8 months, however, only 37% developed secure attachments to their adoptive parents. Further, these late-placed children showed disproportionately high incidences of disorganized attachments and indiscriminately friendly behavior with strangers.

Several possibilities are suggested for the current investigation of children placed in foster care. First, it is possible that the timing of the child's placement in surrogate care is central to the child's ability to organize attachment around the new caregiver's availability. On the other hand, it is possible that the duration of inadequate care, rather than the timing of the new relationship's formation, is most important to the child's ability to organize attachment behavior. Inadequacy of care might best be considered along a continuum (Cicchetti & Barnett, 1991), with Romanian institutional care representing the extreme. The previous care of children placed into foster care falls along the continuum, with no children likely to be as emotionally neglected as most were in the Romanian institutions.

Children's attachments to secondary attachment figures. Findings from day care and kibbutzim settings suggest that children are somewhat less likely to form secure relationships with professional caregivers compared with parents (Howes & Hamilton, 1992; Sagi, 1985; Sagi et al., 1995). Foster parents might be seen as fitting into this general category of professional caregivers. If so, and if this finding of lower levels of secure attachments is robust, foster children might be expected to show disproportionately high levels of insecure attachment to their foster parents. On the other hand, foster parents differ from day care and kibbutzim providers in that they are the primary caregivers for the duration of the child's placement.

Similar to findings with biologically related dyads, responsive and sensitive caregiving on the part of professionals nonetheless predicts the development of a secure infant–caregiver relationship (Goosens & van IJzendoorn, 1990). This finding suggests that children organize their attachment behaviors around the availability of the caregivers currently providing care. For foster children, this finding suggests that foster parent availability should affect children's organization of attachment behaviors with their new caregivers. The limits of this finding, however, have not been explored. It is possible that children with problematic early experiences carry forward their models of relationships in a less flexible way than many other children. In this case, depending on the child's history of caregiving, foster parent availability may not be expected to affect child expectations for new relationships to a great extent.

Howes and Hamilton (1992) reported that day-care children who experienced a change in teachers between 18 and 24 months of age were rated as less secure with teachers at both 24 and 30 months compared with children who did not experience a change. This finding may well have implications for the effects of disruptions in relationships with primary, as well as secondary, attachment figures.

Children's developing attachments to foster parents. In our lab, we examined attachment behaviors that infants displayed toward their foster mothers using a diary methodology (Stovall & Dozier, 2000). Attachment behaviors in a sample of 38 foster mother–infant dyads were examined on a daily basis for a period of 60 days following the child's placement. Infants placed at younger ages (6 to 12 months) showed more secure behaviors than those placed later (12 to 20 months), and children placed with mothers with autonomous states of mind showed more secure behaviors than those placed with nonautonomous foster mothers. Further, younger children's attachment behaviors stabilized more quickly than did those of older children. Stable attachment behaviors emerged within the first 2 weeks of placement for most younger infants, contrasted with up to 2 months for older infants. Foster parents tended to behave in ways that complemented their babies' behavior, with even autonomous foster parents providing little nurturance to children who appeared not to need it. Older infants seemed to take the lead in this "relationship dance" (Stern, 1977), overshadowing foster parents' contributions to the dance. This transactional pattern seemed likely to be self-perpetuating, with older infants continuing to have low expectations for nurturing care and continuing to behave in ways that did not elicit nurturance.

The Present Study

These various findings suggest several possibilities regarding foster children's attachments to their new caregivers. First, after a period of adjustment and consolidation, foster infants may organize their attachments around the availability of their new caregivers. If so, we would expect their newly consolidated attachments to foster mothers to be largely concordant with their foster mothers' state of mind with regard to attachment. A second possibility is that the effects of foster infants' earlier caregiving experiences and disruptions in caregiving may be so potent that current caregiver characteristics are eclipsed. If so, there should be little concordance between caregiver state of mind and foster infant attachment. A third possibility is that there is some concordance between foster mother state of mind and foster infant attachment, but only when children were placed into care early (before about 1 year of age). These possibilities were explored in the present research.

METHOD

Overview

Fifty foster infant–mother dyads participated in this study. All were part of a larger longitudinal study of the effects of interventions for foster parents, but none of the participants had yet received intervention services. Foster mothers completed the Adult Attachment Interview (AAI) in their homes. Foster infants and their foster mothers participated in the Strange Situation between the ages of 12 and 24 months, at least 3 months after placement in the foster home.

Participants

All 50 infants had been placed with their caregivers between birth and 20 months of age, with a mean age at placement of 7.7 months (SD = 6.2). Twenty-nine of the children were males and 21 were females. Most (64%) of the infants were African American, with 28% European American, and 8% Hispanic. Similarly, most (64%) of the foster mothers were African American, with the remaining 36% European American. Most (88%) of the dyads were ethnically matched. Case records indicated that children were placed in foster care for one or more of the following reasons: neglect (62%), parental substance abuse (36%), family instability (16%), abandonment (14%), inadequate housing (10%), parental incarceration (10%), physical abuse (6%), and sexual abuse (2%). Twenty-eight of the children were in their first foster placement, 17 were in their second, and 5 had been in more than two (*range* = 3 to 5 placements).

Foster mothers ranged in age from 26 to 69, with a mean of 47 years (SD = 12). The range in the number of foster children for whom they had cared was from 1 to 80, with a mean of 17, and a median of 6. At the time of participation, the number of foster children in their homes ranged from 1 to 5, with a median of 2. Family income for foster families averaged $36,000, ranging from the lowest income category in our study (less than $10,000; n = 2) to the second highest income category ($60,000 to $100,000; n = 2). Family incomes were rather evenly distributed in the income categories between $10,000 and $50,000. Half (25) of the foster mothers were married or living with a partner, and half (25) were single (widowed, divorced, or never married). None of the foster mothers were biologically related to the foster infants.

Measures

Adult Attachment Interview. The AAI (George, Kaplan, & Main, 1996) is a semistructured interview designed to assess caregivers' state of mind with regard to attachment. In the interview, foster mothers were asked to describe their relationships with their parents when they were young, to instantiate descriptions with specific memories, to recall incidences of distress, and to conceptualize relationship influences. The time required to administer the interview ranged from 45 to 70 minutes. When possible, foster mothers were administered this interview when study children were first placed in their care. For nearly half of the foster mothers ($n = 22$), these interviews had been conducted when a previous child from the larger research project was in their care. Therefore, AAIs were administered between 31 months prior to the study child's placement to 10 months following the study child's placement. The median time of administration was 0.8 months following the study child's placement ($M = 0.8$, $SD = 8.29$ months). Because the stability of state of mind classifications is high (Bakermans-Kranenburg & van IJzendoorn, 1993), differences in timing of administration were not considered important.

Using the Main and Goldwyn (1998) system, foster mothers were classified as autonomous with regard to attachment when they were generally coherent in their discourse and showed a valuing of attachment. Foster mothers were classified as dismissing when they showed a devaluing or dismissing of the importance of attachment, and were likely to show a lack of recall for attachment experiences, and/or an idealization of attachment figures, and/or imperturbability. Foster mothers were classified as preoccupied when their discourse was characterized by angry involvement with attachment figures or by rambling speech. Finally, they were classified as unresolved when they showed lapses in monitoring of reasoning or discourse regarding a loss or trauma.

Dismissing, autonomous, and preoccupied classifications are stable over periods ranging from 1 to 15 months, with the unresolved category showing slightly lower levels of stability than other categories (Bakermans-Kranenburg & van IJzendoorn, 1993; Main, 1996; Sagi et al., 1994). Interrater agreement on classifications is well over 80%, and classifications are independent of interviewer and unrelated to autobiographical memory, verbal or performance measures of intelligence, or social desirability (Bakermans-Kranenburg & van IJzendoorn, 1993; for an overview, see van IJzendoorn, 1995). Mothers' AAI classifications measured both before and after their children's birth predict infant security in ways that are consistent with attachment theory (Benoit & Parker, 1994; Fonagy, Steele, & Steele, 1991; Ward & Carlson, 1995).

Interviews were audiotaped and transcribed by professional transcriptionists. Four raters coded the transcripts using the classification system developed by Main and Goldwyn (1998). All coders had attended the 2-week training course sponsored by Mary Main and Erik Hesse and passed the reliability test with agreement of at least 85% with Main and Hesse. A random set of 12 AAIs was double coded, with agreement on these interviews of 100%, $\kappa = 1.00$, for three-way classification, and 75%, $\kappa = .61$, for four-way classification. Given that reliability for unresolved status was lower than for other categories, all interviews were double coded for unresolved status, and disagreements were conferenced. Coders were blind to child-attachment classification and to other information regarding the participants.

Strange Situation. The Strange Situation (Ainsworth et al., 1978) is a laboratory procedure designed to stress infants, allowing assessment of infants' reliance on the caregiver when they are distressed. Infants are separated from the caregiver on two occasions and then reunited, with attachment behaviors (infants' proximity seeking, contact maintenance, resistance, and avoidance) coded during the reunion episodes. Infants are classified as secure if they seek out whatever contact is needed and are calmed readily by their caregiver; as avoidant if they turn away from their caregiver when distressed; and as resistant if they show an angry resistance to caregivers. Infants in this study were also rated on disorganization, using the criteria developed by Main and Solomon (1990). Disorganization is coded when the infant strategies for dealing with distress break down in the caregiver's presence or when infants appear to lack a strategy for dealing with distress. Examples of disorganization include an infant backing up against the wall when the parent enters the room, wandering around the room aimlessly, or appearing dazed and motionless for a long period of time (Main & Solomon, 1990). The child is classified as disorganized when one or more events meet threshold criteria. Children classified as disorganized are also given a secondary classification of secure, avoidant, or resistant.

At the time the children participated in the Strange Situation they were between the ages of 12 and 24 months ($M = 16.5$, $SD = 4.1$) and had been in the care of their current foster parents between 3 and 21 months ($M = 9.2$, $SD = 5.2$). Three coders, blind to other study data, coded the Strange Situations. All three had attended the training course on coding of organized strategies (secure, avoidant, resistant) offered by Alan Sroufe and the training course on disorganized coding offered by Mary Main. Coders had also passed reliability tests for classifying organized and disorganized strategies offered by Sroufe, reaching at least 80% agreement with expert coders. A random set of 12 Strange Situations was double coded; agreement on these was 100%, $\kappa = 1.00$, for major category and 82%, $\kappa = .73$, when the disorganized category was included. Given the lower reliability for the disorganized classification, all videotapes with indications of disorganized behavior were double coded and disagreements resolved by conference.

Although the Strange Situation was originally developed for use with biologically intact mother–infant dyads, several types of evidence suggest its appropriateness in assessing attachment quality among nonbiologically related dyads. First, kibbutzim infants tended to develop secure attachments with some metapelet and insecure attachments with others, suggesting that the Strange Situation reflects the infants' organization of attachment around the availability of the specific caregiver (Sagi et al., 1995). Second, work by Stovall and Dozier (2000) suggests that infants' attachments to new foster caregivers usually stabilize within 2 months of foster-care placement, making the assessment of attachment quality meaningful at that time.

The Strange Situation was developed for the assessment of attachment of babies between the ages of 12 and 18 months (Ainsworth et al., 1978). The procedure has been used, however, in investigations with older babies, including those up to 24 months of age. Because we were interested in the effects of the timing of foster-care placement on attachment quality, children up to 24 months of age were included in our investigation. To ensure that any results were not attributable to our inclusion of older infants in the study, analyses that included only those children who were younger than 20 months of age, in addition to analyses that included all children, were conducted.

RESULTS

Foster Mother AAI

Slightly more than half (54%) of the foster mothers were coded as having primary classifications of autonomous state of mind, with 22% classified as dismissing and 24% classified as unresolved. (The only mother with a preoccupied classification had a primary unresolved classification.) Of the mothers with unresolved states of mind, 58% had secondary autonomous classifications and 42% had secondary nonautonomous (4 dismissing, 1 preoccupied) classifications, representing 14% and 10% of the total sample, respectively.

Infant Attachment Classification

About half (52%) of the children were classified as secure in the Strange Situation, with most others (34%) classified as disorganized. An additional 6% were classified as avoidant, and 8% were classified as resistant. The results from the van IJzendoorn (1995) meta-analysis were used to provide the expected distribution of attachment classifications. The proportion of children with secure attachments was similar to that reported in the meta-analysis, but the foster care sample had a larger proportion of children with disorganized attachments (Table 1.1).

Associations among Foster Mother State of Mind, Infant Attachment, and Other Variables

Associations among variables of primary interest (foster mother state of mind and infant attachment) and variables that were not of direct interest in this study (e.g., foster mother age, income, racial match) were examined to determine whether variables of secondary interest should be included in subsequent analyses. Foster mother age, marital status, foster family income, the number of foster children in the foster home, the placement cause, the number of previous placements, and racial match of foster mother and child were not

TABLE 1.1
Breakdown of Infant Attachment Classifications for Foster-Care Infants and Infants in the van IJzendoorn (1995) Meta-Analysis

Attachment Classification	Foster-Care Infants		Meta-Analysis Infants	
	%	*n*	%	*n*
Secure	52	26	52	287
Avoidant	6	3	21	116
Resistant	8	4	5	28
Disorganized	34	17	21	117

Note: Organized versus disorganized: $\chi^2(1, N = 50) = 9.42, p < .01$.

significantly related to foster mother state of mind, child attachment, or the concordance between maternal state of mind and child attachment, $p > .05$. Only higher income was associated with higher concordance, $p < .05$. Given the number of comparisons conducted, this single significant finding was unimpressive. With a Bonferroni correction, this finding did not emerge as significant. As a result, these additional variables were not considered in subsequent analyses.

Concordance between Maternal State of Mind and Infant Attachment

On the basis of Schuengel et al.'s (1999) finding that unresolved mothers with secondary autonomous classifications are likely to have secure rather than disorganized babies, unresolved/autonomous mothers were included in the autonomous group in the first analyses. Given that most reports in the literature consider these unresolved/autonomous mothers as nonautonomous, analyses that included these mothers in the nonautonomous group were also conducted. Concordance between foster mother state of mind and foster infant attachment was examined first with the two-way match (autonomous and non-autonomous state of mind matched with secure and insecure attachment, respectively). As can be seen in Table 1.2, there was a 72% match, versus 52% expected on the basis of chance alone, $\kappa = .43$, $\chi^2(1, N = 50) = 10.42, p < .01$. This level of concordance was similar to that found in the van IJzendoorn meta-analysis for biologically intact dyads. When unresolved foster mothers with secondary autonomous ratings were included in the nonautonomous group (rather than in the autonomous group), findings remained significant, with a 68% concordance, $\kappa = .36$, $\chi^2(1, N = 50) = 6.44, p < .05$.

The findings for the 43 infants assessed at 20 months or younger in the Strange Situation were similar to those for the full sample. The two-way correspondence between maternal state of mind and infant attachment was

72%, $\kappa = .45$, $\chi^2(1, N = 43) = 9.92$, $p < .01$, when unresolved/autonomous mothers were included in the autonomous group, and 70%, $\kappa = .40$, $\chi^2(1, N = 43) = 6.75$, $p < .01$, when they were included in the nonautonomous group.

As can be seen in Table 1.3, concordance for the four-way match was 56% when unresolved/autonomous mothers were included in the autonomous group, $\kappa = .27$, $\chi^2(6, N = 50) = 13.77$, $p < .05$. When unresolved/autonomous mothers were included in the nonautonomous group, the concordance was 52%, $\kappa = .24$, $\chi^2(6, N = 50) = 13.06$, $p < .05$. Findings for the smaller sample of infants assessed before 20 months revealed a four-way correspondence of 53%, $\kappa = .25$, $\chi^2(6, N = 43) = 15.99$, $p < .05$, when unresolved/autonomous mothers were included in the autonomous group, and 51%, $\kappa = .23$, $\chi^2(6, N = 43) = 14.25$, $p < .05$, when they were included in the nonautonomous group.

Given that disorganized attachment appears to represent a significant risk for later psychopathology, the link between maternal state of mind and children's development of organized (secure, avoidant, and resistant attachments) versus disorganized attachments was examined. Only 21% of foster mothers with autonomous states of mind had children with disorganized attachments, whereas 62.5% of foster mothers with nonautonomous states of mind had children with disorganized attachments, $\kappa = .41$, $\chi^2(1, N = 50) = 8.52$, $p < .01$.

TABLE 1.2
Concordance Between Foster Mother State of Mind and Infant Attachment for Two-Way Match

	Foster Mother State of Mind	
Infant Attachment	Autonomous	Nonautonomous
Secure	23	3
Insecure	11	13

Note: $\chi^2(1, N = 50) = 10.42$, $p < .01$. Concordance = 72%; $\kappa = .43$.

TABLE 1.3
Concordance between Foster Mother State of Mind and Infant Attachment for Four-Way Match

Infant Attachment	Autonomous	Dismissing	Preoccupied	Unresolved/ Nonautonomous
Secure	23	2	0	1
Avoidant	2	1	0	0
Resistant	2	2	0	0
Disorganized	7	6	0	4

Note: $\chi^2(6, N = 50) = 13.77$, $p < .05$. Concordance = 56%; $\kappa = .27$.

Age at Placement

Age of placement in foster care was not associated with infant attachment, either as a main effect or as an interaction with maternal state of mind. Given that previous findings had suggested that age at placement would be an important predictor of infant security, this null result was explored carefully. Whether considered as a continuous or as a dichotomous variable, placement age did not approach significance as a predictor of organized/disorganized attachment or secure/insecure attachment, or as a predictor of concordance between foster mother state of mind and infant security. The mean age at placement for babies with organized attachments was 7.3 months, and for babies with disorganized attachments, it was 8.6 months. This difference did not approach significance, $p > .40$.

DISCUSSION

Foster infants' attachment security was concordant with foster mothers' state of mind at levels similar to that seen among biologically intact dyads. These results are striking and have important implications both for children placed in out-of-home care and for attachment among intact mother–infant dyads. These results suggest that when placed in the first year and a half of life, foster children can organize their attachment behaviors around the availability of their new caregivers. When placed later than birth, most children in our sample had been exposed to neglect, and some to abuse, as well as up to five changes in caregivers. Nonetheless, when placed with autonomous caregivers, these children often formed secure attachments.

Among biologically intact dyads, it has not been possible to differentiate clearly between a genetic and environmental explanation for the concordance between maternal state of mind and infant attachment. It was plausible that the concordance between maternal state of mind and infant attachment reflected some tendency shared between mother and child to react to stimuli in parallel ways. For example, Fox (1995) suggested that the temperamental (or personality) characteristics of reactivity and affective bias likely represented the mechanism by which state of mind and attachment were associated. Twin and sibling studies (e.g., Ricciuti, 1992; van IJzendoorn et al., 2000) have failed to provide consistent support for a genetic mechanism, although a genetic argument is hard to rule out in the absence of findings from nonrelated dyads. This study's findings provide compelling evidence that it is maternal characteristics, rather than shared temperament or other genetically linked characteristics, that primarily determine children's attachment strategies.

Given our previous findings (Stovall & Dozier, 2000), we had expected age at placement to be a powerful predictor of infant attachment quality. In our previous study, we found that foster mothers reported more insecure behaviors during the first 2 months of placement among babies placed at older ages than among babies placed at younger ages, regardless of foster mothers' state of mind. In this previous study, a diary methodology that relied on the foster mother's report of child and caregiver behaviors was used. This methodology allowed for examination of the process by which children formed new attachments. In the current study, using the Strange Situation, the "consolidated attachment" of infants who had been with their foster mothers for at least 3 months was assessed. The results suggest that when babies are placed in foster care during the first 20 months of life, the age at which they are placed does not affect the quality of attachments formed with new caregivers. It seems that even though late-placed foster infants initially push their caregivers away (as reflected in Stovall and Dozier's diary data), eventually the children organize attachment behavior around the availability of their new caregivers.

There have been relatively few studies of infants' attachments following the disruption of a primary relationship. At some level, therefore, the implications of our current findings are unclear. Essentially, we do not know what attachment reflects in terms of its organizational function and its predictive value for infants who have experienced disrupted attachments. For children from stable, intact dyads, attachment serves to organize experience (Sroufe, 1983) and to generalize to feelings about the self and others (Cassidy, 1988; Matas et al., 1978; Sroufe, 1989). For children with disrupted relationships, it is unclear what role attachments to new surrogate caregivers play in the organization of feelings about self and others. Plausibly, the disruption of previous relationships, or the poor quality of previous relationships, may have made indelible imprints on children. On the other hand, children who form secure attachments to surrogate caregivers following previous relationship failures may be demonstrating the ability to rework models of self and other. These questions can only be addressed by longitudinal studies of the impact of children's new attachments to surrogate caregivers on later representations of self and other.

It is important to note that the proportion of children with disorganized attachments was larger than typically seen among normal samples. It is interesting to note, however, that children were only at increased risk for disorganized attachments when their caregivers had nonautonomous states of mind. Only 21% of children with autonomous caregivers had disorganized attachments, a figure that is not especially large for any sample. The majority of children who had caregivers with nonautonomous states of mind, however, had disorganized attachments. Even caregivers with dismissing states of mind were likely to have children with disorganized attachments. Among biologically intact dyads, mothers with dismissing states of mind are most likely to have babies with avoidant attachments, a status that does not confer substantial risk to a child. Whereas children in biologically intact dyads can organize their attachment behavior around the availability of a somewhat rejecting parent, most children who have experienced relationship disruption appear unable to do so. Rather, children who have experienced relationship disruption are likely to develop disorganized attachment strategies unless they are in the care of nurturing surrogate caregivers. We expect that the experience of relationship disruption is so disorganizing that only with the development of a relationship with a nurturing caregiver can the child begin to develop an organized attachment.

Given that this is the first study in the literature reporting concordance between parental state of mind and child attachment quality among children in foster care, it will be important to replicate these rather startling results. We included a wide age range of children (from 12 to 24 months) in the primary analyses. Because our sample was not large, we must particularly question our null results regarding age at placement. Subsequent studies should further study the importance of age at placement by looking at larger samples of children placed at various ages.

Some might question the use of the infant Strange Situation coding system for children as old as 24 months of age. Although this system was developed for the coding of children 18 months old and younger, the system has been used in a number of studies for the coding of attachment among children as old as 24 months. We chose not to restrict the sample to children 18 months and younger because of our interest in examining the effects of age at placement. To ensure that our findings were not unduly affected by the inclusion of 20- to 24-month-old children, we reanalyzed data including only those children younger than 20 months of age.

Finally, it will be critical that these results be extended longitudinally such that the meaning of attachment can be ascertained for children who have experienced relationship disruption. Although children appear able to form secure attachments to new, nurturing caregivers after several months time, it is unclear what organizational role these attachments play in the development of information processing strategies and in representations of self and other. Longitudinal studies of children placed with surrogate caregivers will clarify the role that new attachments play for these children following relationship disruption.

In summary, we suggest that these results speak to the strength of the human propensity for relatedness. Despite experiences of inadequate care, disruptions in care, or both, young children placed with nurturing caregivers were often able to develop trusting, secure attachments.

ACKNOWLEDGMENTS

Support for this research was provided by National Institute of Mental Health grant 52135 to the first author. The authors thank Denise Berilla, Anna

Nutter, and Diana Eldreth for their help in collecting data. They give their appreciation to Gerri Robinson and Yvonne Gilchrist of the Baltimore City Department of Social Services; to Isaac Palmer, John Bates, and Darlene Lantz of the Delaware Department of Services for Children, Youth, and Their Families, and to caseworkers, foster families, birth families, and children at both agencies. Thanks also go to Mary Main, Annie Bernier, and several anonymous reviewers for helpful comments on the article.

ADDRESSES AND AFFILIATIONS

Corresponding author: Mary Dozier, Department of Psychology, University of Delaware, 220 Wolf Hall, Newark, DE 19716-2579; e-mail: mdozier@udel.edu. K. Chase Stovall is at Cornell University Medical Center, Ithaca, NY; Kathleen E. Albus and Brady Bates are also at the University of Delaware.

REFERENCES

Ainsworth, M. D. S., Blehar, M. C., Waters, E., & Wall, S. (1978). *Patterns of attachment: a psychological study of the strange situation.* Erlbaum, Hillsdale, NJ.

Bakermans-Kranenburg, M. J., & van IJzendoorn, M. H. (1993). A psychometric study of the Adult Attachment Interview: reliability and discriminant validity. *Developmental Psychology, 29,* 870–880.

Benoit, D., & Parker, K. C. H. (1994). Stability and transmission of attachment across three generations. *Child Development, 65,* 1444–1456.

Carlson, E. A. (1998). A prospective longitudinal study of disorganized/disoriented attachment. *Child Development, 69,* 1107–1128.

Cassidy, J. (1988). Child–mother attachment and the self in six-year-olds. *Child Development, 59,* 121–134.

Chisholm, K. (1998). A three-year follow-up of attachment and indiscriminate friendliness in children adopted from Romanian orphanages. *Child Development, 69,* 1092–1106.

Cicchetti, D., & Barnett, D. (1991). Toward the development of a scientific nosology of child maltreatment. In W. M. Grove & D. Cicchetti (Eds.), *Thinking clearly about psychology: personality and psychopathology* (pp. 346–377). Minneapolis: University of Minnesota Press.

Elicker, J., Englund, M., & Sroufe, L. A. (1992). Predicting peer competence and peer relationships in childhood from early parent–child relationships. In R. D. Parke & G. W. Ladd (Eds.), *Family-peer relationships: modes of linkage.* Hillsdale, NJ: Erlbaum.

Fonagy, P., Steele, H., & Steele, M. (1991). Maternal representations of attachment during pregnancy predict the organization of infant–mother attachment at one year of age. *Child Development, 62,* 891–905.

Fox, N. A. (1995). Of the way we were: Adult memories about attachment experiences and their role in determining infant-parent relationships: a commentary on van IJzendoorn (1995). *Psychological Bulletin, 117,* 404–410.

George, C., Kaplan, N., & Main, M. (1996). *Adult Attachment Interview.* Unpublished manuscript, University of California, Berkeley.

Goldsmith, H. H., & Alansky, J. A. (1987). Maternal and infant temperamental predictors of attachment: a meta-analytic review. *Journal of Consulting and Clinical Psychology, 55,* 805–816.

Goldsmith, H. H., & Campos, J. J. (1990). The structure of temperamental fear and pleasure in infants: a psychometric perspective. *Child Development, 61,* 1944–1964.

Goosens, F. A., & van IJzendoorn, M. H. (1990). Quality of infants' attachments to professional caregivers: relation to infant–parent attachments and day-care characteristics. *Child Development, 61,* 832–837.

Howes, C., & Hamilton, C. E. (1992). Children's relationships with child care teachers: stability and concordance with parental attachments. *Child Development, 63,* 867–878.

Juffer, F., & Rosenboom, L. G. (1997). Infant–mother attachment of internationally adopted children in the Netherlands. *International Journal of Behavioral Development, 20,* 93–107.

Juffer, F., Status, G. J. J. M., Bakermans-Kranenburg, M. J., & van IJzendoorn, M. H. (1999, April). *In search of the origins of adopted children's behavior problems.* Paper presented at the biennial meeting of the Society for Research in Child Development, Albuquerque, NM.

Lewis, M., Feiring, C., McGuffog, C., & Jaskir, J. (1984). Predicting psychopathology in six-year-olds from early social relations. *Child Development, 55,* 123–136.

Lyons-Ruth, K., Alpern, L., & Repacholi, B. (1993). Disorganized infant attachment classification and maternal psychosocial problems as predictors of hostile-aggressive behavior in the preschool classroom. *Child Development, 64,* 572–585.

Lyons-Ruth, K., Easterbrooks, A., & Cibelli, C. (1997). Infant attachment strategies, infant mental lag, and maternal depressive symptoms: predictors of internalizing and externalizing problems at age 7. *Developmental Psychology, 33,* 681–692.

Main, M. (1996). Introduction to the special section on attachment and psychopathology: 2. Overview of the field of attachment. *Journal of Consulting and Clinical Psychology, 64,* 237–243.

Main, M., & Goldwyn, R. (1998). *Adult attachment classification system.* London: University College.

Main, M., & Hesse, E. (1990). Parents' unresolved traumatic experiences are related to infant disorganized attachment status: is frightened and/or frightening parental behavior the linking mechanism? In M. T. Greenberg, D. Cicchetti, & E. M. Cummings (Eds.), *Attachment in the preschool years* (pp. 161–182). Chicago: University of Chicago.

Main, M., & Solomon, J. (1990). Procedures for identifying infants as disorganized/disoriented during the Ainsworth Strange Situation. In M. T. Greenberg, D. Cicchetti, & E. M. Cummings (Eds.), *Attachment in the preschool years* (pp. 121–160). Chicago: University of Chicago.

Matas, L., Arend, R. A., & Sroufe, L. A. (1978). Continuity of adaptation in the second year: the relationship between quality of attachment and later competence. *Child Development, 47,* 511–514.

Minde, K., Corter, C., Goldberg, S., & Jeffers, D. (1990). Maternal preference between premature twins up to age four. *Journal of American Academy of Child and Adolescent Psychiatry, 29,* 367–374.

O'Connor, T. G., Bredenkamp, D., & Rutter, M. (1999). Attachment disturbances and disorders in children exposed to early severe deprivation. *Infant Mental Health Journal, 20,* 10–29.

Ricciuti, A. E. (1992). Child–mother attachment: a twin study (University Microfilms No. 9324873). *Dissertation Abstracts International, 54,* 3364.

Sagi, A. (1985). Security of infant–mother, –father, –metapelet attachments among kibbutz-reared Israeli children. In I. Bretherton & E. Waters (Eds.), Growing points in attachment theory and research. *Monographs of the Society for Research in Child Development,* 50(1–2, Serial No. 209).

Sagi, A., van IJzendoorn, M. H., Aviezer, O., Donnell, F., Koren-Karie, N., Joels, T., & Harel, Y. (1995). Attachments in a multiple-caregiver and multiple-infant environment: the case of the Israeli kibbutzim. In E. Waters, B. Vaughn, G. Posada, & K. Kondo-Ikemura (Eds.), Caregiving, cultural, and cognitive perspectives on secure-base behavior and working models: new growing points of attachment theory and research. *Monographs of the Society for Research in Child Development,* 60(2–3, Serial No. 244).

Sagi, A., van IJzendoorn, M. H., Scharf, M., Koren-Karie, N., Joels, T., & Mayseless, O. (1994). Stability and discriminant validity of the Adult Attachment Interview: a psychometric study in young Israeli adults. *Developmental Psychology, 30,* 988–1000.

Schuengel, C., Bakermans-Kranenburg, M. J., & van IJzendoorn, M. H. (1999). Frightening maternal behavior linking unresolved loss and disorganized infant attachment. *Journal of Consulting and Clinical Psychology, 67,* 54–63.

Singer, L. M., Brodzinsky, D. M., Ramsay, D., Steir, M., & Waters, E. (1985). Mother–infant attachment in adoptive families. *Child Development, 56,* 1543–1551.

Sroufe, L. A. (1983). Infant–caregiver attachment and patterns of adaptation in preschool: the roots of maladaption and competence. In M. Perlmutter (Ed.), *The Minnesota Symposia on Child Psychology, 16,* 41–83.

Sroufe, L. A. (1989). Relationships and relationship disturbances. In A. J. Sameroff & R. N. Emde (Eds.), *Relationship disturbances in early childhood* (pp. 97–124). New York: Basic.

Stern, D. (1977). *The first relationship.* Cambridge, MA: Harvard University Press.

Stovall, K. C., & Dozier, M. (2000). The evolution of attachment in new relationships: single subject analyses for ten foster infants. *Development and Psychopathology, 12,* 133–156.

van IJzendoorn, M. H. (1995). Adult attachment representations, parental responsiveness, and infant attachment: a meta-analysis on the predictive validity of the adult attachment interview. *Psychological Bulletin, 117,* 387–403.

van IJzendoorn, M. H., Moran, G., Belsky, J., Pederson, D., Bakersman-Kranenburg, M. J., & Kneppers, K. (2000). The similarity of siblings' attachments to their mothers. *Child Development, 71,* 1086–1098.

Vandell, D. L., Owen, M. T., Wilson, K. S., & Henderson, V. K. (1988). Social development in infant twins: peer and mother–child relationships. *Child Development, 59,* 168–177.

Ward, M. J., & Carlson, E. A. (1995). Associations among adult attachment representations, maternal sensitivity, and infant–mother attachment in a sample of adolescent mothers. *Child Development, 66,* 69–79.

2

Child–Parent Attachment and Children's Peer Relations: A Quantitative Review

Barry H. Schneider, Leslie Atkinson, and Christine Tardif

The central premise of attachment theory is that the security of the early child–parent bond is reflected in the child's interpersonal relationships across the life span. This meta-analysis was based on 63 studies that reported correlations between child–parent attachment and children's peer relations. The overall effect size (ES) for child–mother attachment was in the small-to-moderate range and was quite homogeneous. ESs were similar in studies that featured the Strange Situation and Q-sort methods. The effects were larger for peer relations in middle childhood and adolescence than for peer relations in early childhood. ESs were also higher for studies that focused on children's close friendships rather than on relations with other peers. Gender and cultural differences in ESs were minimal. The results for the few studies on father–child attachment were inconclusive.

Bowlby (1969) proposed that the infant constructs models of the world, significant persons within it, and the self. These *internal working models*, or states of mind that guide behavior, become more sophisticated with age and are applied to the child's broadening social world. On the basis of these models, the child predicts the behavior of others and makes motivational attributions. Although internal working models are amenable to change with change in the environment, they cannot be modified easily. This is because they involve intrinsically conservative expectancies (later experience is interpreted in light of earlier experience) and because these expectancies influence behavior such that expectations are confirmed, or at least not disconfirmed (e.g., someone who expects a rebuff may invite it, thereby confirming expectations, or she or he may avoid interaction, thereby precluding disconfirmation of expectations). Models of others' behavior are brought from the home and may resist change even when they do not accurately reflect the reality of new playmates.

However, several investigators have questioned the theory linking attachment security to subsequent child adjustment. Grusec and Lytton (1988) queried the assumption that attachment acts causally. They speculated that attachment is an indicator of the child's overall resilience and adjustment, which may have other sources. Hinde (1988) argued that the construct of internal working models has become a catchall explanation of stability within attachment theory. Hinde suggested that other, nonattachment constructs, such as temperament, might serve this purpose equally well (see also Kagan, 1995) and that no convincing evidence exists for the causal role, or even the existence, of internal working models. Remarking that the empirical support for attachment falls short of theory-based expectation, Lewis and Feiring (1989) argued that theorists fail to consider important socialization agents other than parents that influence children's social relationships. Belsky and Cassidy (1995) concluded that "the notion of internal working models as the causal process explaining the associations between attachment security and the developmental sequelae remains a useful interpretive heuristic in need of empirical evaluation" (p. 383).

Basic data on the strength of the association between attachment security and peer relations are a prerequisite to the resolution of this controversy. Quantitative synthesis of research results facilitates the objective comparison of results across studies that have used a common metric. It is particularly useful in synthesizing results when there are a substantial number of studies but modest sample sizes in each, as in the case of the present meta-analysis. The provision of such an estimate was the first purpose of this meta-analysis. The derivation of an overall effect size (ES), however, represents only the starting point of this meta-analysis. To avoid the pitfalls of "combining multiple studies involving specific, exotic, and diverse procedures, participants, and hypotheses and then generalizing to people in general" (Lepper, Henderlong, & Gingras, 1999, p. 671), we discuss the specifics of particular studies in a narrative format when there are few studies addressing a particularly relevant hypothesis or population and especially when samples are small or procedures flawed.

POTENTIAL MODERATING FACTORS

The second purpose of this meta-analysis was to identify variables that moderate the relation between attachment security and peer relations. Many possible moderating factors exist.

Assessment of Attachment

Most studies of attachment and peer relations have relied on Ainsworth and Wittig's (1969) Strange Situation to measure attachment security. Lamb and Nash (1989) argued that this laboratory task lacks ecological validity. Clarke-Stewart (1989) and Thompson (1988) argued that independent behavior in the Strange Situation has been mistakenly interpreted as (insecure) avoidance of the caregiver.

The second commonly used measure of attachment in this literature is the Attachment Q-set (Waters & Deane, 1985). Designed as an ecologically valid alternative to the Strange Situation, the Attachment Q-set involves observation of the caregiver–child dyad in and around the home. However, one might wonder whether the instrument truly measures attachment behavior (which is a response to stressful circumstances, such as are incorporated into the Strange Situation) or whether it measures some correlate(s) of that behavior. The Q-set provides a continuous metric representing the *degree* to which a relationship is secure. However, it has been argued that attachment theory pertains to quality of attachment, not quantity (Ainsworth, Blehar, Waters, & Wall, 1978). On the other hand, the continuous metric of the Attachment Q-set may provide more statistical power than the categorical metric of the Strange Situation. For whatever reasons, meta-analytic results indicate only modest convergence between the Attachment Q-set and the Strange Situation ($r = .26$; van IJzendoorn, Vereijken, & Ridsen-Walraven, in press).

Investigators have also developed a variety of other techniques to assess attachment security. Cassidy and Marvin (1992) and Crittenden (1988) developed separation–reunion systems for preschoolers, although Goldberg, Washington, et al. (1999) questioned the continuity of the former with respect to infant attachment classifications. Bretherton, Ridgeway, and Cassidy (1990) constructed a doll story play task for preschoolers, but the task may not be well suited to clinical samples (Greenberg, DeKlyen, Speltz, & Endriga, 1997). George, Kaplan, and Main (1996) developed the Adult Attachment Interview, but it may have limitations where adolescents are concerned (Cobb, 1996). This proliferation of attachment instruments, many with putative short-comings, suggests the need for a comparative and integrative approach to the literature.

Assessment of Peer Relations

Most of the major instruments for assessing children's peer relations have been used in attachment studies, including sociometrics, direct observation, and reports from parents and teachers. In addition, some studies have included self-report measures of peer relations, which are of questionable validity as measures of actual social behavior, especially in the case of youngsters with externalizing disorders (Kupersmidt & Patterson, 1991). The various assessment methods vary greatly in terms of validity and reliability; they often provide divergent pictures of the same child's peer relations (e.g., Bierman & Welsh, 1997).

Virtually every conceivable aspect of peer relations has been included in attachment research, but it is not clear that all are equally relevant. Admittedly, there are "broad" views of attachment (see discussion by Thompson, 1998) according to which child–parent attachment could be expected to predict many if not most aspects of children's cognitive and social development, in contrast to "narrow" views in which child–parent attachment is assumed to predict only close, intimate relationships. Nevertheless, even the broad views of attachment do not provide any basis for assuming that all aspects of social development will be affected to the same extent.

Accordingly, the most meaningful contrast that could emerge from a synthesis of the literature is between measures of friendship and measures of peer relations in larger groups. This contention is consistent with the relationship perspective (e.g., Belsky & Cassidy, 1995; Hinde, 1979; Sroufe & Fleeson, 1986; Waters & Sroufe, 1983) that advocates going beyond conceptualizations of social competence in terms of constructs that pertain mostly to large-group interaction, such as popularity/rejection (Belsky & Cassidy, 1995; Fox, 1995; Kerns, 1994; Shulman, 1995). These theorists argue that the intense, intimate experience of family life is more closely associated with the child's success in forming intense, intimate relationships with friends. On the basis of their qualitative review, for example, Belsky and Cassidy (1995) concluded, "In thinking about the sequelae of attachment security … there seems to be a clear need to distinguish intimacy or intimacy-like relations from mere sociability" (p. 394).

This argument implies that the influence of attachment on relationships must be summarized separately from its impact on social exchanges with peers who are not close friends, and that time-lagged correlations should be compared with concurrent correlations between attachment and social relations. Sroufe (1988) implored theorists to respect the boundaries of attachment theory in making predictions about children's functioning in later life. He argued for limiting predictions to such domains as inner confidence, self-worth, and intimacy and closeness in interpersonal relationships. There is a growing consensus that both acceptance in large groups and involvement in satisfying close relationships have implications for adjustment, though possibly in different ways (Asher, Parker, & Walker, 1996). Perhaps, as Sullivan (1953) theorized, interaction with intimate friends during childhood and adolescence provides the best foundation for satisfying, close relationships later on.

We are not suggesting that attachment security is unrelated to aspects of social competence other than intimacy in close friendship. Social competencies in large groups and in close relationships are conceptually and empirically related. First, acceptance in a large group expands the network of potential friends, thereby increasing the opportunity to form intimate friendships. Popularity affords friendship (Bukowski, Pizzamiglio, Newcomb, & Hoza, 1996). Second, success in social relations at the large-group level requires some of the same skills as are involved in forming and maintaining close friendships. Bukowski et al. discussed some of these common skills; they emphasized the ability to resolve conflict, to share positive affect, and to reciprocate liking. Some of these elements, especially the exchange of positive affect and of sentiments of liking, are important elements of early parent–child bonds and thus may relate to early attachment security. However, there are important differences in addition to the commonalities between the constructs, especially with regard to the exchange of intimacy, which is central in friendship but not in popularity. Hence, the working model for relationships that is based on the first intimate relationship should be most (although not uniquely) relevant to later intimate relationships, such as close friendship.

Obstacles to global peer acceptance may also be impediments to intimacy in close relationships. Aggression and shyness/withdrawal are the major obstacles to peer acceptance. Attachment can be seen as an antecedent to both. As noted by Troy and Sroufe (1987), children with insecure "avoidant" parents may expect hostility from others and relate to peers on the basis of that expectation with preemptive displays of hostility. According to Rubin, LeMare, and Lollis (1990), such avoidant attachment patterns are more likely to arise under adverse "setting conditions," such as the child being of a difficult temperament or the mother being socially isolated and/or under financial stress. The interpersonal aggression that arises from expectations of hostility should logically affect both close and casual social relationships. However, it is logical to expect that the hostility is transferred most directly from the parent–child relationship to the peer relationship most similar to it—namely, the bond between close friends. Furthermore, aggressive behavior alienates peers (Asher & Coie, 1990), which restricts the network of potential friends. Aggressive children tend to form relationships with other aggressive children (Dishion, Andrews, & Crosby, 1995); these friendships between antisocial children and youth are often superficial ones lacking in intimacy (Selman & Schultz, 1990).

The same reasoning applies to social withdrawal. Infants who display insecure, ambivalent patterns of attachment expect to be rejected by others. They remain passive in peer contexts in order to avoid rejection (Rubin, Bukowski, & Parker, 1998). This ambivalent pattern is seen as more probable if the child is biologically predisposed to become less aroused in novel social situations and if the family system is already vulnerable because of external stresses (e.g., unemployment) and/or inadequate provision of social support (Rubin et al., 1990). From early adolescence on, shyness or withdrawal alienates peers (Hodgens & McCoy, 1989). This alienation restricts the pool of candidates for close friendships; signs of social withdrawal are evident in relationships with close friends as well as in large-group social interaction. For example, withdrawn children are less talkative and less competitive with their friends than are nonwithdrawn children (Schneider, 1999). Thus, there are reasons to believe that child–parent attachment may affect many aspects of children's social transactions with peers who are not close friends. Furthermore, acceptance or rejection in large groups and the behaviors (e.g., aggression and social withdrawal) that may lead to acceptance or rejection may function as regulators of access to close friendships. Although there may be reasons why attachment may differentially affect such variables as popularity, aggression, and social withdrawal, we focus herein on what we consider the most important distinction from a conceptual standpoint: the comparison of more and less intimate relationships.

The major tools of peer-relations research—namely, observation, sociometrics, and third-party ratings—can all be used to measure both general peer acceptance and close friendships, but their content would differ dramatically. For example, direct observations of children's play during recess have been used to quantify frequency or duration of contacts with peers in comparison with frequency or duration of solitary play. It is also possible, although not always easy, to use direct observation to assess such aspects of intimate friendship as mutual affection, emotional support, and intimacy, even in young children (Howes, 1996). Unfortunately, such direct observation has not typically been used in studies of attachment and peer relations, perhaps because many of the critical moments in friendship occur out of range of observational technology.

There are developmental differences in the relative importance of many of the salient features of friendship. Harry Stack Sullivan, who emphasized the pivotal importance of intimate friendship for psychosocial development, argued for the importance of friendship at only one period of development: right before and during adolescence (Berndt, 1996; Sullivan, 1953). It is difficult, though possible, to assess affection and intimacy in the friendships of young children, but their friendships are not characterized by mutual emotional support, self-disclosure, or frequent expressions of acceptance (Howes, 1996). The exchange of intimacy is acknowledged in children's comments about their friendships from preadolescence on (Berndt, Hawkins, & Hoyle, 1986); it becomes the central feature of friendship only in adolescence (Aboud & Mendelson, 1996; Clark, Mills, & Corcoran, 1989). The differentiation between friendship and social interactions with nonfriends is the central distinction of this article. We also investigated several other variables that may serve to moderate the relation between attachment security and peer relations, as described in the following sections.

Gender of Parent and Child

Because of the mother's primary caregiving role in Western societies, one might expect that child–mother attachment is of greater consequence for future relationships (Belsky, 1996). Nevertheless, it is possible that the quality of father–child attachment is strongly related to children's social relations, especially for boys in the preschool and early school years, when same-sex friendships are the norm (e.g., Daniels-Beirness, 1989).

Age at Assessment

Age at assessment of both attachment and peer relations may be important. With respect to attachment, theorists have argued that internal working models become more stable with age (Bowlby, 1969). De Wolff and van IJzendoorn (1997) offered this argument as an explanation for their meta-analytic finding that the ES linking maternal sensitivity to attachment security is stronger in older than in younger samples (although the explanation has been questioned; see Atkinson et al., 2000). On the basis of such theory and data, one would expect that the later attachment is assessed, the more predictive of subsequent peer relations it would be. Further, as introduced earlier, the aspects of friendship that parallel most directly many of the central features of secure attachment—especially intimacy, security, and trust—do not emerge as major dimensions of children's peer relationships until preadolescence and adolescence.

Time between Assessments of Attachment and Peer Relations

Given strong claims made about the long-term effects of attachment quality (e.g., Bowlby, 1973), it is important to consider the strength of associations between measures of attachment and peer relations as a function of the time lapse between them. Bowlby's theory implies that disturbances of early attachment are reflected in relationships over the entire life course, though it emphasizes that favorable experiences in later years may mitigate the negative effects of early attachment problems and vice versa (Main, Kaplan, & Cassidy, 1985; van IJzendoorn & Bakermans-Kranenburg, 1997). Accordingly, longitudinal data spanning several developmental stages provide more convincing support of the theory than do concurrent correlations between attachment and peer relations. Nevertheless, Youngblade, Park, and Belsky (1993) speculated that correlations might be higher in studies featuring concurrent assessment of attachment and peer relations, which represent the effects of the child–parent relationship at the time it was measured rather than the effects of the child–parent bond as it was years earlier.

Risk Status

Many longitudinal studies in attachment have been faulted for their use of nonrepresentative, middle-class samples (Lamb & Nash, 1989), although some studies of attachment and peer relations have been conducted with participants of lower socioeconomic status (SES; e.g., Troy & Sroufe, 1987). Many protective aspects of middle-class homes may attenuate the sequelae of early attachment insecurity (e.g., Bates, Maslin, & Frankel, 1985; Belsky, Rosenberger, & Crnic, 1995). Therefore, it would be useful to compare the effects of attachment on peer relations for samples differing in SES.

Beyond low SES, several studies involve samples at risk for psychiatric disorder and the children of parents who have psychiatric diagnoses. The question arises as to the comparative impact of attachment in vulnerable child populations versus low-risk populations. Furthermore, it would be heuristically useful to establish the relative contribution of underlying relationship disturbances to disorders that are diverse in phenomenology (Rutter, 1995). In addition to nonclinical populations, data are available regarding children referred for psychiatric services (Wright, Binney, & Smith, 1995) and for children with known risk factors such as a history of maltreatment (Lyons-Ruth, Alpern, & Repacholi, 1993) and low birth weight (Rose-Krasnor, Rubin, Booth, & Coplan, 1996).

Culture

Concepts of attachment-related secure-base behavior are applicable in diverse cultures (Waters, Vaughn, Posada, & Kondo-Ikemura, 1995), but it is not clear that attachment is equally crucial to children's peer relationships in all cultures. In many cultures, for example, siblings, extended family members, and neighbors are more active in child socialization than they are in North America (Stanton, 1995). Hence, one might expect that child–parent attachment might be more predictive of peer relations in North American samples than in samples in which the child-rearing responsibility is shared more diversely.

INTEGRATIVE CHALLENGES

There has been little attempt to integrate findings in the literature that address attachment and peer relations. Quite apart from the disparate approaches outlined above, or perhaps because of this diversity, there are apparent contradictions in the literature that have never been addressed. For example, some investigators reported significant associations between attachment security and later interaction with unfamiliar age-mates (Pastor, 1981) and adults (Main & Weston, 1981; Plunkett, Klein, & Meisels, 1988). Other studies failed to show significant associations between attachment security and interaction with unfamiliar peers (Jacobson & Wille, 1986) and adults (Frodi, 1983; Lamb, Hwang, Frodi, & Frodi, 1982; Thompson &

Lamb, 1984). No attempt has been made to reconcile these inconsistencies. This integrative failure also manifests in a lack of even basic strategies for organizing the literature. Belsky and Cassidy (1995) observed, for example, "In view of the fact that attachment theory is a theory about the characteristics, consequences, and determinants of close relationships, it is surprising that efforts to conduct or even review research linking attachment history and social development have not attended to distinctions among the partners (e.g., familiar vs. unfamiliar peers) whose interactions with children are being studied" (p. 393). Meta-analytic techniques are ideal for resolving such issues.

Our major hypotheses were (a) that the overall ES for studies on the link between child–parent attachment and children's peer relations would be significantly different from zero, (b) that the ESs would be significantly larger in studies of close friendships than in studies focusing on less intimate peer relationships, and (c) that the ESs would be larger in studies conducted with participants in middle childhood and adolescence than in studies conducted with preschoolers. In addition, we explored the other distinctions outlined above.

METHOD

Retrieval of Studies

We conducted computerized searches of PsycLIT, MedLine, and Dissertation Abstracts International to locate relevant studies that appeared between 1970 and 1998. We used the following keywords in different combinations: *attachment, child–mother interaction, child–parent relations, peer/social competence, interpersonal interaction, friendship,* and *peer relations.* We also scanned manually the abstracts of the Society for Research in Child Development and the International Conference of Infant Studies as well as the more recent issues of *Child Development, Developmental Psychology, Psychological Review,* and *Psychological Bulletin* to ensure the inclusion of studies that had not yet been included in the computerized databases. Finally, we searched the reference lists of each article that had been retrieved.

Inclusion and Exclusion Criteria

The search procedures generated approximately 200 studies. Given this substantial number, we imposed relatively stringent inclusion criteria. To be included, a study had to (a) describe original data; (b) include a measure of attachment to a parent, other than self-report, that was (c) collected before the child reached age 18; (d) include a quantitative measure of children's peer relations that was other than self-report; (e) feature assessment of attachment security and children's peer relations before age 18; (f) include data on both securely and insecurely attached participants or a continuous measure of attachment; and (g) be written in English or another language understood by a member of our research team (French, Italian, or Spanish). If studies meeting these criteria did not include sufficient data for statistical analysis, we contacted the authors. Additional data were received from 19 of the 32 authors contacted.

In some cases, the same data were reported in more than one publication. To avoid duplication, we used the more recent publication and added any data from the earlier versions that were not included. In three other instances, more than one publication described the same longitudinal study, but the articles published after the first one contained reports of new follow-up data. Two of these studies featured two follow-up points each, for a total of four articles. Another longitudinal study by Sroufe and colleagues was reported in nine different publications covering nine different follow-up points. We felt it was important not to assign disproportionate weight to these three longitudinal studies in computing the overall ESs. Therefore, the data pertaining to all follow-up points were combined in those calculations. However, we considered it more meaningful when calculating ESs for specific age groups and for specific types of measures to separate the data pertaining to different follow-up points within these three longitudinal studies. Therefore, in those ancillary analyses, the number of effects exceeds the number of studies.

Sixty-three studies, with a combined sample of 3,510 children, met the inclusion criteria. An independent graduate research assistant, not involved in any other aspect of the coding or analyses, co-rated the articles in the original pool to establish interrater reliability regarding inclusion decisions. He agreed with 98% of the original raters' decisions. Disagreements were resolved by consensus.

Although studies were excluded for a variety of reasons, our criteria led to the systematic exclusion of one relatively coherent group of studies that were conducted with adolescents and that used self-reports of both attachment and peer relations. Despite their heuristic value, those studies are limited because the findings may be inflated by shared method variance.

Coding of Study Features

Each study was coded on (a) attachment measure (e.g., Strange Situation or Q-sort; this feature was also expanded to include a categorization of all studies as employing either dichotomous or continuous attachment measures); (b) source of information about children's peer relations (e.g., direct observation, peer report, teacher report); (c) dimension(s) of peer relations considered (e.g., peer-directed aggression, peer-directed withdrawal, quality of friendship); (d) familiarity of play partners to focal child participants (i.e., friends, unfamiliar peers, etc.); (e) information about close friendships (existence, stability, quality, whether information was available about the characteristics of the friend or his or her attachment with parents); (f) gender of child and parent participants; (g) mean age of participants when attachment and (h) peer relations were measured; (i) time between the measurement of attachment and peer relations; (j) risk status of the sample (e.g., low SES, parents with psychiatric disorder); (k) publication date; and (l) dissemination medium (i.e., journal article, thesis, conference presentation). A second coder independently classified half the studies. The kappa coefficient for interrater reliability exceeded .80 for each of the categories.

Calculation of Effect Sizes

Weighted ES correlations (*rs*) were computed with Schwarzer's (1988) meta-analytic software. When necessary, we calculated estimates of *r* directly using means and standard deviations reported in the original articles or supplied by the authors. The ESs used in the analyses pertain to differences in peer relations between children classified as securely and insecurely attached.

Results reported as nonsignificant and unaccompanied by relevant test statistics accounted for 28% of the total number of ESs and came from 38% of the studies. In these cases, we substituted the mean ES of nonsignificant results that were reported within the data set, $r = .07$, based on 94 ESs from 38 studies. We believe this is preferable to Rosenthal's (1984) suggestion of substituting an estimate based on $p = .50$, which would also distort findings because of the inclusion of ESs that are considerably lower than those typically found in this literature for nonsignificant effects. Nevertheless, we report mean ESs based on both Rosenthal's practice and the method we propose.

To avoid assigning disproportionate influence to studies that included multiple measures of attachment and/or peer relations, we averaged ESs within each study to yield a single correlation for the assessment of overall strength of the relationship between attachment and peer relations. However, in many of the analyses performed to identify moderators of ESs, we allowed the number of ESs to exceed the number of studies. This was necessary, for example, to compare the ESs for the various aspects and measures of social competence because multiple measures of social competence were included in almost all of the studies.

RESULTS

Attachment to Mothers

Overall Predictive Strength. The average global ES was .20 ($SE = .16$). This effect is significantly different from zero ($Z = 11.91$, $p < .001$). Rosenthal and Rubin's (1982) binomial ES display suggests that if secure attachment were a treatment and if peer relations had a dichotomous outcome (successful vs. unsuccessful), then 59% of securely attached children would have successful peer relations compared with 41% of those insecurely attached. The fail-safe *n* indicates that 165 additional studies (2.6 times the number of studies identified in this meta-analysis) with nonsignificant results would be needed to reduce the overall ES to the just-significant level. This figure (165) falls short of Rosenthal's (1991) critical value, $5k+10$ (which equals, in this case, 325). Therefore, we cannot be reasonably sure that the significance of the effect under consideration will not be negated by as yet unpublished null findings. The mean ES would drop to .16 if calculated according to Rosenthal's convention of estimating the ESs for unspecified nonsignificant findings at $p = .50$; it would increase to .27 if undetailed nonsignificant effects were deleted.

Chi-square tests indicated that the ES distribution was homogeneous, $\chi^2(62, N = 63) = 68.8$, *ns*; this was confirmed by disjoint cluster analysis, which indicated that all ESs except for a single outlier chi-square (Troy & Sroufe, 1987, $r = .69$) were part of a single cluster ($p < .05$). This is best interpreted as indicating that the ESs can be treated as estimates of the same parameter, with sampling error the most likely explanation for differences among estimates (Cooper & Hedges, 1994, p. 432). Nevertheless, we followed the injunction of Johnson, Mullen, and Salas (1995) and Rosenthal (1995) to explore for potential moderators regardless of the results of tests of homogeneity. Skew (.688; $SE = .277$) and kurtosis (.484; $SE = .548$) statistics were well within acceptable limits. Therefore, parametric statistics were used in many of the comparisons reported below.

Analysis of variance (ANOVA) revealed no significant differences between concurrent and longitudinal studies. There were also no significant differences among the dissemination media (journal, thesis, convention paper, book chapter). The descriptive statistics appear in Table 2.1.

Moderators of the Association Between Child–Mother Attachment and Children's Peer Relations

Close friendship. Table 2.2 summarizes the data from the original studies of close friendships. The diversity of friendship measures used precluded meaningful quantitative comparison of the implications of these features for ES. To test our hypothesis that the ESs pertaining to friendship would be higher than the ESs for other types of peer relationships, we matched each of these studies on friendship with a randomly selected study conducted with unfamiliar peers, as described above. ESs pertaining to friendship ($n = 10$,

TABLE 2.1
Average Effect Size (*r*) by Source of Study

Source	*M*	*k*	*SD*
Studies featuring concurrent measurement of attachment and social competence			
Journal article	.223	27	.147
Thesis	.193	7	.134
Chapter	.210	2	.038
Convention paper	.167	3	.165
Studies featuring measurement of social competence at follow-up			
Journal article	.215	27	.192
Thesis	.181	2	.156
Chapter	.003	4	.108

$M = .24$, $SD = .14$) were significantly higher than those of the comparison group ($n = 10$, $M = .14$, $SD = .11$), $F(1, 18) = 4.33$, $p < .05$.

Assessment of attachment. ESs were not significantly different when Strange Situation and Q-sort findings were compared. Nor were findings significantly different when the analysis was extended to compare dichotomously scored and continuous variables (see Table 2.3).

Assessment of peer relations. We borrowed the dimensional structure of the Revised Class Play method (Masten, Morison, & Pellegrini, 1985) to distinguish among three types of peer-related behavior: aggression, withdrawal, and sociability/leadership. We added a fourth dimension, sociometric choice, which measures the extent to which peers accept a child as a potential companion. Mean ESs for these dimensions, and the different sources of information about them, are listed in Table 2.4. ANOVA revealed that the difference in ESs among the dimensions of peer relations was significant: $F(3, 94) = 3.51$, $p < .05$. Post hoc Tukey's honestly significant difference (HSD) tests indicated that the ESs for sociability/leadership were higher ($p < .05$) than the ESs for the other dimensions.

ANOVA also revealed a significant difference among the sources of information, $F(3, 94) = 9.22$, $p < .01$. Post hoc Tukey tests indicated that the ESs for maternal ratings of children's peer relations were significantly ($p < .05$) higher than the ESs for all the other sources, which did not differ from each other.

Child gender. Separate data for boys and girls were available for only 14 studies and are summarized in Table 2.5. The difference between the ESs for boys and girls was not significant.

TABLE 2.2
Studies Pertaining to Children's Close Friendships

Study	*n*	Age(s) in years		Attachment measure(s)	Friendship measure(s)	Effect size for friendship (*r*)	Dyadic analysis of friendship
		Attachment	Friendship				
Booth, Rubin, & Rose-Krasnor (1998)	58	4	8	Reunion Rating Scale	Social support from best friend	.11	No
Freitag et al. (1996)	40	1–1.5	10	Strange Situation	Parent interview regarding child's competence in friendship	.43 (mother attachment); .07 (father attachment)	No
Howes, Matheson, & Hamilton (1994)	84	1 and 4	4	Strange Situation	Friendship Quality Q-set	.07	No
Kerns (1994)	42	4	5	Attachment Q-set	Observation of dyadic interaction	.20	Yes
Kerns & Gruys (1995)	86	4	4	Attachment Q-set	Observation of "progress toward forming a friendship"	.09	Yes
Kerns, Klepac, & Cole (1996)	74	10	10	Security Scale (parent self-report)	1. Reciprocal friendship nominations 2. Ratings of relationship quality	.28	Yes
Park (1992)	41	4.5	4.5	Attachment Q-set	Mothers' ratings of children's reaction to friend moving away	.31	No
Park & Waters (1989)	66	4	4	Attachment Q-set	Observations of pairs of friends during free play	.27	Yes

Pierrehumbert, Iannotti, & Cummings (1985)	48	2	5	Strange Situation	Mothers' reports of the number of child's friends and degree of friendship	.47	No
Shulman, Elicker, & Sroufe (1994)	32	4	11	Strange Situation	1. Observations of interactions of friends at summer camp 2. Camp counselors' ratings 3. Children's ratings of friendship quality 4. Sociometric nominations of friends	.18	No
Youngblade, Park, & Belsky (1993)*	164	1	5	1. Strange Situation	1. Mothers' reports of children's friendships	.01 (mother attachment); .02 (father attachment)	No
				2. Attachment Q-sort	2. Observation of dyadic interaction		

* Some of the findings from this study were published in Youngblade and Belsky (1992).

TABLE 2.3
Average Effect Sizes (*r*) by Attachment Measure

Attachment measure	*M*	*k*	*SD*
Strange Situation	.124	26	.140
Q-sort	.219	17	.134
Continuous	.205	28	.166
Categorical	.160	35	.151

TABLE 2.4
Average Effect Sizes (*r*) by Aspect of Social Competence and Source of Information

Aspect and source	*M*	*k*	*SD*
Social withdrawal			
Observed	.147	14	.164
Teacher rated	.077	4	.093
Peer rated	.068	2	.308
Parent rated	.070	1	
Aggression			
Observed	.137	17	.167
Teacher rated	.110	7	.093
Peer rated	.170	3	.145
Parent rated	.194	2	.405
Sociability/leadership			
Observed	.147	35	.166
Teacher rated	.129	8	.133
Peer rated	.120	4	.066
Parent rated	.313	3	.260
Sociometric choice	.133	13	.087
All aspects			
Observed	.144	66	.158
Teacher rated	.111	19	.102
Peer rated	.129	22	.066
Parent rated	.233	6	.314

Note: The mean of the effect sizes in the table is not the same as the mean effect size for the data set because the latter was calculated on the basis of one effect size per study. Ratings of friendship quality are not included in the peer-rated totals.

Age at assessment. The correlation ($n = 63$) between the average age of participants at the time of the first attachment measure in each study and the overall ES was .23 ($p < .05$). The correlation between attachment security and the average age of participants at the time of the last peer-relations measure was also significant, $r(63) = .22$, $p < .05$.

Confirmation of our hypothesis that the ESs would be significantly larger for participants in middle childhood or adolescence than for younger children was complicated by the fact that a disproportionate number of the studies involved young children. A cutoff of 8 years represents the transition to middle childhood in a meaningful way. We also considered a cutoff of 10 years, but that would have left too few studies in the older block for meaningful analysis. ANOVA revealed that the ESs for the 16 studies conducted with participants 8 years old and older ($M = .26$, $SD = .16$) were significantly higher than the ESs of the 59 studies conducted with younger participants ($M = .17$, $SD = .16$), $F(1, 73) = 4.14$, $p < .05$.

Time between assessments of attachment and peer relations. There is no evidence that the time separating assessments influences the strength of association between attachment and peer relations, $r(63) = .04$.

Risk status. No significant differences emerged when at-risk samples were compared to samples with no known risk and when samples at risk because of psychological disturbance were compared with low-SES samples (see Table 2.5). Disentangling the effects by type of risk is complicated because a

TABLE 2.5
Average Effect Sizes (*r*) by Participant Characteristics

Characteristic	*M*	*k*	*SD*
Gender			
Boys—concurrent	.295	8	.139
Boys—follow-up	.162	6	.096
Girls—concurrent	.163	8	.259
Girls—follow-up	.238	6	.322
Age (in months) at time of attachment measurement			
< 13	.137	11	.130
13–24	.126	20	.145
25–36	.167	7	.175
37–48	.252	10	.173
> 48	.227	18	.126
Age (in years) at time of social-competence measurement			
3 or < 3	.155	19	.175
4–5	.185	32	.142
6–9	.201	9	.140
> 9	.297	9	.142
Risk status			
No known risk	.166	45	.154
Low SES	.201	8	.101
At risk for disorder	.234	8	.168

Note. SES = socioeconomic status.

disproportionate number of individuals with psychological disturbances are of low socioeconomic status (SES) (Hollingshead & Redlich, 1958). Therefore, although we had no choice but to follow the original source in designating a sample as at risk because of either low SES or psychiatric disturbance, there may be considerable overlap not taken into consideration in the design. There was wide fluctuation among the ESs for studies conducted with samples identified only as low in SES; the ESs ranged from .02 through .49. Studies conducted with children experiencing psychological disturbances were few and very heterogeneous in terms of the nature and severity of the problems.

Culture. In addition to the 54 studies with North American samples, there were three studies from the highly collective societies (see Hofstede, 1984) of East Asia (Nakano, Usui, & Miyake, 1984–1985, conducted in Japan; Sull, 1995, conducted in Korea; and Wu, 1992, conducted in China), with ESs of .15, .16, and .19, respectively. There were four studies conducted with Western European samples, all from countries classified by Hofstede as individualistic. Two were from Germany (Freitag, Belsky, Grossmann, Grossmann, & Scheurer-Englisch, 1996; Suess, Grossmann, & Sroufe, 1992), with ESs of .43 and .47, and two were from the United Kingdom (Turner, 1991; Wright et al., 1995), with ESs of .18 and .59. Granot and Mayseless (1996) studied Israeli city children; the ES for that study was .28. Oppenheim, Lamb, and Sagi (1988) studied kibbutz children raised in communal sleeping arrangements; the ES for child–mother attachment was .07. The average ES for these nine studies was .27 (SD = .16), compared with a mean of .18 (SD = .16) for the 54 studies conducted in North America; the difference was not significant. This finding is qualified, however, by the small number of studies conducted outside of North America.

Attachment to Fathers

Only seven studies involved attachment to fathers. In two of these (Kobak & Sceery, 1988; Moore, 1997), the data on mothers and fathers were combined and indiscriminable. The average ES for the remaining five studies was .10 and was homogeneous, $\chi^2(4, N = 5) = 5.15$, *ns*. The best comparison for these is with the data on child–mother attachment from the same studies. The average ES for those was .08; the difference between the data on mother and father attachment in the same studies was not significant. Unfortunately, only one of the studies (Marcus & Mirle, 1990) provided separate data on father–son and father–daughter attachment. Marcus and Mirle found that attachment to fathers was correlated only with the social competence of boys. However, it is difficult to generalize the results of that study because of the idiosyncratic measure of attachment used, its specific focus on children seen for custody evaluation during parental divorce proceedings, and the limited peer-relations measures.

DISCUSSION

Interpreting the Overall Effect Size

In this meta-analysis, we studied the relation between attachment security and peer relations. In terms of attachment to mothers, the ES was a significant .20. To put this ES in perspective, consider Cohen's (1988) proposal to regard correlations of .10, .30, and .50 as small, medium, and large ESs, respectively. Cohen acknowledged, however, that these figures are arbitrary. It would be helpful to compare the ESs found here with ESs characterizing other predictors of peer relations, for example, parental regulation of autonomy or child temperament. In that way, we could derive a sense of the *relative* contribution of attachment security to peer relations. However, the requisite meta-analyses have not been published, a fact that limits the interpretability of ESs found here and that also represents a profound lacuna in the study of peer relations in general. Here we discuss the implication of the overall .20 ES before scrutinizing the implications of the limited heterogeneity within the data set.

The focus on relative ESs is all the more important because the file drawer statistic suggested that the number of identified studies precludes confident acceptance of the significance of the link between attachment security and peer relations. That is, 165 studies averaging null results would render the .20 ES just significant. This falls short of the fail-safe 325 studies required by Rosenthal's (1991) criteria. Given that much new research is needed in the area, it is imperative that we identify the strongest methodologies at this juncture. This will permit accurate estimation of the ES linking attachment and peer relations. Furthermore, if this ES is actually larger than the overall .20 identified here, use of stronger methods will reduce the critical fail-safe *n*, the number of studies requisite for confident acceptance of the hypothesis in question.

The .20 ES provides some evidence for the predictive power of attachment theory. However, the size of the effect seems incongruous with strong causal claims made in the literature. Whatever their magnitude, correlation-based ES estimates do not indicate causation (Cooper, 1984). However, the absence of a significant correlation would preclude a causal link. Current knowledge does not provide a basis for reconciling causal reasoning with findings that reach statistical significance but explain little variance. The low correlation is, at best, consistent with a modest influential role of attachment security on peer relations.

This possible incongruity between theory and data may indicate that the theory is faulty. This possibility is almost never acknowledged among the original articles, many of which claim support for the theory on the basis of data that pertain to a subset of measures or samples. At best, the small ES is consistent with the notion that attachment is only one among many influences on peer relations. As mentioned above, other parental influences may include affective bonds, disciplinary practices, modeling, and regulation of the child's autonomy and contact with peers. Genetics may also play a role. Needed at this point is a multivariate approach exploring the relative, cumulative, and interactive impact of multiple influences on peer relations.

Measurement Problems as Possible Constraints on Effect Size

Explanations other than erroneous theory involve poor methodology or weaknesses in operationalizing one or both of the constructs in question. Although we mentioned some possible shortcomings of the various measures of attachment in the introduction, our meta-analysis did not reveal significant differences between the Strange Situation and Attachment Q-set measures nor between classificatory and continuous measures. Nevertheless, the fact that the Strange Situation and the observer-rated Attachment Q-set show modest convergent validity ($r = .26$, as mentioned earlier) implies the possibility that these and other attachment instruments assess different constructs or different aspects of the same construct. If this is the case, then it is possible that many or most of the attachment measures used in studies of peer relations do not, in fact, reflect those attachment processes that are most relevant to the study of peer relationships.

It should also be mentioned, with respect to the possible constraining influence of attachment measurement, that early attachment measures may be unstable. Belsky, Campbell, Cohn, and Moore (1996), for example, found no reliable stability in Strange Situation classifications among three samples of infants assessed twice within 6 or 7 months. Similarly, Goldberg and Washington et al.'s (1999) prediction of attachment security from 1 to 4 years did not exceed chance (based on the Strange Situation and a preschool separation procedure, respectively). In a qualitative review, Thompson (1998) pointed out that the stability of attachment security depends on numerous contextual factors (as yet insufficiently explored) such as family SES, changing life circumstances (e.g., mothers' return to work; nonmaternal care), and maternal personality variables of particular relevance here. Justifiability of attachment, whether explained by known environmental change or merely attributable to measurement error, may attenuate the link between attachment and other social relations, especially in longitudinal studies.

Similarly, issues with respect to the assessment of peer relations may also attenuate the association between attachment and other relationships. Some peer relations measures may assess aspects of peer relationships that are more strongly associated with attachment than are other aspects. Our inclusion criteria excluded what may be the least valid source of information on children's peer relations, at least in terms of convergent validity: their self-reports (Bierman & Welsh, 1997). Nevertheless, this exclusion downplays the child's own perspective, which some regard as distinct from that of external sources but not necessarily inaccurate (e.g., Hymel & Franke, 1985). The decision to eliminate these self-report studies reflected a desire to base our inferences on the best data. Nevertheless, it may be of heuristic value to consider those studies briefly because they complement the database of this meta-analysis with a large number of adolescent studies. Although we did not calculate meta-analytic statistics for the discarded studies, our impression is that the ESs probably vary as much as those of the studies that qualified for inclusion and may not be excessively inflated by shared method variance. Some of the samples did yield significant correlations between self-reports of peer relations and self-reports of attachment to parents (Kobak & Sceery, 1988; Soble, 1987). However, Lapsley, Rice, and FitzGerald (1990) did not find a significant association between parent–adolescent attachment and social adjustment in the first year of college. Rice, Cunningham, and Young (1997) found that attachment to fathers was associated with social competence at college but that attachment to mothers was not. Schneider and Younger (1996) found that self-reported attachment to both fathers and mothers was inconsistently correlated with self-report and parent-report measures of peer relations in high school.

Similar mixed results characterize the relatively few studies conducted in which self-reports were used with children rather than adolescents. For example, Toth and Cicchetti (1996), working with child victims of abuse by parents, found that self-reports of relatedness with parents correlated with self-perceptions of social competence. However, in following into elementary school a sample of children who had participated in intensive observational research during preschool, Howes, Hamilton, and Philipsen (1998) found that early attachment bonds with teachers correlated with children's perceptions of the quality of their friendships but that earlier mother–child attachment was unrelated.

Many researchers chose peer and teacher reports, which are valid measures of peer relations but perhaps not optimal for the purpose of assessing the implications of early child–parent attachment bonds. Peer and teacher reports on children's peer relations do provide information that is useful, for example, in identifying children who are rejected by their peers or who are aggressive and disruptive in their classrooms. However, both peer and teacher reports are subject to positive and negative halo effects, which might lead to the designation as socially competent of children who are physically attractive, proficient at sports, excellent at academics, and compliant with school routines. There is little reason to believe that the more distal predictors of peer acceptance or teacher-rated social competence are linked closely to child–parent attachment.

Child–Parent Attachment as a Predictor of Children's Friendship

We predicted a stronger ES for friendship studies because the bonds of family life are more similar to the trust and intimacy of close friendships than to the social skills involved in negotiating peer relations with other classmates and acquaintances. This proved to be the case (*r*s = .24 and .14 for studies of friendship and of relations with nonfriends, respectively), confirming the conclusions of an earlier qualitative review (Belsky & Cassidy, 1995). Therefore, we posit that the subset of friendship studies provides the best estimate available of the ES between attachment and peer relations, although we acknowledge that there are few such studies in the literature ($n = 10$). Hence, the .24 ES must be interpreted with caution pending further research. It should also be noted that the comprehensive measurement of friendship that has been advocated recently (e.g., Furman, 1996) is rarely evident in the 10-study data set. Most of the many facets of friendship are absent from the original data (see Table 2.2). Friendships are almost always measured at a single time point, often from the perspective of only one of the two friends. Information about the attachment status of both friends was gathered in only four studies (Kerns, 1994; Kerns & Gruys, 1995; Kerns, Klepac, & Cole, 1996; Park & Waters, 1989). No investigator assessed the prosociality of the friend, although an antisocial friend can do more harm than good to a child's overall social competence. These issues both limit the generalizability of extant studies and suggest a direction for future work.

Two other findings are consistent with the finding that attachment is more strongly related to friendship than to relations with peers who are not close friends. The first involves the fact that the link between attachment and peer relations strengthens with the age at which peer relations are measured. This may account for the higher ESs for samples older than 8 years, because the processes inherent in forming and maintaining friendships—such as intimacy, conflict resolution, and reliable alliance—are related more closely to the overall social competence of children from the middle elementary-school years onward (Aboud & Mendelson, 1996; Berndt et al., 1986). It is important to note that the critical studies in which follow-up continued into the early adolescent years, when close friendships crystallize and affect overall psychosocial adjustment (e.g., Sullivan, 1953), are not numerous. The promise of this direction is indicated by the relatively large ESs in the studies conducted on friendship with children in preadolescence and adolescence (see Table 2.2: Freitag et al., 1996, ES = .43; Kerns et al., 1996, ES = .28; and Pierrehumbert, Iannotti, & Cummings, 1985, ES = .18). Furthermore, the effects of attachment for adolescents may have been underrepresented in the present calculations because we consolidated the multiple articles from Alan Sroufe's laboratory to avoid assigning weight to multiple studies from the same laboratory. Nevertheless, those articles describe the data that are probably the most comprehensive, the longest, and the most relevant to the purposes of the present review. Thus, despite many drawbacks, there are some patterns in the present findings that are perfectly consistent with attachment theory.

Consistent with the comparatively large ES linking attachment and friendship is the significant difference between ESs based on parent-rated social interaction and those based on information obtained from peers or teachers or by direct observation. One explanation for this finding is that mothers have a more extensive and relevant perspective on their children's social interaction: They see their children with friends during more informal interactions that portray the children's relationship styles. However, it is also possible that the mothers' own attachment representations and their own relationships with their children may color their perception of their children's peer relationships. This issue exemplifies the need for multiple assessment approaches within any given study of peer relationships.

Age and Cultural Differences

Another finding of interest in the present meta-analysis was the significant correlation ($r = .23$) showing that the older the sample is when assessed for attachment security, the stronger the ES linking attachment and peer relations. Bowlby (1969) argued that internal working models become more stable with age. The broad range of ages incorporated here may render this meta-analysis particularly sensitive to the development of stable working models through infancy, childhood, and adolescence. The increasing stability of these models may account for the increasing power of prediction. The upper limit of validity is constrained by reliability; hence, a more stable predictor potentially has greater power than a less stable predictor. Another possibility is that as children age, child–parent and peer–peer relations become more similar.

However, we cannot rule out the possibility that the ES discrepancy between older and younger participants is attributable to methodological differences. Unfortunately, our ability to detect such artifacts is limited by the small number of studies conducted with children older than 8 years. We did find a significant ($p < .05$) cultural difference: More studies in the older block were conducted outside of North America (42% vs. 12%). Several other differences between the studies conducted with older and younger children were marginal ($.10 > p > .05$): More studies in the older block involved children at risk (25% vs. 10%); in studies featuring follow-up components, the interval was longer ($M = 5.0$ years [$SD = 4.5$] vs. 2.9 years [$SD = 1.9$]), $F(1, 33) = 3.56$, $p = .068$. However, these differences (i.e., culture, risk status, and follow-up interval) were not significant predictors of ES in the full data set. Furthermore, there were no significant differences in the proportions of studies featuring follow-up; the use of Strange Situation or Q-sort methods as the original measure of attachment; or the relative frequency of direct observations and peer, parent, and teacher reports to assess peer relations. It is true that Q-sort measures tend to be used with older participants ($M = 48$ months, compared with 17 months for the Strange Situation in the current sample). This fact may account for some of the age differences because, as reported above, the ESs for Q-sort findings were somewhat higher than those for Strange Situation findings, although the difference was not significant. However, many of the highest ESs were in follow-up studies by Sroufe and his colleagues, in which early adolescents were followed for many years after the initial attachment measurement, which was based on the Strange Situation technique. Furthermore, although ESs for studies using Q-sort methods were somewhat larger than those for studies using the Strange Situation, the difference was not significant. Hopefully, the reasons for the correlations between age and ES will become clearer as more studies are conducted with older children and adolescents.

With respect to cross-cultural issues, the number of studies conducted outside of North America is limited, but within-culture variation in ESs appears as great as cross-cultural variation. These data provide no reason to doubt the cross-cultural replicability of the hypothesis that attachment is linked to peer relations. However, many of the studies were conducted in societies similar to the United States in terms of the major dimensions of cultural variation: The United States, Germany, the United Kingdom, and the urban Jewish population in Israel are all classified as relatively individualistic within the spectrum of societies (Hofstede, 1984). The mostly collectivistic societies of Latin America and Africa are not represented at all in the literature. Comparisons between Northern and Southern Europe could also be revealing because of the greater orientation toward extended family in the Mediterranean European countries (Georgas et al., 1997). Thus, although there is evidence for the applicability of attachment theory across cultures, its pertinence to much of the world's population has yet to be explored.

Examination of the individual studies provides clues as to why the ESs within cultures vary as widely as ESs across cultures. In Europe, the most probable explanation for the ES in the Suess et al. (1992) study, which is much higher than the ESs in the other two German studies, is that Suess et al. measured the friendships of early adolescents, whereas the other studies focused on the less intimate relations of younger children. The three studies conducted in East Asia do represent collectivistic countries in which the extended family assumes a predominant role in children's upbringing. One of these, however, was conducted in China after the implementation of the one-child policy. Its ES, higher than those of the studies from Japan and Korea, may reflect the external constraints on child–parent bonds that result from the one-child policy, because only children may receive particularly high levels of responsiveness and attention from their parents (Wu, 1992). The one study conducted with kibbutz children (Oppenheim et al., 1988) had a lower ES for child–parent attachment than the Israeli study by Granot and Mayseless (1996), which was conducted with city children. This finding may reflect the compensatory effect of attachment to the kibbutz *metapelet*. Thus, although the discrepant findings among studies conducted in Europe and Asia can be reconciled to some extent, corroboration of the utility of attachment theory in non-Western countries depends on new research.

Possible Moderators Requiring Additional Investigation

There was no significant difference between groups according to risk status, and there was as much variability within low-risk and high-risk groups as there was between them. These findings may be attributable to the failure to differentiate varied forms of disturbance when studying clinical populations (e.g., Wright et al., 1995) and may render it impossible to respond to Rutter's (1995) plea for clarification of the implications of attachment theory for a typical child development. Nevertheless, there were very high ESs in the few studies conducted with atypical child samples, such as Troy and Sroufe's (1987) study on bully victims, which emerged as an outlier, as well as the Wright et al. (1995) study of a mixed clinical sample, which had the second highest ES in the data set (.59). These high ESs may or may not be coincidental. Further research with atypical populations will determine whether attachment bonds are particularly crucial for the peer relations of children experiencing psychological distress.

Although the diversity of the child–mother attachment literature lends itself to rich speculation, little can be established about the implications of child-father attachment for children's peer relations. The ES is small but is similar to the ES found in comparable data on maternal attachment and peer relations. Beyond this, we can say little. The ES is based on only five studies. Moreover, all but one of these studies (Freitag et al., 1996) focused on children's large-group interactions to the neglect of close interpersonal relationships and did not distinguish between the effects of paternal attachment on the peer relations of sons and daughters. Thus, we conclude that the implications of paternal attachment for children's peer relations remain largely unexplored.

About 25% of the studies in the current data pool considered other family or child variables in addition to parent–child attachment as predictors of children's peer relations. Unfortunately, the calculation of meta-analytic estimates of these additional contributions was precluded by the heterogeneity of the variables. In none of these studies was attachment the sole significant predictor of children's peer relations. In most studies, variables other than attachment accounted for substantial additional variance: child temperament (Bates et al., 1985; Sull, 1995), child-rearing practices (Fagot, 1997; Youngblade & Belsky, 1992), attitudes toward parenting (Adams, 1994; Kavesh, 1991), maternal depression (Rubin, Both, Zahn-Waxler, Cummings, & Wilkinson, 1991), maternal psychosocial adjustment (Lyons-Ruth et al., 1993), child's attachment to teachers (Howes & Wu, 1990), child's prior day-care experience (Howes, 1991), and observed maternal warmth (Christopoulou, 1988). In two studies of preschoolers, Lieberman (1977) found that attachment and other variables predicted different aspects of child social competence: Attachment correlated with nonverbal indicators of social competence, such as sharing, whereas the childen's previous experience with peers better predicted verbal interactions. In a few cases (e.g., Silverman, 1990, on child-rearing styles, and Denham, 1987, on mothers' display of emotion), both attachment and other variables were found to be linked to children's peer relations, but the analyses were not designed to compare their relative contributions.

In closing, we suggest that relatively little will be gained with new correlational studies linking mother–child attachment with the mainstays of peer-relations assessment (i.e., observations and sociometrics) during early childhood. More comprehensive studies exploring multiple dimensions of mothering and fathering as predictors of children's close interpersonal relationships across the life span would complement the existing data meaningfully. Although the data presented in this article do illustrate that child–parent attachment is correlated with children's peer relations, none of the studies provides a suitable rejoinder to Hinde's (1988) contention that there is no evidence for the existence or causal role of internal working models. It is very conceivable that the attachment bond facilitates children's peer relations in other ways. For example, mothers of securely attached children have been found to encourage reciprocity and cooperativeness in child–mother interactions (see Russell, Pettit, & Mize, 1998), which may transfer to peer relations. Secure attachment may lead to positive, authoritative child-rearing, which may account for its effects on peer relations (Goldberg, Grusec, & Jenkins, 1999). Hopefully, the next generation of research on child–parent attachment and children's peer relations will improve more substantially on the hypothesis that "all good things go together" (Youngblade & Belsky, 1992).

REFERENCES

References marked with an asterisk indicate studies included in the meta-analysis.

Aboud, F. E., & Mendelson, M. J. (1996). Determinants of friendship selection and quality: developmental perspectives. In W. M. Bukowski, A. F. Newcomb, & W. W. Hartup (Eds.), *The company they keep: friendship in childhood and adolescence* (pp. 87–136). New York: Cambridge University Press.

*Adams, B. L. (1994). *An investigation of the interrelationships among security of attachment, parenting attitudes, and the development of competence.* Unpublished doctoral dissertation, Virginia Consortium for Professional Psychology, Virginia Beach, VA.

*Adamson, L. (1990). *The relationship between attachment and social competence in peer relations in early childhood.* Unpublished doctoral dissertation, Boston University, School of Education.

Ainsworth, M. D. S., Blehar, M. C., Waters, E., & Wall, S. (1978). *Patterns of anachment: a psychological study of the strange situation.* Hillsdale, NJ: Erlbaum.

Ainsworth, M. D. S., & Wittig, B. A. (1969). Attachment and exploratory behavior of one-year-olds in a strange situation. In B. M. Foss (Ed.), *Determinants of infant behavior IV* (pp. 111–136). London: Methuen.

*Allen, J. P., Moore, C., Kuperminc, G., & Bell, K. (1998). Attachment and adolescent social functioning. *Child Development, 69,* 1406–1419.

Asher, S. R., & Coie, J. D. (1990). *Peer rejection in childhood.* New York: Cambridge University Press.

Asher, S. R., Parker, J. G., & Walker, D. L. (1996). Distinguishing friendship from acceptance: implications for intervention and assessment. In W. M. Bukowski, A. F. Newcomb, & W. W. Hartup (Eds.), *The company they keep: friendship in childhood and adolescence* (pp. 366–405). New York: Cambridge University Press.

Atkinson, L., Niccols, G. A., Paglia, A., Coolbear, J., Parker, K. C. H., Poulton. L., Guger, S., & Sitarencos, G. (2000). A meta-analysis of time between maternal sensitivity and attachment assessments: implications for internal working models in infancy/toddlerhood. *Journal of Social and Personal Relationships, 17,* 791–810.

*Bates, J. E., Maslin, C. A., & Frankel, K. A. (1985). Attachment insecurity, child–mother interaction, and temperament as predictors of behavior-problem ratings at age three years. In I. Bretherton & E. Waters (Eds.), *Monographs of the Society for Research in Child Development, 50,* 167–193.

Belsky, J. (1996). Parent, infant, and social-contextual antecedents of father–son attachment security. *Developmental Psychology, 32,* 905–913.

Belsky, J., Campbell, S. B., Cohn, J. F., & Moore, G. (1996). Instability of infant–parent attachment security, *Developmental Psychology, 32,* 921–924.

Belsky, J., & Cassidy, J. (1995). Attachment theory and evidence. In M. Rutter & D. Hay (Eds.), *Development through life* (pp. 373–402). London: Blackwell.

Belsky, J., Rosenberger, K., & Crnic, K. (1995). Maternal personality, marital quality, social support and infant temperament: their significance for infant–mother attachment in human families. In C. R. Pryce, R. D. Martin, & D. Skuse (Eds.), *Motherhood in human and nonhuman primates* (3rd Schultz-Biegert Symposium, Kartause Ittingen, 1994; pp. 115–124). Basel, Switzerland: Karger.

Berndt, T. J. (1996). Exploring the effects of friendship quality on social development. In W. M. Bukowski, A. F. Newcomb, & W. W. Hartup (Eds.), *The company they keep: friendship in childhood and adolescence* (pp. 346–365). New York: Cambridge University Press.

Berndt, T. J., Hawkins, J. A., & Hoyle, S. G. (1986). Changes in friendship during a school year. Effects on children's and adolescents' impressions of friendship and sharing with friends. *Child Development, 57,* 1284–1297.

Bierman, K. L., & Welsh, J. A. (1997). Social relationship deficits. In E. J. Mash & L. G. Terdal (Eds.), *Assessment of childhood disorders* (pp. 328–365). New York: Guilford Press.

*Booth, C. L., Rose-Krasnor, L., McKinnon, J., & Rubin, K. H. (1994). Predicting social adjustment in middle childhood: the role of preschool attachment security and maternal style. *Social Development, 3,* 189–204.

*Booth, C. L., Rose-Krasnor, L., & Rubin, K. H. (1991). Relating preschoolers' social competence and their mothers' parenting behaviors to early attachment security and high-risk status. *Journal of Social and Personal Relationships, 8,* 363–382.

*Booth, C. L., Rubin, K. H., & Rose-Krasnor, L. (1998). Perceptions of emotional support from mother and friend in middle childhood: links with social-emotional adaptation and preschool attachment security. *Child Development, 69,* 427–442.

*Bost, K. K., Vaughn, B. E., Washington, W. N., Cielinski, K. L., & Bradbard, M. R. (1998). Social competence, social support, and attachment: demarcation of construct domains, measurement, and paths of influence for preschool children attending Head Start. *Child Development, 69,* 192–218.

Bowlby, J. (1969). *Attachment and loss: Vol. 1: Attachment.* Harmonsworth, Middlesex, England: Penguin.

Bowlby, J. (1973). *Attachment and loss: Vol. 2: Separation.* New York: Basic Books.

Bretherton, L. Ridgeway, D., & Cassidy, J. (1990). Assessing internal working models of the attachment relationship. In M. T. Greenberg, D. Cicchetti, & M. Cummings (Eds.), *Attachment in the preschool years: theory, research and intervention* (pp. 273–308). Chicago: University of Chicago Press.

Bukowski, W. M., Pizzamiglio, M. R., Newcomb, A. F., & Hoza, B. (1996). Popularity as an affordance for friendship: the link between group and dyadic experience. *Social Development, 5,* 189–202.

Cassidy, J., & Marvin, R. (1992). *Attachment organization in preschool children: procedures and coding manual.* Unpublished manuscript, Pennsylvania State University and University of Virginia.

Christopoulou, C. (1988). *Familial antecedents of peer social competence in second graders.* Unpublished doctoral dissertation, University of Virginia.

Clark, M. S., Mills, J. R., & Corcoran, D. M. (1989). Keeping track of needs and inputs of friends and strangers. *Personality and Social Psychology Bulletin, 15,* 533–542.

Clarke-Stewart, K. (1989). Infant day care: maligned or malignant? *American Psychologist, 44,* 266–273.

Cobb, C. L. H. (1996). Adolescent–parent attachments and family problem-solving styles. *Family Process, 35,* 57–82.

Cohen, J. (1988). *Statistical power analysis for the behavioral sciences* (2nd ed.). Hillsdale, NJ: Erlbaum.

*Cohn, D. A. (1990). child–mother attachment of six-year-olds and social competence at school. *Child Development, 61,* 152–162.

Cooper, H. M. (1984). *The integrative research review: a social science approach.* Beverly Hills, CA: Sage.

Cooper, H. M., & Hedges, L. V. (1994). *The handbook of research synthesis.* New York: Russell Sage Foundation.

*Copeland-Mitchell, J., Denham, S. A., & DeMulder, E. K. (1997). Q-sort assessment of child-teacher attachment relationships and social competence in the preschool. *Early Education and Development, 8,* 27–36.

Crittenden, P. M. (1988). Relationships at risk. In J. Belsky & T. Nezworski (Eds.), *Clinical implications of attachment theory* (pp. 136–174). Hillsdale, NJ: Erlbaurn.

Daniels-Beirness, T. (1989). Measuring peer status in boys and girls: a problem of apples and oranges. In B. H. Schneider, G. Attili, J. Nadel, & R. P. Weissberg (Eds.), *Social competence in developmental perspective* (pp. 107–120). Dordrecht, The Netherlands: Kluwer.

*Denham, S. A. (1987, August). *Child competence and maternal emotion socialization correlates of attachment Q-Sort variables.* Poster presented at the 95th Annual Convention of the American Psychological Association, New York, NY.

De Wolff, M. S., & van IJzendoorn, M. H. (1997). Sensitivity and attachment: A meta-analysis on parental antecedents of infant attachment. *Child Development, 68,* 571–591.

Dishion, T. J., Andrews, D. W., & Crosby, L. (1995). Antisocial boys and their friends in early adolescence: relationship characteristics, quality, and interactional process. *Child Development, 65,* 139–151.

*Elicker, J., Englund, M., & Sroufe, L. A. (1992). Predicting peer competence and peer relationships in childhood from early child–parent relationships. In R. D. Parke & G. W. Ladd (Eds.), *Family–peer relationships: models of linkage* (pp. 77–106). Hillsdale, NJ: Erlbaum.

*Erez, T. (1995). Predicting preschoolers' social coping from early attachment history. In S. Shulman (Ed.), *Close relationships and socioemotional development: human development* (pp. 1–34). Norwood, NJ: Ablex.

*Erickson, M. F., Sroufe, L. A., & Egeland, B. (1985). The relationship between quality of attachment and behavior problems in preschool in a high-risk sample. *Monographs of the Society for Research in Child Development, 50* (1–2, Serial No. 209).

*Fagot, B. I. (1997). Attachment, parenting, and peer interactions of toddler children. *Developmental Psychology, 33,* 489–499.

*Fagot, B. I., & Kavanagh, K. (1990). The prediction of antisocial behavior from avoidant attachment classification. *Child Development, 61,* 864–873.

*Fagot, B. I., & Pears, K. C. (1996). Changes in attachment during the third year: consequences and predictions. *Development and Psychopathology, 8,* 325–344.

Fox, N. A. (1995). Of the way we were: Adult memories about attachment experiences and their role in determining infant–parent relationships: a commentary on van IJzendoorn. *Psychological Bulletin, 117,* 404–410.

*Freitag, M. K., Belsky, J., Grossmann, K., Grossmann, K. E., & Scheurer-Englisch, H. (1996). Continuity in child–parent relationships from infancy to middle childhood and relations with friendship competence. *Child Development, 67,* 1437–1454.

Frodi, A. (1983). Attachment behavior and sociability with strangers in premature and full-term infants. *Infant Mental Health Journal, 4,* 14–22.

Furman, W. (1996). The measurement of friendship perceptions: conceptual and methodological issues. In W. M. Bukowski, A. F. Newcomb, & W. W. Hartup (Eds.), *The company they keep: friendship in childhood and adolescence* (pp. 41–65). New York: Cambridge University Press.

*Galluzo, D. C., Matheson, C. C., Moore, J. A. & Howes, C. (1990). Social orientation to adults and peers in infant child care. In N. Fox & G. Fein (Eds.), *Infant day care: the current debate* (Vol. 4, pp. 183–192). Norwood, NJ: Ablex.

Georgas, J., Chirstakopoulou, S., Poortinga, Y. H., Angleitner, A., Goodwin, R., & Charalambous, N. (1997). The relationship of family bonds to family structure and function across cultures. *Journal of Cross-Cultural Psychology, 28,* 303–320.

George, C., Kaplan, N., & Main, M. (1996). *Adult Attachment Interview* (3rd ed.). Unpublished manuscript, University of California, Berkeley, Department of Psychology.

Goldberg, S., Grusec, J. E., & Jenkins, J. M. (1999). Confidence in protection: arguments for a narrow definition of attachment. *Journal of Family Psychology, 13,* 475–483.

Goldberg, S., Washington, J., Myhal, N., Janus, M., Simmons, R. J., MacLusky, I., & Fowler, R. S. (1999). *Stability and change in attachment from infancy to preschool.* Manuscript submitted for publication.

*Granot, D., & Mayseless, O. (1996, July). *The relation between attachment patterns and adaptive functioning in the school environment amongst children in middle childhood.* Paper presented at the meeting of the International Society for the Study of Behavioral Development, Quebec City, Quebec, Canada.

Greenberg, M. T., DeKlyen, M., Speltz, M. L., & Endriga, M. C. (1997). The role of attachment processes in externalizing psychopathology in young children. In L. Atkinson & K. Zucker (Eds.), *Attachment and psychopathology* (pp. 196–222). New York: Guilford Press.

Grusec, J., & Lytton, H. (1988). *Social development.* New York: Springer-Verlag.

*Hellstrom, L. A. (1994). *The relationship between preschoolers' attachment, social competence, and parenting stress in two types of child care arrangements.* Unpublished master's thesis. Concordia University, Montreal, Quebec, Canada.

Hinde, R. A. (1979). *Towards understanding relationships.* London: Academic Press.

Hinde, R. A. (1988). Continuities and discontinuities: conceptual issues and methodological considerations. In M. Rutter (Ed.), *Studies of psychosocial risk: the power of longitudinal data* (pp. 95–122). Cambridge, England: Cambridge University Press.

Hodgens, J. B., & McCoy, J. F. (1989). Distinctions among rejected children on the basis of peer-nominated aggression. *Journal of Clinical Child Psychology, 18,* 121–128.

Hofstede, G. (1984). Hofstede's culture dimensions: an independent validation using Rokeach's Value Survey. *Journal of Cross-Cultural Psychology, 15,* 417–433.

Hollingshead, A. B., & Redlich, F. C. (1958). *Social class and mental illness,* New York: Wiley.

*Howes, C. (1991). A comparison of preschool behaviors with peers when children enroll in child-care as infants or older children. *Journal of Reproductive and Infant Psychology, 9,* 10–115.

Howes, C. (1996). The earliest friendships. In W. M. Bukowski, A. F. Newcomb, & W. W. Hartup (Eds.), *The company they keep: friendship in childhood and adolescence* (pp. 66–86). New York: Cambridge University Press.

Howes, C., Hamilton, C. E., & Philipsen, L. C. (1998). Stability and continuity of child–caregiver and child–peer relationships. *Child Development, 69,* 418–426.

*Howes, C., Matheson, C. C., & Hamilton, C. E. (1994). Maternal, teacher, and child care history correlates of children's relationships with peers. *Child Development, 65,* 264–273.

*Howes, C., Rodning, C., Galluzzo, D. C., & Myers, L. (1990). Attachment and child care: relationships with mother and caregiver. In N. Fox & G. Fein (Eds.), *Infant day care: the current debate* (pp. 169–181). Norwood, NJ: Ablex.

Howes, C., & Wu, F. (1990). Peer interactions and friendships in an ethnically diverse school setting. *Child Development, 61,* 537–541.

Hymel, S., & Franke, S. (1985). Children's peer relations: assessing self-perceptions. In B. H. Schneider, K. H. Rubin, & J. E. Ledingham (Eds.), *Children's peer relations: issues in assessment and intervention* (pp. 75–92). New York: Springer-Verlag.

*Jacobson, J. L., Tianen, R. L., Wille, D. E., & Aytch, D. M. (1986). Infant–mother attachment and early peer relations: the assessment of behavior in an interactive context. In E. C. Mueller & C. R. Cooper (Eds.), *Process and outcome in peer relationships* (57–78). Orlando, FL: Academic Press.

*Jacobson, J. L., & Wille, D. E. (1986). The influence of attachment pattern on developmental changes in peer interaction from the toddler to the preschool period. *Child Development, 57,* 338–347.

Johnson, B. T., Mullen, B., & Salas, E. (1995). Comparison of three meta-analytic approaches. *Journal of Applied Psychology, 80,* 94–106.

Kagan, J. (1995). On attachment. *Harvard Review of Psychiatry, 3,* 104–106.

*Kavesh, L. B. (1991). *Antecedents of peer competence in childhood.* Unpublished doctoral dissertation, University of Illinios at Chicago.

*Kerns, K. A. (1994). A longitudinal examination of links between child–mother attachment and children's friendships in early childhood. In S. Shulman (Ed.), *Close relationships and socioemotional development: human development* (Vol. 7, pp. 379–381). Norwood, NJ: Albex.

*Kerns, K. A., & Barth, J. M. (1995). Attachment and play: convergence across components of child–parent relationships and their relations to peer competence, *Journal of Social and Personal Relationships, 12,* 243–260.

*Kerns, K. A., & Gruys, A. (1995, April). *child–mother attachment and friendship formation in preschoolers.* Paper presented at the meeting of the Society for Research in Child Development, Indianapolis, IN.

*Kerns, K. A., Klepac, L., & Cole, A. (1996). Peer relationships and preadolescents' perceptions of security in the child–mother relationship. *Developmental Psychology, 32,* 457–466.

*Klein, R. P., & Durfee, J. T. (1979). Prediction of preschool social behavior from social emotional development at one year. *Child Psychiatry and Human Development, 9,* 145–151.

*Kobak, R. R., & Sceery, A. (1988). Attachment in late adolescence: working Models, affect regulation, and representations of self and others, *Child Development, 59,* 135–146.

Kupersmidt, J., & Patterson, C. J. (1991). Childhood peer rejection, aggression, withdrawal, and perceived competence as predictors of self-reported behavior problems in adolescence. *Journal of Abnormal Child Psychology, 19,* 427–449.

*LaFreniere, P. J., & Sroufe, L. A. (1985). Profiles of peer competence in the preschool: interrelations between measures, influence of social ecology, and relation to attachment history. *Developmental Psychology, 21,* 56–69.

Lamb, M. E., Hwang, G. P., Frodi, A., & Frodi, M. (1982). Security of the mother- and father-infant attachment and its relation to sociability with strangers in traditional and non-traditional Swedish families. *Infant Behavior and Development, 5,* 3–367.

Lamb, M. E., & Nash, A. (1989). Infant–mother attachment, sociability, and peer competence. In T. J. Berndt & G. W. Ladd (Eds.), *Peer relationships in child development* (pp. 219–246). New York: Wiley.

Lapsley, D. K., Rice, K. G., & FitzGerald, D. P. (1990). Adolescent attachment, identity, and adjustment to college: implications for the continuity of adaptation hypothesis. *Journal of Counseling and Development, 68,* 561–565.

Lepper, M. R., Henderlong, J., & Gingras, I. (1999). Understanding the effects of extrinsic rewards on intrinsic motivation: uses and abuses of meta-analysis; comment on Deci, Koestner, and Ryan. *Psychological Bulletin, 125,* 669–676.

Lewis, M., & Feiring, C. (1989). Infant, mother and mother–infant interaction behavior and subsequent attachment. *Child Development, 60,* 831–837.

*Lieberman, A. F. (1977). Preschoolers' competence with a peer: relations with attachment and peer experience. *Child Development, 48,* 1277–1287.

*Lyons-Ruth, K. Alpern, L., & Repacholi, B. (1993). Disorganized infant attachment classification and maternal psychosocial problems as predictors of hostile-aggressive behavior in the preschool classroom. *Child Development, 64,* 572–585.

Main, M., Kaplan, N., & Cassidy, J. (1985). Security in infancy, childhood, and adulthood: a move to the level of representation. *Monographs of the Society for Research in Child Development, 50* (1–2, Serial No. 209).

Main, M., & Weston, D. (1981). The quality of toddler's relationship to mother and father: related to conflict behavior and readiness to establish new relationships. *Child Development, 52,* 923–940.

*Malatesta-Magai, C., Leak, S., Tesman, J., Shepard, B., Culver, C., & Smaggia, B. (1994). Profiles of emotional development: individual differences in facial and vocal expression of emotion during the second and third years of life. *International Journal of Behavioral Development, 17,* 239–269.

Marcus, R. F., & Mirle, J. (1990). Validity of a child interview measure of attachment as used in child custody evaluations. *Perceptual and Motor Skills, 70,* 1043–1054.

Masten, A. S., Morison, P., & Pellegrini, A. (1985). A revised class play method of peer assessment. *Developmental Psychology, 21,* 523–533.

*Moore, C. W. (1997). *Models of attachment, relationships with parents, and sexual behavior in at-risk adolescents.* Unpublished doctoral dissertation, University of Virginia, Department of Psychology.

*Moss, E., Parent, S., Gosselin, C., Rousseau, D., & St-Laurent, D. (1996). Attachment and teacher-reported behavior problems during the preschool and early school-age period. *Development and Psychopathology, 8,* 511–525.

*Nakano, S., Usui, H., & Miyake, K. (1984–1985). Individual differences in responses to unfamiliar objects at twenty-three months of age. *Research and Clinical Center for Child Development,* 8 (Annual Report), 43–55.

Oppenheim, D., Lamb, M. E., & Sagi, A. (1988). Infant-adult attachments on the kibbutz and their relation to socioemotional development 4 years later. *Developmental Psychology, 2224,* 427–433.

*Park, K. A. (1992). Preschoolers' reactions to loss of a best friend: developmental trends and individual differences. *Child Study Journal, 22,* 233–252.

*Park, K. A. & Waters, E. (1989). Security of attachment and preschool friendships. *Child Development, 60,* 1076–1081.

*Pastor, D. L. (1981). The quality of mother–infant attachment and its relationship to toddlers' initial sociability with peers. *Developmental Psychology, 17,* 326–335.

*Pierrehumbert, B., Iannotti, R. J., & Cummings, E. M. (1985). Mother–infant attachment, development of social competencies and beliefs of self-responsibility. *Archives de Psychologie, 53,* 365–374.

*Pierrehumbert, B., Iannotti, R. J., Cummings, E. M., & Zahn-Waxler, C. (1986). Attachment Maternel et dependance. Quelque apports de la psychologie experimentale [Maternal attachment and dependency: some contributions of experimental psychology]. *Neuropsychiatrie de l'Enfance, 34,* 409–420.

*Pierrehumbert, B., Iannotti, R. J., Cummings, E. M., & Zahn-Waxler, C. (1989). Social functioning with mother and peers at 2 and 5 years: the influence of attachment. *International Journal of Behavioral Development, 12,* 8–100.

Plunkett, J. W., Klein, T., & Meisels, S. J. (1988). The relationship of preterm infant–mother to stranger sociability at 3 years. *Infant Behavior and Development, II,* 83–96.

Rice, K. G., Cunningham, T. J., & Young, M. B. (1997). Attachment to parents, social competence, and emotional well-being: a comparison of Black and White late adolescents. *Journal of Counseling Psychology, 44,* 89–101.

*Rose-Krasnor, L., Rubin, K. H., Booth, C. L., & Coplan, R. (1996). The relation of maternal directiveness and child attachment security to social competence in preschoolers. *International Joournal of Behavioral Development, 19,* 309–325.

Rosenthal, R. (1984). Interpersonal expectancy and psi: some commonalties and differences. *New Ideas in Psychology, 2,* 47–50.

Rosenthal, R. (1991). *Meta-analytic procedures for social research.* London: Sage.

Rosenthal, R. (1995). Writing meta-analytic reviews. *Psychological Bulletin, 118,* 183–192.

Rosenthal, R., & Rubin, D. B. (1982). A simple, general-purpose display of magnitude of experimental effect. *Journal of Educational Psychology, 74,* 166–169.

*Rubin, K. H., Both, L., Zahn-Waxler, C., Cummings, E. M., & Wilkinson, M. (1991). Dyadic play behaviors of children of well and depressed mothers. *Development and Psychopathology, 3* 243–251.

Rubin, K. H., Bukowski, W., & Parker, J. E. (1998). Peer interactions, relationships, and groups. In W. Damon (Series Ed.) & R. N. Eisenberg (Vol. Ed.), *Handbook of child development: Vol. 3, Social, emotional, and personality development* (5th ed., pp. 619–700). New York: Wiley.

Rubin, K. H., LeMare, L., & Lollis, S. (1990). Social withdrawal in childhood. In S. R. Asher & J. D. Coie (Eds.), *Peer rejection in childhood* (pp. 217–249). New York: Cambridge University Press.

Russell, A., Pettit, G. S., & Mize, J. (1998). Horizontal qualities in parent–child relationships: parallels with and possible consequences for children's peer relationships. *Developmental Review, 18,* 313–352.

Rutter, M. (1995). Clinical implications of attachment concepts: retrospect and prospect. *Journal of Child Psychology and Psychiatry and Allied Disciplines, 36,* 549–571.

Schneider, B. H. (1999). A multi-method exploration of the friendships of children considered socially withdrawn by their school peers. *Journal of Abnormal Child Psychology, 27,* 115–123.

Schneider, B. H., & Younger, A. J. (1996). Adolescent–parent attachment and adolescents' relation with their peers: a closer look. *Youth & Society, 28,* 95–108.

Schwarzer, R. (1988). Meta-analysis programs. *Behavior Research Methods, Instruments & Computers, 20,* 338.

Selman, R. L., & Schultz, L. H. (1990). *Making a friend in youth.* Chicago: University of Chicago Press.

Shulman, S. (1995). *Close relationships and socioemotional development.* Norwood, NJ: Ablex.

*Shulman, S., Elicker, J., & Sroufe, L. A. (1994). Stages of friendship growth in preadolescence as related to attachment history. *Journal of Social and Personal Relationships, 11,* 341–361.

Silverman, N. (1990). *Attachment, maternal behavior and preschool competence at age three.* Unpublished doctoral dissertation, Boston University.

Soble, J. E. (1987). *The relationship between past and current attachment and current emotional functioning during late adolescence.* Doctoral dissertation. California School of Professional Psychology, Los Angeles, 1987. *Dissertation Abstracts International, 48,* 1821-B (Order No. DA8713198).

*Sroufe, L. A. (1983). Infant–caregiver attachment and patterns of adaptation in preschool: the roots of maladaptation and competence. In M. Perlmutter (Ed.), *Minnesota Symposium on Child Psychology* (Vol. 16, pp. 41–81). Hilsdale, NJ: Erlbaum.

Sroufe, L. A. (1998). The role of infant–caregiver attachments in development. In J. Belsky & L. Nezworski (Eds.), *Clinical implications of attachment* (pp. 18–38). Hillsdale, NJ: Erlbaum.

*Sroufe, L. A., Carlson, E., & Shulman, S. (1993). Individuals in relationships: development from infancy through adolescence. In D. C. Funder, R. D. Parke, C. Tomlinson-Keasey, & K. Widaman (Eds.), *Studying lives though time: personality and development* (pp. 315–342). Washington, D.C.: American Psychological Association.

Sroufe, L. A., & Fleeson, J. (1986). Attachment and the construction of relationships. In W. Hartup & Z. Rubin (Eds.), *Relationships and development* (pp. 51–71). Hillsdale, NJ: Erlbaum.

*Sroufe, L. A., Schork, E., Motti, E., Lawroski, N., & Lafreniere, P. (1984). The role of affect in social competence. In C. Izard, J. Kagan, & R. Zajonc (Eds.), *Emotion, cognition and behavior* (pp. 289–319). New York: Plenum Press.

Stanton, M. E. (1995). Patterns of kinship and residence. In B. B. Ingoldsby & S. Smith (Eds.), *Families in multicultural perspective: perspectives on marriage and the family* (pp. 97–116). New York: Guilford Press.

*Suess, G. J., Grossmann, K. E., & Sroufe, L. A. (1992). Effects of infant attachment to mother and father on quality of adaptation in preschool: from dyadic to individual organisation of self. *International Journal of Behavioral Development, 15,* 43–65.

*Sull, I. (1995). *Temperament, child–mother attachment, and peer relationships in Korean preschool children.* Unpublished doctoral dissertation. Temple University.

Sullivan, H. S. (1953). *The interpersonal theory of psychiatry.* New York: Norton.

Thompson, R. A. (1988). The effects of infant day care through the prism of attachment theory: a critical appraisal. *Early Childhood Research Quarterly, 3,* 273–282.

Thompson, R. A. (1998). Early sociopersonality development. In W. Damon (Series Ed.) & N. Eisenberg (Vol. Ed.), *Handbook of child psychology* (5th ed., pp. 25–104). New York: Wiley.

Thompson, R. A., & Lamb, E. E. (1984). Infants, mothers, families, and strangers. In M. Lewis (Ed.), *Beyond the dyad* (pp. 195–222). New York: Plenum Press.

Toth, S. L., & Cicchetti, D. (1996). Patterns of relatedness, depressive symptomatology, and perceived competence in maltreated children. *Journal of Consulting and Clinical Psychology, 64,* 32–41.

*Troy, M., & Sroufe, L. A. (1987). Victimization of pre-schoolers: role of attachment relationship history, *Journal of the American Academy of Child and Adolescent Psychiatry, 26,* 166–172.

*Turner, P. J. (1991). Relations between attachment, gender, and behavior with peers in preschool. *Child Development, 62,* 1475–1488.

*Urban, J., Carlson, E., Egeland, B., & Sroufe, A. (1991). Patterns of individual adaptation across childhood. *Development and Psychopathology, 3,* 445–460.

*Vandell, D. L., Owen, M. T., Wilson, K. S., & Henderson, V. K. (1988). Social development in infant twins: peer and child–mother relationships. *Child Development, 59,* 168–177.

van IJzendoorn, M. H., & Bakermans-Kranenburg, M. J. (1997). Intergenerational transmission of attachment: state of the art in psychometric, psychological and clinical research. In L. Atkinson & K. Zucker (Eds.). *Attachment and Psychopathology* (pp. 135–170). New York: Guilford Press.

van IJzendoorn, M. H., Vereijken, C. M. J. L., & Ridsen-Walraven, J. M. A. (in press). Is the Attachment Q-sort a valid measure of attachment security in young children? In B. E. Vaughn & E. Waters (Eds.), *Patterns of secure base behavior: Q-sort perspectives on attachment and caregiving,* Mahwah, NJ: Erlbaum.

*Wartner, U. G., Grossmann, K., Fremmer-Bombik, E., & Suess, G. (1994). Attachment patterns at age six in south Germany: predictability from infancy and implications for preschool behavior. *Child Development, 65,* 1014–1027.

Waters, E., & Deane, K. E. (1985). Defining and assessing individual differences in attachment relationships: Q-methodology and the organization of behavior in infancy and early childhood. *Monographs of the Society for Research in Child Development, 50* (1–2, Serial No. 209).

Waters, F., & Sroufe, L. A. (1983). Social competence as a developmental construct, *Developmental Review, 3,* 79–97.

Walters, E., Vaughin, B. E., Posada, G., & Kondo-Ikemura, K. (Eds.). (1995). Caregiving, cultural and cognitive perspectives on secure-base behavior and working models: new growing points of attachment theory and research. *Monographs of the Society fro Research in Child Development, 60* (2–3, Serial No. 244).

*Walters, E., Wippman, J., & Sroufe, L. A. (1979). Attachment, positive affect, and competence in the peer group: two studies in construct validation. *Child Development, 50,* 821–829.

*Weinfield, N. S., Ogawa, J. R., & Sroufe, L. A. (1997). Early attachment as a pathway to adolescent peer competence. *Journal of Research on Adolescence, 7,* 241–265.

Wright, J. C., Binney, V., & Smith, P. K. (1995). Security of attachment in 8–12-year-old: a revised version of the Separation Anxiety Test, its psychometric properties and clinical interpretation. *Journal of Child Psychology and Psychiatry, 36,* 757–774.

Wu, F. (1992). *Social competency of only-children in China: associations among maternal attachment, teacher attachment, and peer relationships.* Unpublished doctoral dissertation, University of California, Los Angeles.

*Youngblade, L. M., & Belsky, J. (1992). Child–parent antecedents of 5-year-olds' close friendships: a longitudinal analysis. *Developmental Psychology, 28,* 700–713.

*Youngblade, L. M., Park, K. A., Belsky, J. (1993). Measurement of young children's close friendship: a comparison of two independent assessment systems and their associations with attachment security. *International Journal of Behavioral Development, 16,* 563–587.

3

Separation Anxiety in Parents of Adolescents: Theoretical Significance and Scale Development

Ellen Hock, Mary Eberly, Suzanne Bartle-Haring, Pamela Ellwanger, and Keith F. Widaman

Parents of adolescents commonly face separation-related issues associated with children's increasing independence and imminent leave-taking. The aims of this investigation were (1) to develop a reliable and valid measure of parental emotions associated with separation and (2) to validate the measure by relating it to other attributes (attachment relationship quality, parent–child communication, and parent–adolescent differentiation) assessed in mothers, fathers, and their adolescents. The newly constructed, 35-item Parents of Adolescents Separation Anxiety Scale (PASAS) was administered to 686 parents of teenagers in grades 6, 8, 10, and 12 or college-bound freshmen and seniors. Factor analyses supported formation of two subscales: Anxiety about Adolescent Distancing (AAD) and Comfort with Secure Base Role (CSBR); both subscales showed distinctive patterns of change with child age. Parents' reports indicated that healthy adult attachment styles were associated with lower AAD and higher CSBR scores; children of parents who had higher AAD scores reported lower quality of attachment to both mothers and fathers.

INTRODUCTION

Research on parents' separation from infants and young children is abundant (Deater-Deckard, Scarr, McCartney, & Eisenberg, 1994; DeMeis, Hock, & McBride, 1986; Fein, Gariboldi, & Boni, 1993; Hock & Schirtzinger, 1992; McBride & Belsky, 1988; Stifter, Coulehan, & Fish, 1993); yet, little research exists on parents' feelings about separation from their adolescent children. This is somewhat surprising because their children's adolescence is a time when parents face challenges that focus on separation-related issues. Society places expectations on both adolescents and their parents for increasing adolescent self-reliance and autonomy from parents; separation of adolescents from their parents is imminent and represents a major life transition. During this developmental transition, adolescents are highly engaged in the process of relationship renegotiation (Grotevant & Cooper, 1986; Youniss & Smollar, 1985). Parents, too, are active participants in renegotiation; to understand the course and outcome of this interactive process, parents' feelings and experiences need to be identified. The primary goal of the present investigation is to document comprehensively the presence and developmental course of parents' concerns about separation from their adolescent children.

Psychologists from many theoretical perspectives agree that issues associated with parent–child separation are central to understanding psychosocial development across the life span. Responses to actual separation events or threats of separation relate to relevant characteristics of important relationships such as the level of trust or the quality of attachment. Separation responses include many diverse feelings, such as anxiety associated with being apart from the significant other, sadness with the imminent or existing loss, and anger or frustration about the inability to remain in close proximity (Hock, McBride, & Gnezda, 1989). The anxiety or concern that mothers and fathers experience associated with separation from a child is referred to as parental separation anxiety and is defined as "an unpleasant emotional state tied to the separation experience" (Hock, McBride, & Gnezda, 1989).

Parents' separation anxiety is distinctly different from that experienced by children. Prior research on attachment tended to focus almost exclusively on separation anxiety and associated separation behaviors of infants and young children. That research noted the adaptive function of separation anxiety and behaviors for the survival of the individual and the species. Attachment theory (Bowlby, 1969, 1973, 1980), however, can also provide a conceptual base for understanding parental anxiety that is associated with separation experiences. When activated by a separation event or impending danger, feelings associated with separation impel parents to provide protection and to increase physical proximity to their children (Bowlby, 1973, pp. 92, 253). Furthermore, in Volume 3 of *Attachment and Loss,* Bowlby (1980) discussed individual differences in the ways in which adults react to loss or threats of loss of close relationships. Drawing on ideas about representational models, Bowlby argued that an individual's response to a threat of loss is a function of the representational models of attachment figures and of the self that were built during the individual's own childhood. Thus, parents' mental representations of their own attachment relationships impact the way in which they react, behaviorally and emotionally, to separation events.

If the emotional experience of separation is associated with parents mental representations of attachment relationships (Bowlby, 1973; Bloom-Feshbach

& Bloom-Feshbach, 1987), then parents reporting secure mental representations of attachment should perceive separation events as healthy components of adolescent development and provide security by being accessible to their children. Parents who have secure mental representations of attachment relationships would be comfortable providing a "secure base." In a similar vein, Crowell and Waters (1999) recently reported findings from their study of married adults that clearly demonstrate the linkage between healthy mental representations of attachment and individuals' provision of secure base behavior for their partners. In the current study, such a linkage was also expected to exist between parents' attachment security and provision of a secure base for their teenagers. Considering the increasing autonomy of the adolescent, parents would be expected to experience a level of anxiety commensurate with monitoring adolescent activities (Patterson, Reid, & Dishion 1992), but the experienced anxiety would not compel parents to act in a manner that would be intrusive or inhibiting of the adolescent's exploration of new environments and relationships (Armsden & Greenberg, 1987). Moreover, such parents would be inclined to successfully balance intimacy and distance in their relationship with adolescent children. In contrast, parents reporting insecure mental representations of attachment might view separation as rejection or a threat to the integrity of their relationship with their child; in these families, one might expect more anger and conflict. On the other hand, other insecure parents might find that being accessible to their child is draining or depleting and look forward to being relieved of such parental responsibilities.

The Structure of Parental Separation Anxiety

Prior research on parental separation anxiety has focused almost exclusively on parents of infants or young children. For example, a factor analytic study by Hock et al. (1989) found that parental separation anxiety in parents of infants could be represented by a three-factor structure. The first factor, Maternal Separation Anxiety, represented a global dimension consisting of a mother's reports of anxiety and discomfort when away from her child. The second dimension was named Perception of Separation Effects on the Child, which subsumed concerns about the child's well-being in the mother's absence. The third factor, Employment-Related Separation Concerns, comprised items that targeted separation associated with work/career demands. In later studies, Hock and her colleagues found theoretically consistent differential relations of the separate dimensions of parental separation anxiety with other variables. Variables associated with dimensions of parental separation anxiety represented both child characteristics, such as health problems (Humphry & Hock, 1989), and parental attributes such as depressive symptoms (Hock & Schirtzinger, 1992) and role-related beliefs (Hock & Lutz, 1998).

The three-dimensional structure discussed earlier for parental separation anxiety may represent well this domain for parents of infants and young children. When offspring are in the infancy and early childhood periods, parents appropriately may be quite concerned about how separations from the child, particularly separations associated with maternal employment, may affect the child. But, when children reach the adolescent period, many of the concerns from the earlier period in the children's life no longer apply, and new and different concerns arise in and impinge on the parent–adolescent relationship. No longer are parents likely to be overly concerned about how routine absences from their children affect the children emotionally. Instead, parents of adolescents must face a variety of issues stemming from the movement of adolescents toward adulthood, issues such as adolescent autonomy, conflict, decision making, personal responsibility, peer affiliation, dating relationships, and other extrafamilial relationships (cf. Feldman & Elliot, 1990; Montemayor, Adams, & Gullota, 1990). As the nature of the parent–offspring relationship is altered during adolescence, the structure of parental separation anxiety concerning the adolescent is likely to change in response to the evolving relationship between parent and child. Representing the structure of separation anxiety for parents of adolescents is therefore an important research objective.

Relation of Parental Separation Anxiety to Other Constructs

Once the dimensional structure of parental separation anxiety toward adolescent children is determined, exploring the nomological network of these dimensions—or the relations of these dimensions to measures of other constructs—is a relevant concern. Dimensions of parental separation anxiety should be related to other aspects of the parent–child relationship, particularly to conflict behavior, attachment relationships, and family differentiation.

Separation anxiety and conflict behavior. As parents and adolescents renegotiate their relationships, an increase in the frequency and intensity of conflict between parent and adolescent often occurs (Montemayor, 1982). This increase in conflict and the expression of negative emotion might be related to increasing psychological and physical distance between parents and adolescents that occurs as adolescents mature (Flannery, Montemayor, Eberly, & Torquati, 1993; Larson & Ham, 1993; Steinberg, 1989). On a more positive note, some research suggests that the ability to discuss disagreements, resolve conflicts, and reach compromises is rooted in the security of the attachment relationship (Kobak, Cole, Ferenz-Gillies, & Flemming, 1993; Kobak & Sceery, 1988). Research by Kobak and colleagues revealed that adolescents and mothers who were securely attached were able to resolve problem-solving tasks in ways that were characterized by low levels of conflict; that is, securely attached mother–adolescent dyads exhibited low levels of dysfunctional anger and high levels of constructive engagement. Relatedly, a recent investigation of dating partners by Simpson, Rholes, and Phillips (1996) found that couple problem solving was characterized by more anger and less warmth when a partner was insecure-ambivalent or insecure-avoidant, respectively. In the present study, conflictual communication patterns reported by parents and teens were expected to be linked to concerns about separation in parents and, specifically, to be related to lower levels of comfort with issues surrounding autonomy and separation.

Separation anxiety and attachment relations. Theoretically, the psychological and emotional experience of parental separation anxiety should be linked to parents' representations of attachment relationships (Bloom-Feshbach & Bloom-Feshbach, 1987) and witnessed in adolescents' perceptions of attachment to parents. Response to separation is a reflection of the security of the attachment representation. Thus, parents who experience less separation anxiety with their adolescents' increasing self-reliance, while providing a sense of felt security when required by the adolescent, were expected to be most comfortable with others' dependency, need for closeness, and need for independence. Moreover, those parents who were less anxious about separation, in comparison with parents who were more anxious about separation, might be more responsive to adolescent needs for psychological security and exploration. Thus, parental separation anxiety was expected to be inversely related to adolescents' reports of quality of attachment to mothers and fathers.

Separation anxiety and family differentiation. In addition to physical separation, parents and adolescents also must negotiate the psychological process of differentiation. Differentiation—a family-systems-level attribute—is a family's characteristic tolerance for intimacy and individuality or distance among family members and between the family and the outside world (Allison & Sabatelli, 1988; Anderson & Sabatelli, 1990; Bowen, 1978). Consistent with the major tenets of attachment theory, differentiation was hypothesized to be systematically associated with parental separation anxiety. Low differentiation should be linked to attachment representations in which separation experiences would invoke high anxiety and contribute to disputes in family relationships. In contrast, high family differentiation should be more indicative of secure attachment and low separation anxiety; members of highly differentiated families would be flexible and comfortable with their feelings of intimacy and would be able to cope with age-appropriate separation.

The Present Study

The present study had two general aims. The first aim, consisting of instrument development, focused on operationalizing parents' feelings about separation from their adolescent children. Similar to the Maternal Separation Anxiety Scale, which assesses parental feelings about physical separation during infancy (Hock et al., 1989), the new scale—called the Parents of Adolescents Separation Anxiety Scale (PASAS)—asks parents of adolescents to report on their feelings about separation (i.e., worry, sadness, and tension about adolescent distancing for current and impending separation events). The term parental separation anxiety is used in this study of parents of adolescents in much the same way that it was used in previous studies of parents of infants that employed the Maternal Separation Anxiety Scale (Hock et al., 1989; Hock & Schirtzinger, 1992). Simply put, the term describes a state of apprehension experienced by parents associated with separation events involving children. Although the word "anxiety" often connotes a pathological, clinical entity, in this case it reflects concerns about separation that can be quite "normal" and may not be unhealthy or dysfunctional.

To examine parental anxiety across all phases of adolescent development, data were collected from parents of early, mid, and late adolescents (including college students); data from parents in all three age groups were combined to select items and assess the psychometric properties of the new scale. Parent gender, child gender, and developmental differences also were examined.

The second general aim of this study was to evaluate the validity of the new structure of separation anxiety by examining the relation of dimensions of parental separation anxiety to other psychological constructs that assess aspects of functioning in close interpersonal relationships. This approach to validity reflects the approach to construct validity described by Cronbach and Meehl (1955); it further defines the meaning of dimensions of separation anxiety by positioning them within the context of a meaningful nomological network. In this regard, confirming expected correlations between parental separation anxiety and the child's reports of relationship quality is necessary. Parental feelings associated with separation were hypothesized to be related to aspects of adolescents' relationships with their parents, and attributes describing quality of the relationship were investigated from the perspectives of both parents and adolescents. By relating data from different respondents, this study sought to circumvent problems associated with potential bias due to shared variance among measures associated with shared respondent effects.

Data were collected in three samples of participants. Variables used examined aspects of parent–adolescent relationships that are conceptually linked with mental representation of the attachment relationship, particularly perceptions of conflictual communication patterns, attachment quality, and levels of differentiation (i.e., balance of distance and connectedness). In participating families, fathers, mothers, and adolescents were assessed.

METHOD

Samples

Sample 1. Adolescents, $N = 129$, in the 6th, $n = 23$ boys, $n = 23$ girls; 8th, $n = 22$ boys, $n = 22$ girls; and 10th, $n = 20$ boys, $n = 19$ girls, grades were recruited from enrollment lists of one middle school and two high schools in large Midwestern suburban school districts. Requests for study participants resulted in 41% agreeing to participate. Average age for boys was 14.2 years, $SD = 1.6$, and average age for girls was 14.1 years, $SD = 1.6$. Mothers, on average, were 42.9 years old, $SD = 3.8$ years, and fathers, on average, were 45.0 years old, $SD = 4.9$. Seventeen percent were from single-parent homes. Most mothers (75.6%) and fathers (85.7%) had obtained college degrees and were employed full-time (55% of mothers, 93.3% of fathers). Using the income categories, median annual family income fell in the $90,000–$99,999 category.

Sample 2. Adolescents were recruited from enrollment lists of two suburban high schools in a large Midwestern school district; mailed requests for study participation successfully recruited 30% of those on the enrollment lists. In this lower- to middle-income school district most families report incomes of between $20,000 and $60,000. Participants in this study were mothers, $n = 85$, fathers, $n = 74$, and their adolescent children, $n = 35$ boys, $n = 43$ girls. On average, boys were 17.7 years old, $SD = .6$, and girls were 17.4 years old, $SD = .58$. Fourteen percent of the children were from single-parent homes. The average age of mothers was 43.4 years, $SD = 4.5$; fathers, on average, were 45.1 years old, $SD = 6.3$. Approximately 33% of mothers and 50% of fathers had completed undergraduate degrees. Most mothers (76%) and fathers (92%) were employed full time. Using the income categories, median annual family income fell in the $40,000–$49,999 category.

Sample 3. Mothers, $n = 168$, and fathers, $n = 130$ of college-bound freshmen, $n = 34$ males, $n = 55$ females, or college seniors, $n = 24$ males, $n = 50$ females, were recruited from the registrar's list of freshmen and seniors at a large Midwestern university; 38% of those contacted by mail agreed to participate. Eighteen percent were from single-parent homes. On average, college men were 19.7 years old, $SD = 2.2$, and college women were 19.9 years old, $SD = 2.3$; as expected, this recruitment of college seniors included individuals who were ages 20 to 22. These older participants were still functioning in the "student" role, so their parents' beliefs about separation were considered to reflect feelings of parents of older, but not fully independent, adolescents. The college students' mothers were 47.1 years old, SD = 4.9, and their fathers were 48.9 years old, SD = 5.5. Thirty-five percent of mothers and 51.9% of fathers had received college degrees, professional degrees, or both. Using the income categories, median annual family income fell in the $70,000–$79,999 category.

Total sample. For certain analyses, parents from all three samples were combined. This total sample included mothers, n = 378, and fathers, n = 308, who completed the PASAS, and adolescents, n =159 boys, n = 213 girls, ranging in age from 12 years to 25 years. On average, mothers were 44.9 years old; most were employed full-time (63.4%), some were employed part-time (19.7%), and the remaining were homemakers or unemployed (16.9%). Approximately 35% of mothers had attained college degrees, and the remaining mothers had attained at least a high-school education (64%). Fathers were 46.7 years old on average, and 92.7% of fathers were employed full-time. About half of the fathers (53.2%) had college degrees, and the remaining fathers had received at least a high school education (46.8%). The family incomes ranged from $10,000–20,000 to greater than $100,000. Although the sample is generally described as middle class, all income levels were represented and cell sizes were adequate for assessing the relationship between income levels (as indicators of socioeconomic status) and parental separation anxiety. Analyses using family income levels, parental education levels, and parental separation anxiety revealed no significant relationships, so no further analyses of these data are reported or discussed. Families were primarily European-American; participants who were not of European-American descent composed 3%, 6%, and 9% of samples 1, 2, and 3, respectively.

Instruments and Procedures

All samples. Mothers and fathers in all three samples were asked to complete a pilot version of the PASAS. Two areas of literature guided the development of items for the PASAS, namely attachment theory and research in adolescent socioemotional development, to identify issues of relevance to parents of adolescents. Forty-seven Likert-type statements asked parents to rate (on a 5-point scale, with 1 = strongly disagree to 5 = strongly agree) their feelings associated with important parameters of the parent–adolescent attachment relationship. The actual content or subject matter of the items was derived from areas of study emphasized in the adolescent development literature; areas included adolescent autonomy, conflict, decision making, personal responsibility, peer affiliation, dating relationships, and other extrafamilial relationships (cf. Feldman & Elliot, 1990; Montemayor et al., 1990).

Items were constructed to cover selected parameters associated with separation in the attachment literature. The construction was guided, in part, by Weiss (1982), who proposed three characteristics of an attachment relationship: accessibility, physical proximity seeking under stress, and diminished anxiety in the presence of the child. Physical closeness was represented through items assessing pleasure associated with physical closeness as well as expressions of discomfort at being physically separated for both short and extended time periods. Items also included direct statements about parental provision of protection and safety. In addition to physical closeness and protection, another set of items tapped psychological closeness. These items reflected parental pleasure and comfort associated with being accessible, that is, sharing time, activities, and advice with the teenager as well as contrasting feelings that would include resentment of a teenager's dependency.

It was hypothesized that items referring to the parents' pleasure in providing care, support, and advice to the teenager might well cluster together and load on a distinct dimension. It was also anticipated that the items specifically referring to physical contact might well reflect a dimension distinct from more abstract, psychological referents of closeness.

Sample 1. The focus in Sample 1 was the relation of parental separation anxiety to conflict with the adolescent. To assess conflictual communication patterns, each parent and target adolescent completed 20-item parallel versions of the Conflict Behavior Questionnaire (CBQ) (Prinz, Foster, Kent, & O'Leary, 1979). Adolescents completed separate forms for mothers and for fathers. Answered in a True/False format, each statement was designed to assess positive and negative interaction behaviors of parents, adolescents, and their shared relationships. Higher scores represent greater conflict in the parent–child relationship. The CBQ has been used as a clinical diagnostic tool and has been shown to demonstrate adequate psychometric properties (cf. Foster, Prinz, & O'Leary, 1983; Robin & Weiss, 1980). Cronbach's αs were rather high, ranging from .86 through .92.

Adolescents and their parents in Sample 1 individually completed several questionnaires during two 1-hour in-home visits scheduled about 1 week apart. Parents completed the PASAS, and parents and adolescents completed the CBQ. Families received $20 for their participation.

Sample 2. The focus in Sample 2 was the relation of parental separation anxiety to attachment styles. The first measure of parents' attachment style used in this sample was the Adult Attachment Scale (AAS) (Collins & Reed, 1990). Consisting of 18 items, the AAS includes three dimensions of attachment: comfort with closeness and intimacy, comfort with dependency (feeling that one can depend and rely on others), and anxiety about rejection or abandonment. Each item is answered on a 5-point Likert scale ranging from "1 = not at all characteristic of me" to "5 = very characteristic of me." Higher scores indicate the degree to which a particular dimension is characteristic of the individual. Cronbach's αs ranged from .78 through .87 in this study.

The second parent attachment style measure used was the Inventory of Parent and Peer Attachment (IPPA) (Armsden & Greenberg, 1987), a 53-item self-report measure designed to examine an adolescent's positive and negative affective/cognitive experiences with parents and peers as sources of psychological security. The IPPA consists of two scales, one for attachment to parents (28 items) and one for attachment to peers (23 items). Modified mother and father subscales were used for the purpose of the present investigation. Adolescents were asked to indicate how true each item was for them on a 5-point Likert scale. Higher scores represent greater attachment quality. The IPPA has demonstrated strong psychometric properties (Armsden & Greenberg, 1987; Papini, Roggman, & Anderson, 1991). In the present study, Cronbach's αs were .93 and .92 for mothers and fathers, respectively.

The third attachment style measure used was the Family System Test (FAST) (Gehring & Schultheiss, 1987), a spatial measure assessing cohesion and hierarchical status among family members. The original FAST and its facsimile use 9 × 9 matrices. Adolescents were asked to place figurines (for the original) or different-colored adhesive dots (for the facsimile) on the checkerboardlike matrix to indicate cohesion between self–mother and self–father. A different colored dot represented each family member. All adolescents completed the FAST facsimile; a subset of these adolescents ($n = 43$) later participated in a 5 to 10 minutes, face-to-face interview when the original FAST was administered. A cohesion score was determined by calculating the distance between figurines (or dots). To calculate distance, the number of squares that separate figurines were counted if they were in the same row or column; the Pythagorean Theorem ($a^2 + b^2 = c^2$) was calculated if the figurines were at an angle to one another. The cohesion score was obtained by subtracting the distance between figurines from the board's ultimate distance of 12 (cf. Gehring & Feldman, 1988). Scores ranged from .6 to 11; higher scores represent greater cohesion. The original FAST and its facsimile were found to correlate highly, $r = .97$ for mothers and $r = .98$ for fathers. Gehring and Feldman (1988) found the FAST to demonstrate adequate psychometric properties. For analyses in the present investigation, the facsimile cohesion scores were used.

In Sample 2, families were sent a packet that had three envelopes containing questionnaires, one envelope each for the mother, father, and high-school senior. Mothers and fathers completed the PASAS and the AAS; adolescents were given the Inventory of Parent and Peer Attachment (parent subscale) and a facsimile (two-dimensional) of the Family System Test. As an incentive to participate, family members were offered an opportunity to participate in a raffle drawing.

Additionally, adolescents were invited to participate in an extended study of the original (three-dimensional) FAST by returning, with their questionnaires, a card on which they had written their name and phone number. The original, three-dimensional version of the FAST was administered to 43 seniors who were paid $5 for their participation. The original FAST was used to assess the parallel forms' reliability of the facsimile version.

Sample 3. The focus of Sample 3 was the relation of parental separation anxiety to role differentiation within the family. The Differentiation in the Family System Scale (DIFS) (Anderson & Sabatelli, 1992) was used to assess the patterns of differentiation in the family. This particular scale uses a "circular questioning" format that assesses the individual's perception of how various members of the family interact with one another. The scale consists of 11 Likert-type items that provide information about the respondent's views of the patterns of interaction. Items assess the behavioral patterns among family members that reinforce the individual's sense of self as separate yet also maintain a sense of closeness. High scores indicate higher differentiation. Data on four subscales were used in this study: mother-to-adolescent, father-to-adolescent, adolescent-to-mother, and adolescent-to-father. The DIFS has been shown to demonstrate adequate psychometric properties and construct validity (cf. Anderson & Sabatelli, 1992; Bartle & Sabatelli, 1989; Sabatelli & Anderson, 1991). For the present investigation, Cronbach's αs ranged from .83 through .94 for adolescents' perspectives, .85 through .89 for mothers' perspectives, and .83 through .90 for fathers' perspectives.

For Sample 3, a packet was mailed to each participating family; each packet included an introductory letter and three envelopes containing several questionnaires—a set designated for each family member (mother, father, college student). Mothers and fathers were asked to complete the PASAS and the DIFS. Adolescents were asked to complete the DIFS as well.

Analytic Strategies

Factor analyses. For mothers' and fathers' reports, exploratory principal axis factor analyses, in which squared multiple correlations (SMC) were used as communality estimates, were employed to determine the latent structure of the PASAS and to eliminate low-loading items. Factor analyses were conducted for 0 to 4 factor solutions. Because dimensions of parental separation anxiety might be correlated, an oblique rotation method (Promax) was used to determine simple structure; of course, if factors are orthogonal, Promax will find that orthogonal structure. To examine possible parent gender differences, maternal and paternal data sets were initially analyzed separately as independent samples. Factors with eigenvalues greater than 1 and the scree test (Cattell, 1966) were used to determine the number of factors in each group.

To make decisions about item retention, the criterion of a factor loading of .30 was adopted. For an exploratory factor analysis, according to Floyd and Widaman (1995, p. 294), "factor loadings are generally considered to be meaningful when they exceed .30 or .40"; items that failed to achieve a factor loading of .30 or more were eliminated. Additionally, Cronbach's coefficient α was computed to determine the internal consistency and item-to-total correlation for each factor. Items that failed to correlate above .25 with the total scale also were eliminated.

Validity analyses. Simultaneous multiple regressions were employed in all validity study analyses. To evaluate the relations of the two PASAS scales to other measures, each outcome variable of interest was regressed on the two PASAS subscales, Anxiety about Adolescent Distancing (AAD) and Comfort with Secure Base Role (CSBR). First, total model variance (R^2) was examined to determine the degree to which parental separation anxiety measured by using both scales predicted indices of parent–adolescent conflict, attachment, and differentiation. Second, the amount of variance accounted for uniquely by each subscale (sr^2) and the regression coefficient raw score coefficient B for each scale were examined to assess the unique relationship of AAD and CSBR individually with each dependent variable. For all three studies, adolescent gender was collapsed because significant mean differences between male and female adolescents were not found for the AAD or CSBR.

RESULTS

Factor Analysis and Psychometric Evaluation

Three strategies were employed to determine which items of the original set were to be included in the final version of the PASAS. First, as described earlier, conceptual clarity for each item was evaluated to ensure parsimony and confidence that relevant dimensions were tapped. Second, exploratory principal axis factor analysis was used to determine empirically the latent structure and item inclusion and exclusion. Third, Cronbach's coefficient α was used to examine internal consistency. Given a well-defined factor structure, effects of parent gender, adolescent gender, and adolescent age were evaluated on each factor.

Factor analyses. Factors with eigenvalues greater than 1 and scree tests (Cattell, 1966) indicated that a two-factor solution was present for both mothers' and fathers' reports. Twelve items were discarded because of low factor loadings and low item–scale correlations. The 35 items that were retained were again subjected to the same method of factor analysis to reaffirm the factor structure and to determine final factor loadings. (Factor loadings associated with each item are available from the first author.) As before, results yielded a two-factor solution with a simple structure; each item loaded clearly on only one factor. Interfactor correlations showed that the two factors were relatively independent ($r = .17$ for mothers' reports, $r = .20$ for fathers' reports). Identical patterns of items loading on factors were found for mothers' and fathers' data.

Considering the *a priori* hypotheses about dimensions that might be identified by factor analysis, items that reflected parents' enjoyment of being accessible and providing care, support, and advice to their teenager clustered together, as predicted. The hypothesis about the emergence of a factor that would reflect special interest in physical closeness was not confirmed by the factor analytic analyses: The items referring to hugs and holding were evenly distributed on the two factors. The two factors revealed by factor analysis were interpreted and labeled as AAD and CSBR. The PASAS items and scoring key, showing which items are associated with each factor, are given in the Appendix.

The first factor, AAD, consisted of 21 items reflecting parents' feelings of discomfort or loss associated with their adolescent's increasing affiliation with others and decreasing involvement and time spent with parents. Parents having higher scores on the AAD express "hurt" or "emptiness" in response to the child's increasing self-reliance or affiliation with others, whereas parents having lower scores do not report such anxiety and perhaps experience their child's increasing self-reliance as positive. Examples of items loading on the AAD factor include, "I feel resentful when my child goes to his/her room instead of spending time with me" and "I feel sad when I think that my teenager does not seem to enjoy being with me as much anymore." For mothers ($M = 52.0$, $SD = 9.7$), AAD accounted for 39.7% of the variance in the factor analysis and had an internal consistency of .86. For fathers ($M = 55.1$, $SD = 10.4$), AAD accounted for 40.5% of the variance in the factor analysis and had an internal consistency of .88.

The second factor, CSBR, consisted of 14 items, reflecting parents' contentment with being accessible and serving as a source of security to their adolescents who are expanding their social and physical worlds. Higher scores on CSBR reflect parents' satisfaction in providing emotional support, physical support, and guidance for their adolescents. Not only do these parents enjoy "being there" when needed, but they may expect to experience a sense of loss when they are not so obviously needed. On the other hand, lower scores represent a parents' discomfort and dissatisfaction in being accessible. These parents do not express sadness about loss, nor do they experience enjoyment in providing comfort. They appear to look forward to diminished obligation and responsibility for providing physical, economic, and emotional support. Examples of items in CSBR are "I feel good knowing that my teenager feels that he/she can call on me" and "Life will be so much better when my teenager leaves home for good (reverse scored)." For mothers (M = 59.7, SD = 7.4), CSBR accounted for 29.5% of variance and had an internal consistency of .82. For fathers (M = 56.9, SD = 7.2), CSBR accounted for 27.3% of variance and had an internal consistency of .81 (see Appendix).

Gender and developmental differences. To evaluate the effects of parent gender, adolescent gender, and adolescent age on the parents' separation anxiety scores, $2 \times 2 \times 6$ analyses of variance (Parent Gender × Adolescent Gender × Grade) were used. Analyses are based on only those families for whom both mothers and fathers participated.

For the AAD factor, a significant main effect was obtained for grade, $F(5, 666) = 6.11$, $p < .001$. Using Tukey's studentized range test and an α error rate of .05, results revealed that parents of college seniors (M = 48.1, SD = 9.6) reported significantly less anxiety than parents of sixth graders (M = 54.9, SD = 9.0), eighth graders (M = 52.4, SD = 8.5), tenth graders (M = 52.1, SD = 9.0), twelfth graders (M = 53.6, SD = 10.3), and college-bound freshmen (M = 54.1, SD = 10.5). A main effect for adolescent gender was not obtained, and all interactions were nonsignificant.

For the CSBR, a significant main effect was obtained for parent gender, $F(1, 666) = 22.73$, $p < .001$, where mothers (M = 56.1, SD = 6.8) perceived greater comfort with providing a secure base than did fathers (M = 53.4, SD = 6.7). A main effect for grade, $F(5, 666) = 12.57$, $p < .001$, reflecting a general, though not perfectly linear, decline in scores with advancing grade also was obtained. Parents of sixth (M = 58.2, SD = 5.2) and tenth (M = 58.1, SD = 6.0) graders were significantly more involved in their role of providing a secure base and more likely to express sadness about their adolescents' future home-leaving than parents of twelfth graders (M = 53.5, SD = 7.4) and college seniors (M = 52.5, SD = 7.1). Parents of eighth graders (M = 56.6, SD = 6.5) were not significantly different from parents of sixth graders or tenth graders and college-bound freshmen (M = 54.5, SD = 6.4), and parents of college-bound freshmen did not differ significantly from parents of twelfth graders or college seniors. A main effect for adolescent gender was not obtained, and all interactions were nonsignificant. Figure 3.1 displays means by grade for the AAD and CSBR.

Validity Study 1: Separation Anxiety and Conflict Behavior

Parental reports. Multiple regression analyses showed that parents' separation anxiety from adolescents, as a whole, contributed significantly to

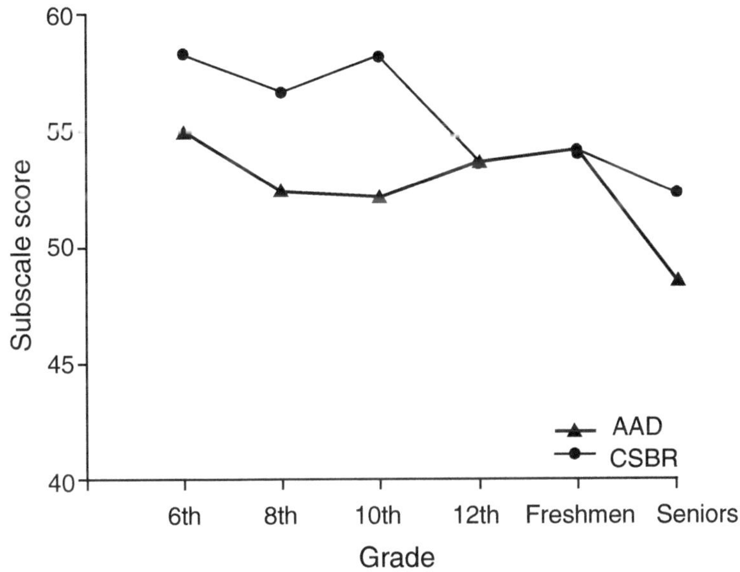

Figure 3.1. Mean scores by grades for each PASAS subscale—Anxiety about adolescent Distancing (AAD) and Comfort with Secure Base Role (CSBR).

parent-reported conflict with the adolescent, for both mothers and fathers (see Table 3.1). The squared semipartial correlations showed that both AAD and CSBR were significantly related to parent-reported conflict for both mothers and fathers. The regression weights revealed that mothers (B = .15) and fathers (B = .16) who reported more AAD also reported more conflictual communication with their adolescents. Conversely, the CSBR scale revealed negative relations with conflict; higher levels of comfort with one's role as a secure base were associated with lower reported communication difficulties for both mothers (B = –.29) and fathers (B = –.20).

Adolescent reports. The regression analyses predicting adolescent-reported conflict with mothers and fathers also showed significant overall relationships for conflict with both mothers and fathers (as shown in the bottom half of Table 3.1). As with the parent-reported conflict, mothers (B = –.17) and fathers (B = –.22) who were comfortable providing a secure base had adolescents who reported less negative, conflictual communication. In contrast, no significant relationships were found between the AAD scale and adolescent reports of negative communication patterns with mothers or fathers.

TABLE 3.1
Summary of Simultaneous Regression Analyses in Validity Study 1: Relating PASAS Scale Scores to Measures of Parent–Child Conflict from the CBQ

			AAD[a]		CSBR[b]	
Dependent Measure	Model R^2	Model *F*	sr^2	B	sr^2	B
Mother report						
Conflict with adolescent (127)	.17***	12.29	.07**	.15	.13***	–.29
Father report						
Conflict with adolescent (104)	.14***	8.47	.11***	.16	.07**	–.20
Adolescent report						
Conflict with mother (127)	.07*	4.63	.03	.08	.06**	–.17
Conflict with father (104)	.10**	5.62	.03	.07	.09**	–.22

Note: Number of participants presented in parentheses.
[a] Anxiety about Adolescent Distancing.
[b] Comfort with Secure Base Role.
*$p < .05$; **$p < .01$; ***$p < .001$.

Validity Study 2: Separation Anxiety and Attachment Relationships

Parental reports. Parents' separation anxiety concerning their adolescents was found to contribute significantly to mothers' and fathers' reports of comfort with closeness (or intimacy), comfort with depending on others, and anxiety surrounding abandonment and rejection (see the first two sections of Table 3.2). Examination of the regression analyses using attachment scores revealed that mothers who experienced greater AAD also reported less comfort with closeness (B = –.11) and less comfort depending on others (B = –.23). Fathers responding with higher scores on the AAD also were less comfortable depending on others (B = –.14) and were more anxious about relationship abandonment and rejection (B = .18). Although no significant relationships were obtained between CSBR and the AAS subscales for mothers' reports, fathers who were more comfortable with providing their adolescents with a secure base were more comfortable with intimacy (B = .28) and less anxious about abandonment or rejection (B = –.30).

Adolescent reports. Regression analyses also revealed that parental separation anxiety significantly contributed to adolescent reports of attachment quality with mothers and fathers and to cohesion with mothers, as shown in the bottom section of Table 3.2. Inspection of the squared semipartial correlations and regression coefficients revealed that higher levels of parental anxiety about adolescent distancing led to lower levels of adolescent-reported quality of attachment for both mothers (B = –.67) and fathers (B = –.52); conversely, the

TABLE 3.2
Summary of Simultaneous Regression Analyses in Validity Study 2: Relating PASAS Scale Scores to Measures of Parent–Child Attachment

Dependent Measure	Model R^2	Model F	AAD[a] sr^2	AAD[a] B	CSBR[b] sr^2	CSBR[b] B
Mother report						
AAS comfort with closeness (85)	.09*	3.85	.06*	–.11	.03	.11
AAS comfort with dependency (85)	.22***	11.53	.20***	–.23	.03	.12
AAS anxiety about rejection (85)	.07	3.07	.05	.13	.02	–.11
Father report						
AAS comfort with closeness (74)	.12**	4.90	.01	–.05	.12**	.28
AAS comfort with dependency (74)	.08*	3.19	.08*	–.14	.00	.05
AAS anxiety about rejection (74)	.24***	10.96	.13***	.18	.15***	–.30
Adolescent report						
IPPA						
Quality of attachment with mother (66)	.23***	9.66	.15***	–.67	.10***	.78
Quality of attachment with father (54)	.24***	8.00	.14***	–.52	.20***	1.06
FAST (facsimile)						
Cohesion with mother (66)	.27***	11.83	.12**	–.07	.17***	.11
Cohesion with father (54)	.05	1.21	.02	–.02	.04	.05

Note: Number of participants presented in parentheses.
[a] Anxiety about Adolescent Distancing.
[b] Comfort with Secure Base Role.
$*p < .05$; $**p < .01$; $***p < .001$.

lower the level of parental anxiety about distancing, the higher the adolescent-reported quality of attachment to the parent. Not surprisingly, high levels of comfort with providing a secure base were associated with higher quality of adolescent-reported attachment to the parent for both mothers (B = .78) and fathers (B = 1.06).

Turning to adolescent-reported cohesion with parents, mothers with higher levels of anxiety about distancing had adolescents who reported lower levels of cohesion with the mother (B = –.07), whereas maternal comfort with providing a secure base was positively related to adolescent-reported cohesion (B = .11). Father reports on the AAD and CSBR scales were unrelated to adolescent-reported cohesion with the father.

Validity Study 3: Separation Anxiety and Family Differentiation

Parental reports. Findings showed that parents' feelings about separating from their adolescents significantly contributed to mothers' and fathers' perceptions of differentiation in their relationships with their adolescents, as shown in the top two sections of Table 3.3. Examination of the unique contribution of each PASAS subscale revealed that higher levels of anxiety about adolescent distancing led to lower levels of parent-reported differentiation from the adolescent for both mothers (B = –.17) and fathers (B = –.15); this inverse relation also means that lower levels of AAD led to higher levels of differentiation from the adolescent. As expected, parents who were more comfortable with their role providing a secure base reported higher levels of differentiation from the adolescent (B = .33 for mothers, and B = .35 for fathers).

Adolescent reports. The influences of parental separation anxiety on differentiation between parent and child were largely replicated by using adolescent reports of differentiation, as shown in the bottom section of Table 3.3. Higher levels of parental anxiety about adolescent distancing were associated with lower adolescent-reported differentiation from both mothers (B = –.18) and fathers (B = –.14). Similarly, parents who were more comfortable with their role providing a secure base had adolescents who reported higher levels of differentiation from the parent (B = .20 for mothers, and B = .11 for fathers), although the coefficient for fathers failed to reach conventional levels of statistical significance.

DISCUSSION

First, considering the psychometric strength of the PASAS, findings supported the belief that separation-related concerns of parents of adolescents can be operationalized and empirically addressed. Two aspects of parents' separation concerns emerged: (1) Anxiety about Adolescent Distancing (AAD) and (2) Comfort with Secure Base Role (CSBR). Each feature was linked to parent–adolescent conflict, attachment representation, and family differentiation in a manner consistent with theoretical predictions.

The AAD dimension reflects parents' anxiety about adolescent distancing, which may be a function of the adolescent's increasing self-reliance and affiliation with peers or other adults. This dimension can be interpreted such that high scores suggest both a reluctance to relinquish control and denial of young persons' autonomy needs and self-functioning. Perhaps parents who score high are unaware of or deny that distancing is normal and appropriate for their children; alternatively, these parents may "personalize" their

TABLE 3.3
Summary of Simultaneous Regression Analyses in Validity Study 3: Relating PASAS Scale Scores to Measures of Parent–Child Differentiation from the DIFS

			AAD[a]		CSBR[b]	
Dependent Measure	Model R^2	Model *F*	sr^2	B	sr^2	B
Mother report Differentiation from adolescent (168)	.17***	16.99	.08***	−.17	.13***	.33
Father report Differentiation from adolescent (120)	.19***	15.29	.08***	−.15	.15***	.35
Adolescent report Differentiation from mother (144)	.11***	8.81	.09***	−.18	.05**	.20
Differentiation from father (115)	.06**	3.44	.05**	−.14	.01	.11

Note: Number of participants presented in parentheses.
[a] Anxiety about Adolescent Distancing.
[b] Comfort with Secure Base Role.
$^*p < .05$; $^{**}p < .01$; $^{***}p < .001$.

adolescents' movement to extrafamilial relationships: that is, they may view such movement as rejection. The tension associated with "losing the child to others" could reflect jealousy and possessiveness. These parents may respond to separation in ways that inhibit their adolescents' age-appropriate autonomous behavior and self-definition. The literature on parenthood has not systematically addressed this negative parental characteristic that may be associated with dysfunction in children. Future investigations must more fully document the incidence of this attribute, its relationship to other parental attributes, and its relevance to the child's independence. In contrast, parents having lower scores on AAD express less tension with adolescents' increasing autonomy; they seem to understand the appropriateness of their adolescents' independence and increased affiliation with others, perhaps overcoming unhealthy tendencies toward jealousy by calling on cognitive interpretations.

The trend analysis shifts our attention to normative matters and suggests that parents' average level of anxiety about adolescent distancing may not significantly decrease until after adolescents move out of the home. The parents of college seniors reported significantly lower scores on this attribute than did the parents of younger adolescents; even parents of college freshmen reported relatively high levels of anxiety about adolescent distancing. Future studies might compare other noncollegiate populations of the same age with college populations. Importantly, these findings from a predominantly middle-class population may differ from other groups defined by distinctive cultural and ethnic identities. As well, populations drawn from urban, inner-city areas may experience harsh, dangerous conditions that would systematically affect some parental concerns in a way that would lead to much higher levels of parental anxiety on this dimension even if the adolescent lives at home. Further research should find it rewarding to use PASAS data to examine parental concerns about separation associated with these differing living environments.

CSBR, the second dimension of the PASAS, reflects parents' commitment to being psychologically and physically accessible to adolescents who are growing more independent and preparing to leave home. Theory would suggest that many parents can and do function in a supportive role, providing unconditional support and guidance to teenagers. High scores on this dimension reflect healthy emotional functioning, even though some anxiety or expressions of sadness are reported. In other words, parents' expression of feelings that reflect missing a child who will grow more independent and leave home is most certainly appropriate. Items included on this scale tap this important dimension.

Recognizing that parents may gear their provision of support to adolescents' need of it is also important. Bowlby (1969) discussed the notion of the goal-corrected partnership, which suggests that mature individuals have the capacity to gear the timing and intensity of their response to their partner's current disposition. Similarly, as the adolescent child moves into young adulthood, parents' provision of secure base behaviors suited to the needs of younger teenagers may decline. Consistent with this expectation, findings reveal a significant decline on this dimension as the children grow older.

This line of thinking about one partner in a dyad gearing responses to the needs of the other also assists our understanding of individual differences in parental separation anxiety. Studies of separation anxiety in mothers of infants show that infant characteristics seem to influence levels of separation anxiety. Temperamentally difficult infants (McBride & Belsky, 1988), infants with colic (Humphry & Hock, 1989), and infants who have experienced health problems (Hock & Lutz, 1998) have mothers who have higher levels of separation anxiety (assessed by the Maternal Separation Anxiety Scale, Subscale 1) than mothers of infants without these problems. Further research is needed to determine, in parents of adolescents, the types of child problems or characteristics that influence parental separation anxiety. In these cases, the direction of influence seems to be from child to parent; however, the patterns of influence associated with parental separation anxiety are complex. Future studies may use models showing transactional effects where the level of functioning of the child colors the parents' feelings and, in turn, the parents' responses influence the child (Marvin & Stewart, 1990).

To summarize the validity studies in this investigation, findings supported the important link between expressions of concern about separation and attachment; results confirmed the belief that response to separation is rooted in the mental representations of attachment relationships (Bloom-Feshbach &

Bloom-Feshbach, 1987; Bowlby, 1973). Data from the PASAS and the AAS revealed expected relationships between healthy attachment reports and less anxiety about adolescent distancing; for fathers, comfort with closeness in attachment relationships also was related to positive feelings about the secure base role. Parents who express healthy feelings about attachment relationships have the capacity to respond to separation from their adolescents in a constructive manner. In contrast, parents characterized by anxiety or a lack of comfort in close relationships are less capable of responding constructively to separation and may even be threatened or feel rejected by the teenagers' interests in interacting with and depending on others.

Complementing the parental attachment findings, adolescents' reports of attachment to mother and father were related in expected directions to both PASAS scales. Higher parental scores on AAD were associated with lower adolescent attachment scores to both mother and father. Similarly, higher scores on CSBR related to teens' healthier reported attachment to mother and father. Thus, if parents can serve as a secure base, adolescents' feelings of connectedness are maintained, which consequently allows adolescents to explore their widening worlds and gain autonomy. This finding is in agreement with Kobak's thinking on the relationship between parental attachment representations and increased adolescent autonomy (Kobak et al., 1993; Kobak, Sudler, & Gamble, 1991). For example, Kobak et al. (1991, p. 463) stated that "Under secure circumstances, teens can successfully assert their autonomy while maintaining a sense of cooperation and partnership with parents."

Findings also revealed that PASAS scores were meaningfully related to levels of conflict and differentiation as reported by adolescents and their parents. Perceptions of negative communication patterns, using the CBQ, were examined from mothers', fathers', and adolescents' perspectives. Findings showed that higher scores on the AAD dimension were related to higher levels of negative communication between parents and adolescents as reported by the parent. Parents who experience more anxiety about adolescent distancing may be experiencing more conflict or may be more inclined to perceive adolescent autonomy gestures as contentious or challenging, thereby reporting greater conflict in communication. Another interpretation would suggest that in families in which the parents' anxiety about distancing is associated with overprotection or overinvolvement, adolescents may increase the intensity and frequency of conflict to feel and be viewed as independent.

The CSBR scores showed an inverse relationship with the CBQ scores for parents and adolescents. Parents who are comfortable in their secure base role may be less upset by their adolescents' attempts at gaining autonomy; if parents consider disagreement on issues to reflect normal growth toward autonomy, disagreements should less likely result in conflict. As Rice (1990) and Hauser et al. (1984) suggest, these parents are able to encourage exploration and ego autonomy. Such parents could provide what Cooper et al. (1983) called an "affective context of compromise and support." As a result, these parents are able to enter into negotiable interchanges, or problem solving, with adolescents before altercations escalate.

Parent–adolescent differentiation was also related to parental separation anxiety. Although most current research on differentiation stems from family systems theory, the concept is highly compatible with the authors' view of separation and attachment theory. In the introduction to his book, *Separating Parents and Adolescents,* Stierlin (1974) cogently addressed the same process of differentiation from a different perspective, that of a traditional psychoanalytic approach. He stated (p. xii), "On all levels, the separation process is shaped by the interaction of centripetal and centrifugal forces which reveal a relational dialectic." His description of these "forces" makes clear that he is speaking about family members distancing from "suffocating closeness" (centripetal) to interpersonal disconnection (centrifugal). Stierlin (p. xii) goes on to point out that these forces shape child–parent interactions, and when they are "out of phase … mutual individuation and separation between parent and child will suffer." Pistole (1994) also addressed differentiation and attachment by arguing that attachment styles can create different distance-regulating patterns within relationships. Results of this study showed that higher levels of self–other differentiation reported by mothers and fathers is positively related to higher parental CSBR. Perhaps parents who are comfortable with the secure base role are able to regulate distance in relationships that allows for both a sense of separateness and connectedness, and such parents likewise are comfortable with others' approaches for more intimacy and needs for individuality.

Also consistent with this interpretation are results revealing that low self–other differentiation between parents and adolescents was related to high levels of AAD. These findings closely reflect the thinking of Cooper et al. (1983) about "individuated relationships." Cooper et al. (p. 56) wrote that an adolescent's leaving process is " … facilitated by individuated family relationships, characterized by separateness, which gives the adolescent permission to develop his or her own point of view, in the context of connectedness, which provides a secure base from which the adolescent can explore worlds outside the family." Findings of the current study demonstrate that the features of parental separation anxiety assessed by the PASAS are related to teenagers' successful transition to young adulthood. Future work with the PASAS should include longitudinal studies that can further document the relationship of the two subscales to adolescent adjustment and the quality of parents' continuing relationships with their adult children.

ACKNOWLEDGMENTS

The authors wish to thank Hyoun Kim and Wilma J. Lutz for their help in the preparation of this manuscript.

ADDRESSES AND AFFILIATIONS

Corresponding author: Ellen Hock, Department of Human Development and Family Science, Ohio State University, 1787 Neil Ave., Columbus, OH 43210; e-mail: hock.1@osu.edu. Mary Eberly is at Oakland University, Rochester, MI; Suzanne Bartle-Haring and Pamela Ellwanger are also at Ohio State University; and Keith F. Widaman is at the University of California at Davis.

APPENDIX

Parents of Adolescents Separation Anxiety Scale: Questionnaire for Parents of Teenagers

The following statements represent matters of interest and concern to parents. Not all people feel the same way about them. Answer the statements as you are feeling now or think you will feel in the near future as your child grows older. Read each statement carefully and circle the number below the item that most closely reflects YOUR degree of agreement or disagreement. Try to answer all statements without skipping items or looking back. Answer all the items without discussing any of them with anyone.

1	2	3	4	5
Strongly Disagree	Somewhat Disagree	Neither Agree nor Disagree	Somewhat Agree	Strongly Agree

1. I am happy when my teenager relies on me for advice about decisions.
2. It will be a sense of relief for me when my teenager moves out of the house permanently.
3. It hurts my feelings when my teenager takes his/her problems to a good friend instead of to me.
4. I like knowing that my teenager will come to me when he/she feels upset.
5. I can't wait for my teenager to leave home for good.
6. I feel most content when I know my child is sleeping under my roof.
7. I feel sad because my teenager doesn't share as much as he/she used to with me.

8. If (When) my teenager goes away to college, I will feel depressed if he/she begins to like school better than home.
9. My teenager is a source of comfort for me when I'm upset.
10. I am relieved to know that the time will come soon when my teenager won't need me any more.
11. It doesn't bother me if my teenager keeps some secrets about himself/herself from me.
12. I feel sad when I think that my teenager does not seem to enjoy being with me as much anymore.
13. I get upset when my teenager takes the advice of another adult more seriously than my advice.
14. I will miss seeing my teenager's belongings around the house after he/she leaves home.
15. Even though it's in the future, I dread the time when my teenager gets married.
16. I really miss holding my teenager like I did when he/she was younger.
17. I feel resentful when my child goes to his/her room instead of spending time with me.
18. I dread thinking about what my life will be like after my teenager leaves home permanently.
19. I am naturally better at keeping my teenager safe than any other person.
20. I feel relieved that my child is a teenager because I don't have to be as concerned about him/her as I used to.
21. I believe that my teenager misses me when he/she is away from me for awhile.
22. I sometimes feel left out because my son/daughter has such close relationships with friends.
23. It makes me feel especially good if my teenager greets me with a hug.
24. I feel sad when I realize my teenager no longer likes to do the things that we used to enjoy doing together.
25. I feel good knowing that my teenager feels that he/she can call on me.
26. I feel very hurt if my teenager pulls away from me when I try to give him/her a hug.
27. Life will be so much better when my teenager leaves home for good.
28. I don't enjoy myself when I'm away from my teenager.
29. I feel uneasy about my teenager going to college because he/she won't need me as much anymore.
30. I would feel hurt if my teenager didn't come to me for comfort.
31. I feel empty inside when I think about my child leaving home for good.
32. I worry that my teenager won't be completely comfortable in an unfamiliar setting if I am not with him/her.
33. When my teenager returns after being away, I feel like giving him/her a big hug.

34. I would feel left out if my teenager asked for advice from another adult such as a teacher, coach, or a parent of a friend.
35. I resent my teenager's need for my help.

Scoring the Parents of Adolescents Separation Anxiety Scale:

1. Reverse the following 7 items so that 1 = 5; 5 = 1; 2 = 4; 4 = 2; (3 = 3): 2, 5, 10, 11, 20, 27, 35.
2. Add the following 21 items to get Anxiety about Adolescent Distancing: 3, 6, 7, 8, 11, 12, 13, 15, 16, 17, 18, 19, 22, 24, 26, 28, 29, 30, 31, 32, 34.
3. Add the following 14 items to get Comfort with Secure Base Role: 1, 2, 4, 5, 9, 10, 14, 20, 21, 23, 25, 27, 33, 35.

REFERENCES

Allison, M. D., & Sabatelli, R. M. (1988). Differentiation and individuation as mediators of identity and intimacy in adolescence. *Journal of Adolescent Research, 3,* 1–16.

Anderson, S. A., & Sabatelli, R. M. (1990). Differentiating differentiation and individuation: conceptual and operational challenges. *The American Journal of Family Therapy, 18,* 32–50.

Anderson, S. A., & Sabatelli, R. M. (1992). The differentiation in the family system scale (DIFS). *The American Journal of Family Therapy, 20,* 77–89.

Armsden, G. C., & Greenberg, M. T. (1987). The Inventory of Parent and Peer Attachment: individual differences and their relationship to psychological well-being in adolescence. *Journal of Youth and Adolescence, 16,* 427–454.

Bartle, S. E., & Sabatelli, R. M. (1989). Family system dynamics, identity development and adolescent alcohol use: implications for family treatment. *Family Relations, 38,* 283–298.

Bloom-Feshbach, J., & Bloom-Feshbach, S. (1987). *The psychology of separation and loss: perspectives on development. Life transitions and clinical practice.* San Francisco: Jossey-Bass.

Bowen, M. (1978). *Family therapy in clinical practice.* New York: Jason Aronson.

Bowlby, J. (1969). *Attachment and loss: Vol. 1. Attachment.* New York: Basic.

Bowlby, J. (1973). *Attachment and loss: Vol. 2. Separation.* New York: Basic.

Bowlby, J. (1980). *Attachment and loss: Vol. 3. Loss, sadness, and depression.* New York: Basic.

Cattell, R. (1966). The scree test for the number of factors. *Multivariate Behavioral Research, 1,* 245–276.

Collins, N., & Reed, S. (1990). Adult attachment, working models, and relationship quality in dating couples. *Journal of Personality and Social Psychology, 58,* 644–663.

Cooper, C., Grotevant, H. D., & Condon, S. (1983). Individuality and connectedness in the family as a context for adolescent identity formation and role-taking skill.

In H. Grotevant & C. Cooper (Eds.), *Adolescent development in the family* (pp. 43–60). San Francisco: Jossey-Bass.

Cronbach, L. J., & Meehl, P. E. (1955). Construct validity in psychological tests. *Psychological Bulletin, 52,* 281–302.

Crowell, J., & Waters, E. (1999, April) *Bowlby's theory in life span development: secure base phenomena in adult partnerships.* Paper presented at the biennial meeting of the Society for Research in Child Development, Albuquerque, NM.

Deater-Deckard, K., Scarr, S., McCartney, K., & Eisenberg, M. (1994). Paternal separation anxiety: relationships with parenting stress, child-rearing attitudes, and maternal anxieties. *Psychological Science, 5,* 341–346.

DeMeis, D., Hock, E., & McBride, S. (1986). The balance of employment and motherhood: a longitudinal study of mothers' feeling about separation from their first born infants. *Developmental Psychology, 22,* 627–632.

Fein, G. C., Gariboldi, A., & Boni, R. (1993). Antecedents of maternal separation anxiety. *Merrill-Palmer Quarterly, 39,* 481–495.

Feldman, S., & Elliot, G. R. (Eds.). (1990). *At the threshold: the developing adolescent.* Cambridge, MA: Harvard University Press.

Flannery, D. J., Montemayor, R., Eberly, M., & Torquati, J. (1993). Unraveling the ties that bind: affective expression and perceived conflict in parent–adolescent interactions. *Journal of Social and Interpersonal Relationships, 10,* 495–509.

Floyd, F. J., & Widaman, K. F. (1995). Factor analysis in the development and refinement of clinical assessment instruments. *Psychological Assessment, 7,* 286–299.

Foster, S., Prinz, R., & O'Leary, D. (1983). Impact of problem-solving communication training and generalization procedures on family conflict. *Child and Family Behavior Therapy, 5,* 1–23.

Gehring, T., & Feldman, S. (1988). Adolescents' perceptions of family cohesion and power: a methodological study of the Family System Test. *Journal of Adolescent Research, 3,* 33–52.

Gehring, T., & Schultheiss, R. (1987). Spatial representations and assessment of family relationships. *The American Journal of Family Therapy, 15,* 261–264.

Grotevant, H., & Cooper, C. (1986). Individuation in family relationships: a perspective on individual differences in the development of identity and role-taking skills in adolescence. *Human Development, 29,* 82–100.

Hauser, S. T., Powers, S. I., Noam, G., Jacobson, A. M., Weiss, B., & Follansbee, D. J. (1984). Familiar contexts of adolescent ego development. *Child Development, 55,* 195–213.

Hock, E., & Lutz, W. (1998). Psychological meaning of separation anxiety in mothers and fathers. *Journal of Family Psychology, 12,* 41–55.

Hock, E., McBride, S., & Gnezda, M. T. (1989). Maternal separation anxiety: mother–infant separation from the maternal perspective. *Child Development, 60,* 793–802.

Hock, E., & Schirtzinger, M. B. (1992). Maternal separation anxiety: its developmental course and relationship to maternal mental health. *Child Development, 63,* 93–102.

Humphry, R., & Hock, E. (1989). Infants with colic: a study of maternal stress and anxiety. *Infant Mental Health Journal, 10,* 263–272.

Kobak, R., Cole, H., Ferenz-Gillies, R., & Fleming, W. (1993). Attachment and emotion regulation during mother–teen problem solving: a control theory analysis. *Child Development, 64,* 231–245.

Kobak, R., & Sceery, A. (1988). Attachment in late adolescence: working models, affect regulation, and representation of self and others. *Child Development, 59,* 135–146.

Kobak, R., Sudler, N., & Gamble, W. (1991). Attachment and depressive symptoms during adolescence: a developmental pathways analysis. *Development and Psychopathology, 3,* 461–474.

Larson, R., & Ham, M. (1993). Stress and "storm and stress" in early adolescence: the relationship of negative events with dysphoric affect. *Developmental Psychology, 29,* 130–140.

Marvin, R. S., & Stewart, R. B. (1990). A family systems framework for the study of attachment. In M. T. Greenberg, D. Cicchetti, & E. M. Cummings (Eds.), *Attachment in the preschool years* (pp. 51–86). Chicago: University of Chicago Press.

McBride, S., & Belsky, J. (1988). Characteristics, determinants, and consequences of maternal separation anxiety. *Developmental Psychology, 24,* 407–414.

Montemayor, R. (1982). The relationship between parent–adolescent conflict and the amount of time adolescents spend alone and with parents and peers. *Child Development, 52,* 1512–1519.

Montemayor, R., Adams, G. R., & Gullota, T. P. (Eds.). (1990). *Advances in adolescent development: Vol 2. The transition from childhood to adolescence.* Newbury Park, CA: Sage.

Papini, D. R., Roggman, L. A., & Anderson, J. (1991). Early-adolescent perceptions of attachment to mother and father: a test of the emotional distancing and buffering hypotheses. *Journal of Early Adolescence, 11,* 258–275.

Patterson, G. R., Reid, J. B., & Dishion, T. J. (1992). *Antisocial boys.* Eugene, OR: Castalia.

Pistole, M. C. (1994). Adult attachment styles: some thoughts on closeness-distance struggles. *Family Process, 33,* 147–159.

Prinz, R., Foster, S., Kent, R., & O'Leary, K. (1979). Multivariate assessment of conflict in distressed and nondistressed mother–adolescent dyads. *Journal of Applied Behavioral Analysis, 12,* 691–700.

Rice, K. G. (1990). Attachment in adolescence: a narrative and meta-analytic review. *Journal of Youth and Adolescence, 19,* 511–538.

Robin, A., & Weiss, J. (1980). Criterion-related validity of behavioral and self-report measures of problem-solving communication skills in distressed and non-distressed parent–adolescent dyads. *Behavioral Assessment, 2,* 339–352.

Sabatelli, R. M., & Anderson, S. A. (1991). Family system dynamics, peer relations, and adolescents' psychological adjustment. *Family Relations, 40,* 363–369.

Simpson, J. A., Rholes, W. S., & Phillips, D. (1996). Conflict in close relationships: an attachment perspective. *Journal of Personality and Social Psychology, 71,* 899–914.

Steinberg, L. (1989). Pubertal maturation and parent–adolescent distance: an evolutionary perspective. In G. R. Adams, R. Montemayor, & T. P. Gullotta (Eds.), *Biology of adolescent behavior and development* (pp. 71–97). Newbury Park, CA: Sage.

Stierlin, H. (1974). *Separating parents and adolescents.* New York: Quadrangle/New York Times.

Stifter, C. A., Coulehan, C. M., & Fish, M. (1993). Linking employment to attachment: the mediating effects of maternal separation anxiety and interactive behavior. *Child Development, 64,* 1451–1460.

Weiss, R. S. (1982). Attachment in adult life. In C. M. Parkes & J. Stevenson-Hinde (Eds.), *The place of attachment in human behavior.* New York: Basic.

Youniss, J., & Smollar, J. (1985). *Adolescent relations with mothers, fathers and friends.* Chicago: University of Chicago Press.

4

"I Got Some Swords and You're Dead!": Violent Fantasy, Antisocial Behavior, Friendship, and Moral Sensibility in Young Children

Judy Dunn and Claire Hughes

Relations between an early interest in violent fantasy and children's social understanding, antisocial and emotional behavior, and interactions with friends were investigated in 40 "hard-to-manage" preschoolers and 40 control children matched for gender, age, and school and ethnic background. Children were filmed alone in a room with a friend and tested on a battery of cognitive tests, including false-belief, executive function, and emotion understanding tasks. Teachers reported on their friendship quality. At age 6 years, the children's understanding of the emotional consequences of antisocial and prosocial actions was studied. The hard-to-manage group showed higher rates of violent fantasy; across both groups combined, violent fantasy was related to poor executive control and language ability, frequent antisocial behavior, displays of anger and refusal to help a friend, poor communication and coordination of play, more conflict with a friend, and less empathic moral sensibility 2 years later. The usefulness of a focus on the content of children's pretend play—in particular, violent fantasy—as a window on children's preoccupations is considered.

INTRODUCTION

Pretend play is central to the lives of many 3- to 5-year olds, and shared pretense is a core feature of their friendships (Gottman, 1986; Howes, Unger, & Mathesen, 1992). A focus on children's pretend play gives us a window on their fantasy worlds, interests, and preoccupations. In pretense, children can take on any identity, role, or activity that they choose. They can be mothers, babies, Cinderella, or Captain Hook. They can make tea or fly to the moon.

Or they can fight, hurt others, or kill or imprison someone. Children's pretend play has received much attention from cognitive developmentalists, who have demonstrated the links between pretense and children's understanding of mind and emotion (Taylor & Carlson, 1997), language development, and ability to differentiate fantasy and reality (Woolley, 1997). In contrast to this active research interest in the development and correlates of pretense, the significance of the *theme* or content of children's fantasies has received much less systematic research attention, although it has long been a focus of clinicians' and educators' interest (e.g., Paley, 1986, 1988). We know that there are broad cultural differences in the themes of fantasy play of children from different communities (e.g., Dunn & Brown, 1991; Farver & Howes, 1993; Farver & Shin, 1997; Martini, 1994), but there is relatively little information on individual differences in the themes of fantasy lives of children growing up within particular cultural communities.

It has been suggested that differences in children's pretend themes may be linked to their personal goals in social situations—that those who are less concerned with harmonious collaborative play and more concerned with pursuing their own interests may choose to enact the more fantastic rather than domestic themes (Connolly, Doyle, & Reznick, 1988; Garvey, 1990). It is also often suggested that some children work through emotional problems and fears through pretend play (see, for example, Gottman, 1986). Are there systematic differences between the fantasies of children with adjustment or interpersonal problems, those at risk for conduct problems or antisocial behavior, and those of other children? In a study of elicited doll play, Howes and colleagues (Howes, Unger, & Mathesen, 1992) found, for example, that children who had been physically abused engaged in pretend play with more aggressive themes than other children. Furthermore, it has been proposed that differences in attachment security may be linked to differences in play themes in young children (Bretherton, 1987). Thus Rosenberg (1983), in a study of 4-year-olds, reported that children who had as 18-month-olds been insecurely attached to their mothers were more likely than securely attached children to engage in pretend play with aggressive, unpleasant themes. There has been a recent revival of interest in the use of directed or elicited doll play as a technique for revealing children's representations of relationships (see Bretherton, 1995; Bretherton, Prentiss, & Ridgeway, 1990) with the presumption that the pretend narratives concerning relationships will differ for disturbed or insecure children, as compared with those of secure and well-adjusted children (Bretherton, 1995; Bretherton & Watson, 1990; Murray, Woolgar, Briers, & Hipwell, 1999).

The study reported here is part of a longitudinal project on children recruited as "hard-to-manage" preschoolers (Hughes, Dunn, & White, 1998). This term is used following Campbell and Ewing (1990) to describe inattentive and restless preschoolers who are reported to be at high risk (approximately even odds) of meeting diagnostic criteria for disruptive disorders at school age (Campbell, 1995). Here the focus is specifically on the children's pretense, and their antisocial, emotional, and social behavior as they played in the company of a friend. Of particular interest were individual differences in violent or aggressive themes in their play. It is known that chronic disruptive behavior can occur in the preschool years (e.g., Campbell & Ewing, 1990; Rose, Rose, & Feldman, 1989) and that early onset of such disruptive behavior is an indicator of high risk for showing "life-course" persistent patterns of antisocial behavior (Moffitt, 1993). Direct observations of disruptive preschool children with their peers are, however, still relatively few (see Alessandri, 1992, for an exception); in part this reflects the problems of applying diagnostic criteria to preschoolers, in whom age-appropriate behavior in response to minor stress can be difficult to distinguish from symptoms of disorder. The "hard-to-manage" children in the sample were found to show significantly higher rates of antisocial behavior and displays of negative emotion, and lower rates of prosocial behavior, than a control group (Hughes, White, Sharpen, & Dunn, 2000). In the present study, the children's pretend play was not elicited or directed as in clinical doll-play studies. Rather, the children were simply left to play in a room alone with a friend and a range of dressing-up materials and toys.

In investigating the relative prominence of violent or aggressive themes in their pretense, a key goal was to understand the correlates of individual differences in the children's interest in violent play. The concern here was not solely with group differences between the "hard-to-manage" group and the control group children, but with the continuities between children labeled as disruptive and other children, the significant individual variation among such difficult children, and individual differences among all the children in the sample, who were recruited from a deprived inner-city area of south London (Hughes, Dunn, & White, 1998). A number of different possible correlates were investigated.

The first set concerned differences in the children's cognitive and language abilities. The role of specific cognitive abilities, such as poor understanding of other people's thoughts, beliefs, and feelings, and of executive control —particularly their planning and inhibitory control—in the interpersonal difficulties and behavior of restless, disruptive children in middle childhood has been highlighted (Arsenio & Fleiss, 1996; Taylor, Sandberg, Thorley, & Giles, 1991; Whalen & Henker, 1992). In this particular sample of younger children there was evidence that, in comparison with the control group, the children had problems in understanding mental states and their connections to human actions, in understanding feelings, and in aspects of executive control; their language abilities were also poorer (Hughes, Dunn, & White, 1998). In the present study, the possibility that the children's interest in violence during their pretend play might be related to such cognitive problems was investigated on the following grounds.

First, individual differences in executive control were related to real-life antisocial behavior in this sample: children who showed poor executive planning and inhibitory control engaged in more bullying, teasing, and violent behavior (Hughes, Dunn, & White, 2000). Therefore, one hypothesis of this study was that violent *fantasies* might also be related to difficulties in such aspects of executive control. Second, as they mature from toddlerhood to preschool age, young children learn to curb their displays of violent behavior, and individual differences in the development of inhibitory control may also contribute to variation in violent fantasy play. Third, individual differences in children's ability to understand the links between mental states and actions (their "theory of mind" abilities) and in their understanding of emotions have been shown to be related to their engagement in shared pretend play (Taylor & Carlson, 1997) and to the frequency and maturity of their shared pretend play with others (Hughes & Dunn, 1997; Youngblade & Dunn, 1995). To share an imaginary world with another person, to cooperate with and contribute to a shared pretend narrative, requires an ability to understand what the other is thinking, feeling, and planning, a grasp of the "possible worlds" (Bruner, 1985) of the fantasy characters. One question of interest was whether children's preoccupations as reflected in the *themes of* their pretend play—the identities that they took on and the stories they enacted—were linked to their ability to understand others' thoughts and feelings.

Also investigated was the possibility that language abilities, which are known to be related to children's engagement in shared pretend play and to their theory of mind abilities (Astington & Jenkins, 1995), might be associated with the themes of the children's fantasies, with more violence and aggression expressed in pretend play by children whose language was less sophisticated. Language problems frequently co-occur with behavioral problems in young children; joint cooperative pretend play clearly involves communicative abilities. In addition to the focus on themes of pretend play, the extent to which the children engaged in pretend play with their friends was investigated: The prediction here was that such ability would be related to the children's sociocognitive skills and language, in particular their understanding of other minds (as assessed in theory of mind tasks), their emotion understanding, and their general linguistic ability. The prediction was that in both the hard-to-manage and control children, extent of shared pretense would be correlated with these abilities. In pursuing these issues, the links between the children's fantasies and their social background, as indexed by maternal education, were also examined.

Another set of possible correlates that was investigated concerned the children's emotional behavior, their responses to emotions in others, and their real-life antisocial actions. The significance of emotional states for children's ability to differentiate fantasy and reality has been explored (Golomb & Galasso, 1995; Samuels & Taylor, 1994; Woolley, 1997); however, little is known about links between emotional expression and responsiveness and the *content* of children's fantasies. The hypothesis was that the children in the sample who were more likely to express anger and irritation, were more easily upset, or were less responsive and helpful when their friends were distressed and those who were more likely to bully and tease would be more likely to engage in violent fantasies.

This brings us to a second key reason for focusing on the themes of children's pretend play: the links between pretend play and close relationships with other children. It has been plausibly argued that it is through social pretend play that young friends express and share concerns and develop intimacy with one another (Gottman & Parker, 1986; Howes, Unger, & Mathesen, 1992). Shared pretend play can be a core feature of close relationships between 4- to 7-year-olds. It has been suggested, however, that some themes in pretend play may be too disturbing for other children to share, or for incorporation into group play in kindergarten (Paley, 1988). For some children who express violence or aggression in their make-believe play, the emotional issues may be too extreme, as Howes and colleagues (1992) noted, to permit joint play and cooperation with others or resolution of conflict. The quality of such children's friendships may then differ. This issue is important to investigate in young children at risk for attentional and disruptive behavior problems. We know that by middle childhood, such children do have problems in their close relationships with peers; in a large-scale longitudinal community study of hyperactive boys, dyadic relationships were found to be more seriously affected than peer group relations (Taylor et al., 1991).

The third reason for the focus on early violent fantasies concerns children's developing moral sensibility. Does an early interest in violent pretend show a relation over time to children's views on the emotions of those who transgress or act violently or unkindly, as well as their views of the emotions of their victims? Individual differences in children's understanding of the emotional consequences of antisocial and prosocial actions are marked, and in those children having difficulty understanding the consequences, have been linked to their disruptive behavior (Arsenio & Fleiss, 1996). There is still little information, however, on the early behavior of children that may be linked to such later differences in moral sensibility. The possibility that violent fantasies are a useful predictor of later moral understanding is investigated here.

In summary, three issues were considered in this study. The first issue was whether the pretend play of young, hard-to-manage children reflected a particular interest in violence. The correlates of the children's interest in violent pretend play, specifically their language, cognitive abilities, emotional expression, and antisocial behavior were assessed, and their age and their mothers' educational level were also considered. The second issue investigated was the relation of children's interest in violent pretend play to their social behavior toward their friends during observations—specifically the frequency of their conflict behavior, quality of communication and cooperation, and engagement in shared pretend play. Teachers' reports on their social behavior with their friends were also examined. The third issue assessed was the relation of children's interest and engagement in violent pretend play to their later moral sensibility.

METHOD

Participants

Participants were 80 children from the London boroughs of Southwark and Wandsworth (Hughes, Dunn, & White, 1998). The 25-item Strengths and Difficulties Questionnaire (SDQ) (Goodman, 1997) was employed as a screening instrument. This is an adaptation of the Rutter scales that shows good agreement with the Achenbach Child Behavior Checklist (Achenbach, 1991), and with observations of behavior (Hughes et al., 2000), and has been found to be preferred by community samples (Goodman & Scott, 1999) and has been extensively used in community samples in the United Kingdom (e.g., Dunn et al., 1998). The SDQ was sent to families of all first-year children attending 15 preschools and nurseries (13 state run, 2 private). Of the 910 questionnaires sent, 487 were completed and returned. Data from a representative U.K. sample of 1,500 4-year-olds in the Avon Longitudinal Study of Pregnancy and Childhood, or ALSPAC (Golding, 1996), were used to establish the 90th percentile for the subscales of hyperactivity and conduct disorder. Maternal ratings for 87 children were above at least one cutoff point; 66 children exceeded both cutoff points. Interviews with teachers corroborated parental ratings for 60 children. Of these, 20 were excluded from the study for the following reasons: not aged between 3,6 and 4,6 (n = 4), no parental consent (n = 9), known language delay or English not first language in the home (n = 3), and family moved away from the area (n = 4). All the remaining 40 children (27 boys, 13 girls; age: M = 51.8 months, SD = 4.7) scored above the 90th percentile for hyperactivity, and 80% also scored above the 90th percentile for conduct disorder.

A control group of 40 children was recruited from the same 15 schools. All control children scored below the 50th percentile for hyperactivity and conduct disorder and were individually matched for gender, age (±2 months; M = 50 months, SD = 4.1), and school/neighborhood. There were no significant differences between the two groups in the number of children from Black or Asian families (18 vs. 12) or from single-parent families (8 vs. 10).

Mothers were interviewed at the start of the study, and three-band codings for occupation (professional/skilled nonmanual/unskilled or manual) and education (university degree/high school qualifications [General Certificate of

Secondary Education—GCSE] or above/no qualifications or low GCSE) were employed. Table 4.1 shows the family background of the families in terms of mothers' occupation and education. Mothers showed a relatively even distribution across the three occupational status categories. There was, however, a marginal group difference in maternal education, with control group mothers having higher levels of education, $\chi^2(2, N = 72) = 5.8, p < .06$).

For the control group, friends were identified on the basis of three criteria: nomination as reciprocal friends by mothers, by teachers, and behavioral identification as friends in two 30-minute observations following Howes and Phillipsen's (1992) observational criteria (children maintain 3-ft proximity to one another, engage in interactive social play, and display positive affect for at least 30% of the combined observations). Because it was unlikely that all of the hard-to-manage preschoolers would meet all of these criteria, friends or "playmates" were identified for this group by nursery teachers and class assistants. Each friend of a hard-to-manage child had to be named by at least two staff members as a regular playmate for the target child before being included in the study. Thirty-five of the 40 children in the hard-to-manage group had an identified reciprocal friendship, and the remaining 5 children were filmed with a "playmate" selected by the teacher. An important aim of the study was to observe children playing with their closest friends, so "boundary crossings" (e.g., friendships within or between the target and control groups) were not excluded. Eleven of the friends of hard-to-manage children scored above the cutoff criterion for hyperactivity; however, there was not a significant difference in the likelihood of children in each group

TABLE 4.1
Family Background for Each Group: Number of Mothers in Each Occupational and Educational Level

	Hard-to-Manage Group Mothers (No.)	Control Group Mothers (No.)
Occupation		
Professional/managerial	10	15
Skilled nonmanual	11	12
Manual/unskilled	12	7
Missing data or not applicable	(9)	(6)
Education		
Postgraduate/college degree	7	18
GCSE or A level	17	12
Low CSE or no qualifications	10	8
Missing data or not applicable	(6)	(2)

Note: GCSE = General Certificate of Secondary Education; CSE = Certificate of Secondary Education.

having a close friendship with a child who scored above the cutoff criterion for hyperactivity, $\chi^2(2, N = 80) = 1.2$, *ns*.

PROCEDURES

Observations

At age 4, two 20-minute observations (on average, 1 week apart) of the child and friend playing alone in a room at school were conducted; the room was equipped with toys and dressing-up clothes, following the procedures of Gottman (1983). The videotaped sessions were then transcribed, with all talk transcribed together with contextual information on physical aggression, intimidating behavior, rule breaking (e.g., stealing candy from the researcher's bags), snatching from the other child, damage to toys, and sexual behavior, as well as helpful actions and expression of positive or negative affect. Coding systems for pretend play, interactive behavior directed at the friend, and antisocial behavior were developed and are described in later sections.

Task Assessments and Interviews

At age 4 a battery of tasks assessing language and cognitive abilities was administered to each child, alone in a room at the school. Half the tests were administered on one visit, and the remaining tests on the second visit 1 week later (see Hughes, Dunn, & White, 1998, for details). Parents completed the Colorado Temperament Inventory (CCTI). At the second school visit, teachers were given a short, semistructured interview that included items related to the quality of the child's friendships. At age 6, children were visited at school, and the moral understanding assessment of Arsenio and Fleiss (1996) was administered to each child, alone in a quiet room.

MEASURES

Observational Measures

The children's pretend play and their interactive behaviors were coded on the basis of their talk and actions during the two observations, transcribed with context notes from the videotaped recording. The coding was based on speaker turns. The transcription included contextual information from the videotapes, such as pretend actions; nonverbal behavior such as helping actions and shaking head ("no") or nodding ("yes"); the joint focus of attention or disagreement over toys; and the expression of positive or negative affect. The mean number of child's audible conversational turns was 170.0 (*SD* = 63.7) for the hard-to-manage group and 165.1 (*SD* = 46.8) for the control group.

Pretend play. Pretend play was coded when the child was pretending to be someone else, speaking within the framework of a fantasy, or discussing the pretend framework or plan. Two measures of pretend were considered here, both based on speaker turns (a turn was all of a speaker's utterances that were bounded by the utterances of another speaker or by a pause of more than 20): the total pretend speaker turns and the theme of each pretend turn. Only one theme was assigned for each speaker turn, and the categorization was mutually exclusive. The following themes were distinguished: (1) domestic, which included pretend play about shopping, feeding, preparing meals, cleaning up, putting babies to bed, and routine real-life experiences for the child, such as visiting the doctor and going to school; (2) monsters, which included play about sharks, spiders, and TV monster characters; (3) violence, which included sword fights, arresting and police narratives, killing, and battles; (4) fairytale/magic, which included fairy stories, "magicking" people, spells, Cinderella and other fairy tales, and princesses; and (5) sex, which included playing at sexual encounters and marriage. If within a speaker turn the child's fantasy included more than one of these themes, the following rules for superseding were applied: violence superseded other themes, sex superseded themes other than violence. Note that these measures of pretend turns included children's comments as they played both solitary pretend and shared or joint pretend; the latter was coded as part of the coding of interaction with the friend (discussed in the next section).

Two coders rated 20% of the transcripts independently to estimate intercoder agreement; Cohen's modified κ for agreement on total pretend was .85; κ for agreement on the theme categories was .81.

Interactive behavior toward a friend. Measures were expressed as proportion of speaker turns (with the exception of amity). The coding system was developed to assess the frequency with which the following features were present in the children's interactive behavior (Dunn & Cutting, 1999; Gottman, 1983; Maguire & Dunn, 1997): (1) cooperative pretend play: discussing a joint pretend plan or game, taking a pretend role as part of a joint pretend narrative, or following a pretend suggestion of the other child; (2) coordinated play: explicitly or implicitly agreeing with the other child's action suggestion, enquiring what the other child wanted to do, agreeing with a "we" demand, or joining in a game initiated by the other child (this category did not include joint pretend play, which was coded as cooperative pretend play); and (3) conflict: prohibiting another's action, disagreeing, protesting, threatening, insulting, or refusing a request. Two further measures reflected communication failure or success: (4) failed bids for attention or response: making explicit demands for attention or requests to the other child to look, help, cooperate, or respond, or turns that included the other child's name that were ignored by that child; and (5) unresponsive: failing to respond to a comment or bid directed toward the child by the friend. The codes for interactive behavior were mutually exclusive.

One final event was coded separately: Amity was explicitly validating or approving the friend, affirming the friendship, expressing affection, joining in joking or shared deviance with amusement, or joint singing or shouting. Amity was coded as an event rather than as a speaker turn because these episodes were of variable length and expressed as a proportion of time the children were together.

Agreement on coding of transcripts (assessed by two coders independently rating transcripts of 24 children) was as follows: cooperative pretend play: $\kappa = .82$, $rs = .95$; coordinated play: $\kappa = .63$, $rs = .81$; conflict: $\kappa = .77$, $rs = .88$; failed bids: $\kappa = .79$, $rs = .81$; unresponsive: $\kappa = .80$, $rs = .85$; and amity: $rs = .92$ (κ was not appropriate for this category because it was an event coding of variable length).

Antisocial behavior. Five mutually exclusive categories of antisocial behavioral events were coded from the videotaped observations: (1) not sharing (refusing to share, or snatching); (2) teasing and bullying (name calling, intimidating behavior); (3) violence (hurting peer, deliberately damaging property); (4) rule breaking (actual or planned rule breaking); and (5) sex play (with self or peer). Rules for superseding were that violence superseded not sharing. Event boundaries were defined by either a clear change in children's activity or a break of at least five speaker turns; this was an arbitrary rule, but important in establishing reliability between coders. For example, two refusals to share within four speaker turns were coded as a single event if the children were clearly referring to the same toy, but were coded as two separate events if the refusals were focused on two different objects. Each event was then expressed as an hourly rate and as a proportion of speaker turns. In the analyses that follow, an aggregate measure of antisocial behavior—the total number of antisocial actions by the child—was employed. Intercoder agreement was assessed by double coding of 25% of transcripts by two independent coders. Cohen's modified κ were as follows: not sharing, 1.0; teasing/bullying, .70; violence, .93; rule breaking, .71; and sex play, .85.

Expression of emotion, response to emotion, and prosocial behavior. Expression of affect was coded positive affect (smiling or laughing) or negative affect (anger or distress). A coding system was developed to focus on the interactional setting in which negative affect was expressed. This system categorized the event type and the child's response to the affect expressed by the friend. For event type, anger/distress events were coded in terms of three mutually exclusive categories: (1) in response to an intentional act by the other, (2) in response to an accidental action by the other, or (3) unrelated to the actions of the other. Response to each event was coded in terms of five mutually exclusive categories: (1) ignored, (2) neutral response (e.g., starts different game), (3) exacerbation of problem for the other, (4) helpful response, or (5) no relevant response (e.g., in two exceptional cases, the emotional event occurred at the end of the session, an adult had reentered the room, and the child requested adult intervention). Event boundaries were defined as described for antisocial events. Agreement between two coders, assessed on 25% of transcripts, was 81% for total number of events, with Cohen's κ of 1.0 for event type, and .91 for response to event.

Task and Interview Assessments

Verbal ability. Receptive verbal ability was assessed with the British Picture Vocabulary Scale (BPVS) (Dunn, Dunn, Whetton, & Pintillie, 1982) at ages 4 and 6 years.

Theory of mind tasks. Children received a comprehensive battery of standard experimental tasks that included counterbalanced forced-choice questions designed to tap their ability to recall their own false beliefs and to predict or explain a character's action (or emotion) on the basis of a mistaken belief. In total, children received four "unexpected identity" questions (Hughes, Dunn, & White, 1998), four "unexpected location" tasks (based on Bartsch & Wellman, 1989), two emotion inference questions (based on a story developed by Harris et al., 1989), and two deception tasks (based on Sodian & Frith's, 1992 procedures—one a penny-hiding game). For each task, children received credit on the test question only if they also responded correctly to all corresponding control questions (e.g., memory for story, reality check, understanding contingency between emotion and desire-outcome match/mismatch). Procedural details for these tasks are available in Hughes, Dunn, & White, (1998). Children were awarded 1 point for each false-belief task passed, except for the explanation tasks. In those tasks, they were awarded 2 points for spontaneous explanations and 1 point for prompted explanations. Children were awarded up to 2 points in the deception tasks. Intertask correlations were high (Cutting & Dunn, 1999), Cronbach's α for all tasks was .80. An aggregate score on theory of mind/deception was calculated as the number of points scored divided by the maximum number of points that the child could have scored (excluding tasks in which the child failed the control).

Executive function tasks. From the set of executive function tasks used by Hughes, Dunn, & White, (1998), two were selected for these analyses of violent pretense activities as being particularly sensitive to young, hard-to-manage children's impairments in inhibitory control and planning ability. As reported in Hughes (1998), these two tasks were discriminators for the hard-to-manage group, who showed intact performance on the other executive function tasks that tapped attentional flexibility and working memory. The first (the detour-reaching box) was a marble-retrieval game, described fully elsewhere (Hughes & Russell, 1993), in which children attempted to reach a marble within an apparatus with a circular hole. In one condition the marble could be retrieved directly with the use of a knob; this procedure was modeled for the child. After three consecutive correct trials, in the next phase of the task, the marble could be obtained only by flicking a switch before reaching in for the marble; hard-to-manage and hyperactive children found this "switch-route" procedure difficult to master. Again this procedure was modeled for the child. Following the procedures described by Hughes and Russell (1993), the criterion for success was three consecutive "switch-route" trials. Performance was rated by subtracting the number of trials to criterion from a maximum of 15 trials.

The second executive function task was Shallice's (1982) Tower of London. This involves high-level skills such as focused and sustained attention, generation of plans, and inhibition of maladaptive responses. The apparatus includes two wooden pegboards, one for the child and one for the examiner, with three pegs of different sizes and three balls. The child was shown simple one-move problems and asked to copy the target arrangement by moving the balls on the pegs one at a time. On each problem the child was told how many moves were needed to copy the target and asked to think about how to solve the problem before beginning. After a "warm-up" of three one-move problems, children were given a set of three problems at each of three levels (two-, three-, and four-move problems). On each subproblem, the child was given 2 points for a perfect solution, 1 point for solutions within the allowed number of moves ($n + 1$), and 0 points for any other response. A child could therefore score a maximum of 18 points.

Emotion understanding within relationships. In an interview based on that used by Cassidy and colleagues (Cassidy, Parke, Butkovsky, & Braungart, 1992), children were asked about the causes of emotions in their mothers, themselves, and their friends (Dunn & Hughes, 1998). Children were shown faces representing four emotions (happy, angry, sad, and scared). After children had correctly identified each emotion, they were asked what made themselves, their friends, and their mother feel each emotion (see Dunn & Hughes, 1998, for details). The adequacy of children's responses was coded on a 5-point scale in which 0 = no response, refusal; 1 = poor response, which consisted of irrelevant remarks or failure to understand causal nature of question; 2 = adequate response, which consisted of one word or simple clauses only, but appropriate and plausible responses; 3 = good response, which consisted of relevant, appropriate sentences, or two or more adequate responses; and 4 = excellent, which consisted of elaborate response or evidence of insight (e.g., mention of mixed emotions or of transient emotional experience).

Teacher interview on children's friendship. Teacher interviews included 14 items that related to the child's friendship with the friend. Each item was coded on a 4-point scale (1 = rarely, 2 = sometimes, 3 = often, 4 = very often). These data were subjected to a principal components analysis with varimax rotation. Three major factors resulted: companionship, affectionate involvement, and helping/sharing. These three factors accounted for 71% of the variance in friendship quality. Scores were transformed into z scores and summed for each scale.

CCTI. Children's temperament was reported by mothers, using the CCTI (Rowe & Plomin, 1977), a 20-item questionnaire in which each item is rated on a scale of 1 (not characteristic or typical of child) to 5 (characteristic or typical of child); there are four subscales (five items each): activity, negative emotionality, shyness, and sociability. Cronbach's αs for these subscales were .60, .80, .75, and .59, respectively.

Moral understanding. At age 6, children were given a shortened version of the task used by Arsenio and Fleiss (1996) to tap their understanding of the emotional consequences of sociomoral events, using the story vignettes for transgressions and prosocial acts (see Hughes & Dunn, 2000). Two different story vignettes were given for each category of sociomoral event. Stories were depicted in three-frame sequences of line drawings, with a brief narrative accompanying each drawing. Two characters, an actor (A) who initiated an action and a recipient (R) of the action, were included in each story. Characters were drawn with affectively neutral expressions, and there was no mention of affective states in the text. Two sets of stories were used, one with male and one with female characters. In the first transgression story, A pushes R off a castle of blocks. In the second story, A breaks a jug and then threatens to hit R if R does not pick up the pieces. In the first prosocial story A lends A's bike to R (and thus A can't ride it). In the second story, A helps R to tidy up a game that R has dropped (unsolicited help). The order of these four stories was counterbalanced across children.

As a familiarization task, the children were first asked to label line drawings of happy, sad, angry, scared, and neutral faces; all children were able to do so accurately. Children were then told that they would hear some short stories and that after each story they would be asked how each story character felt. After each emotion attribution, the children were asked "Why do you think he would feel like that?"

Children's justifications for how the actor and recipient would feel were coded as follows for each of the four stories: 0 = no response; 1 = hedonistic (e.g., in response to labeling A in the first transgression story as happy, "because he's got where he wanted to go"); 2 = conventional/external (e.g., in response to labeling A in the first transgression story as sad, "because the teacher'll be cross with him"); 3 = empathic (e.g., in response to labeling A in the first story as sad, "because the boy who fell off the castle will be hurt"). An aggregate morality score was calculated by summing across the four stories and the two characters (actor and recipient); possible scores thus ranged from 0 to 24. Cronbach's α for this eight-item aggregate was .46. Although this was low, the measure was retained due to its conceptual interest in this particular sample.

RESULTS

Results are reported as follows: First, group and gender differences in total pretend play and in the proportion of pretend play on violent themes are described. Second, the relations between individual differences in total pretend and proportion of violent pretend play, and child characteristics (age, maternal education, cognitive and language abilities, emotional expression and responsiveness, and child temperamental characteristics) are described. Third, the relation of the children's violent pretend play to their observed antisocial behavior, anger, and interactive behavior toward their friends is reported; the relation between child and friend behavior is also described. Fourth, differences in categories of violent pretend play are discussed in relation to the two groups of children. Finally, the relation between children's violent pretend play at 4 years and their moral sensibility as 6-year-olds is investigated.

Group and Gender Differences in Pretend Play Themes

Table 4.2 presents the mean total number of pretend play speaker turns and the mean turns on various themes of pretend play for the two groups (hard-to-manage and control).

ANOVAs were next conducted on the measures of total pretend turns and proportion of pretense with each of the five themes (arcsine transformations were conducted on proportion measures) for effects of group (hard-to-manage vs. controls) and gender, with vocabulary scores treated as covariate. Note the significant group differences in both violent themes, which were higher in the hard-to-manage group, $F(1, 79) = 24.28$, $p < .001$, and magic

TABLE 4.2
Mean Frequencies of Total Pretend Speaker Turns and Pretend Speaker Turns on Different Themes, by Group

	Hard-to-Manage Group		Control Group	
	M	*SD*	*M*	*SD*
Total pretend turns	52.9	38.4	50.9	28.4
Turns on different themes				
Domestic	30.8	24.6	35.3	23.2
Monsters	3.2	4.5	1.7	2.6
Violence	14.1	10.7*	4.8	4.9
Magic	1.4	2.6*	7.6	10.1
Sex	3.4	8.8	1.5	2.3

*Difference between groups significant at $p < .05$.

TABLE 4.3
Mean Frequencies of Total Pretend Turns and Proportion of Violent Turns by Group and Gender

	Hard-to-Manage Group				Control Group			
	Boys ($n = 27$)		Girls ($n = 13$)		Boys ($n = 27$)		Girls ($n = 13$)	
	M	*SD*	*M*	*SD*	*M*	*SD*	*M*	*SD*
Total pretend turns	51.67	40.50	55.54	34.98	48.93	26.14	55.15	33.42
Proportion of violent pretense	.36	.21	.23	.15	.16	.16	.05	.05

themes, which were significantly higher in the control group, $F(1, 79) = 17.37$, $p < .001$.

For total pretend play, there was no significant effect for group, gender, or verbal IQ and no significant interactions (Table 4.3). For the proportion of violent pretend, there was a main effect for group and for gender, $F(1, 79) = 3.91$, $p < .001$, with no significant interaction. The hard-to-manage children and the control-group boys engaged in a higher proportion of violent pretend play; as Table 4.3 shows, the proportion of pretend play with a violent theme was twice as high in the boys in the "hard-to-manage" group as in the control-group boys, and such play was rarely shown by the girls in the control group.

There was no significant group difference in the number of children who engaged in at least one turn of violent pretend (37 and 38 children in the control and hard-to-manage groups, respectively). There was no significant effect for gender or verbal IQ in the proportion of pretend play on magic themes.

Relation between Pretend Play and Proportion of Violent Pretend Play and Child Characteristics

In the analyses that follow, correlations between child characteristics and total pretend play turns and proportion of violent pretend play turns for the total sample of children are reported, given this study's interest in individual variation across both groups. Table 4.4 shows these correlations and the correlations for each group separately. Note that total pretend play turns and proportion of violent pretend play turns were significantly negatively correlated, $r(80) = -.29$, $p < .05$.

The measure of total pretend play turns was positively correlated with age, higher maternal education, the interview measure of emotion understanding, and the aggregate measure of understanding other minds. The combined sample of the proportion of violent themes in pretend, in contrast, was significantly negatively correlated with the children's language ability, theory of mind understanding, and measures of executive control (the detour-reaching box task and the Tower of London planning task). Correlations were also run with the CCTI scales and the pretend measures (not shown in Table 4.4). Activity, emotionality, shyness, and sociability scores were not significantly correlated with the pretend or violent pretend measures for the whole sample, the hard-to-manage group, or the control group; correlations ranged from $r\ (80) = .00$ to .03 for the whole sample, and from $r(40) = -.04$ to .02 for the other groups.

The correlation between proportion of violent themes in the children's pretend play and the cognitive measures controlling for the language ability scores were run next. After controlling for language ability, the correlation between the proportion of violent pretend and each of the executive function measures remained significant, $rs(74) = -.23$, $p < .05$ for both; however, the correlation between theory of mind performance and violent pretend was no longer significant.

Relation between Total Pretend and Proportion of Violent Pretend and Observational Measures of Emotional and Interactive Behavior with Friends

Table 4.4 shows the correlations between total pretend play turns and proportion of violent pretend play and children's observed emotional and antisocial behavior and their interactions with their friends. The pattern of correlations was very different for total pretend play turns and for violent pretend play turns. Whereas the total number of pretend play turns was unrelated to the children's expression of anger, antisocial actions, or unhelpful response to the other child's distress or upset, the proportion of violent pretend play was positively correlated with each of these measures. Children who engaged in a high frequency of pretend were relatively unlikely to fail in their bids for

TABLE 4.4
Correlations Between Pretend Measures and Child Characteristics, and Observational Measures of Children's Interaction with Friends (*n* = 80 for Both Groups Combined)

	Pretend Play Turns			Proportion of Violent Pretend Play		
	H2M	Controls	Combined	H2M	Controls	Combined
Child characteristics/background						
Age	.28	.16	.24*	.13	.15	.20
Maternal education	.16	.41**	.25*	–.09	–.13	–.22
Verbal ability (BPVS)	.03	.33**	.15	–.29	–.15	–.36*
Emotion understanding	.30	.22	.26*	.15	–.28	–.03
Theory of mind aggregate	.25	.50**	.33*	–.14	–.18	–.26*
Executive function						
Detour reaching	.18	.13	.11	–.22	–.20	–.29*
Tower of London	.24	.24	.21	–.35*	–.20	–.23*
Observation of interaction						
Antisocial behavior	–.29	.03	–.18	.29	.05	.44*
Anger	.07	.09	.03	.36*	.19	.37*
Refusal to help	–.14	–.21	–.04	.53**	.33	.33*
Cooperative pretend	.81**	.82**	.80**	–.31*	–.28	.08
Coordinated action	–.03	–.08	.04	.08	.23	–.31*
Conflict	–.41**	–.11	–.28*	.46*	–.17	.23*
Failed bids	–.20	–.60**	–.38*	.11	.40**	.21
Unresponsive	–.43**	–.23	–.34*	.03	–.05	–.07
Amity	.51**	–.07	.27*	–.22	–.03	–.15

Note: H2M = hard-to-manage; BPVS = British Picture Vocabulary Scale.
**p* < .05; ***p* < .01.

social interaction, or to fail to respond to their friends' communicative moves, but they were more likely to show high scores on the amity measure and fewer conflict moves against their friends. These "frequent pretenders" were particularly likely to share successfully in cooperative pretend—that is, they "picked up" and responded appropriately to pretend suggestions and play moves by their friends. In contrast, the children who scored high on proportion of violent pretend play were less likely than their peers to coordinate their activities with those of their companions and more likely to be in conflict with them.

The Behavior of the Friends of the Hard-to-Manage Children

The finding of the relative lack of coordination and cooperative sharing of pretend play between the children who scored high on violent pretend play and their friends is relevant to the issue of how far the friends themselves had contributed to the high rates of violent pretend play displayed by the children in the hard-to-manage group. Associations between violent pretend play by child and by friend within the hard-to-manage group were tested for; there was no significant correlation between child and friend in the proportion of violent pretend play, $r(40) = -.14$. That is, there was no evidence for reciprocal influences playing a major role in young hard-to-manage children's violent fantasies. There were, in fact, several incidents in which the friends refused to join in the violent pretend play, even when incited to join, as in the example that follows, in which a child in the hard-to-manage group and his friend are playing with swords.

Child, brandishing sword: "Kill! Kill! Kill me!"
Friend: "No!" and drops his weapon.

Control Group

Within the control group, the incidence of violent pretend play was too low to expect significant correlations between individual differences in proportion of violent pretend play and the various cognitive and behavioral measures. As Table 4.4 shows, however, the correlations with executive functions, verbal ability, theory of mind, anger, refusal to help, and lack of cooperative pretend are similar in direction to those in the hard-to-manage group, although they do not reach significance.

Themes within Violent Pretend

The broad category of violent pretend play included a range of different types of violent action and story; the interest was in whether the children in the hard-to-manage group differed from the control group children in the extent to which their violent play involved hurting others. Therefore, the children in the two groups were compared in the occurrence of the following different types of violent pretend: (1) violence that involved killing or inflicting pain on another, in pretend fighting or arrests (example: "Chop chop chop, you're dead!"); (2) play in which monsters, dinosaurs, or sharks attacked and hurt the other child; and (3) dramatic play concerning doctors and hospitals that involved physical investigations described as painful, as in the example that follows:

Child as doctor giving injection: "I give you an infection [*sic*] ... where would you like it? In your arm or your bottom?"
Friend: "In my shoe."

Child: "No, in your arm then."
Friend: "In my bottom."
Child: "Ok then."
Friend (Patient) bends over, child (Doctor) pretends to inject into bottom, patient pretends that it hurts. Friend (Patient): "Aah!"
Child (Doctor): "Oh it hurted, didn't it?"
Friend (Patient): "Yeah!"
Child (Doctor): "Shall I carry you?" Both laugh. Doctor pretends to cut patient open: "I'm just gonna cut you open to see if you've got germ inside."

(4) play that involved enacting "cops and robbers" dramas with arrests and jailing, without deliberate infliction of pain or hurt; (5) enactment of "fairy stories" that referred to death or violence (example: a princess is being sent away from the royal court: "You must go and find your fortune"; "Why?"; "Because your mother is going to be killed in a minute"); and (6) incidents in which a toy spider or insect was killed or attacked. The occurrence of these different categories in the hard-to-manage and control groups was investigated (see Table 4.5).

The significance of the group difference in numbers of children engaging in pretend play that involved violent attacks on the other child (Categories 1 and 2 combined) in the two groups was highly significant, with more children in the hard-to-manage group engaging in pretend play that involved hurting or killing with violent attacks or fighting, $\chi^2(2, N = 80) = 13.65, p < .001$).

Relation of Violent Pretend at 4 Years and Moral Sensibility at 6 Years

The final issue addressed was the relation of children's violent pretend play at age 4 to their age 6 justifications for emotional attributions in the moral stories (which involved actors and recipients in incidents that included

TABLE 4.5
Number of Children Engaging in Different Themes within the Category of Violent Pretend Play in the Two Groups

	Number of Children					
Group	Violent Fighting, Attacking the Other	Monsters Hurting/ Attacking the Other	Doctors, etc., Involving Hurt	Police/ Arresting without Hurt	Fairy Stories with Violence	Violence to Animals
Hard-to-manage	23	8	3	1		1
Control	5		7	2	2	3

both transgressions and prosocial actions). There was a significant negative correlation between the proportion of violent pretend play observed at 4 years of age and children's moral-emotion justification scores at age 6: $rs(70) = -.27$, $p < .05$. Children who had engaged in a high proportion of violent pretend play as 4-year-olds were, as 6-year-olds, less likely than their peers to give explanations of the feelings of the actors and recipients in these stories in terms that were empathetic and were more likely to do so in "hedonistic" or selfish terms, or with reference to external punishment. To investigate the predictive power of violent pretend when considered independently of the other 4-year variables with which it was correlated, a series of multiple regression analyses was conducted. In these analyses the following variables were included as three steps: (1) group status (hard-to-manage vs. control); verbal ability at 6 years, because it was correlated with the moral measure, $rs\ (70) = .26$, $p > .05$; (2) antisocial behavior, angry displays, and friendship quality (teachers' report of companionship) at age 4 years, entered as a single step; and (3) proportion of violent pretend in observations. The combined variance and the unique variance explained by each step were investigated. The results are shown in Table 4.6.

The combined variance in the moral-emotions measure explained by all variables together was 22%. The proportion of violent pretend play engaged in by the children at age 4 years made a significant independent contribution to the variance of 12%, beyond the contribution made by the other 4-year-old variables, and 6-year-old verbal ability.

DISCUSSION

In this sample of children from a deprived urban community in south London, those who engaged in frequent pretend were especially good at

TABLE 4.6
Regression Analyses Predicting Moral-Emotion Justification Scores at 6 Years

	ΔR^2	β	t
Background	.05		
Group status		.12	.74
Vocabulary (6 years)		.20	1.48
4-year measures	.06		
Antisocial behavior		.27	1.82**
Anger displays		–.10	–.66
Friendship quality (teacher report)		–.39	–2.59*
Proportion of violent pretend play (4 years)	.12*	–.37	–2.21*
Final $R^2 = .22$, $F\ (6, 50) = 2.31$, $p < .05$			

*$p < .05$; **$p < .10$.

understanding others' thoughts as assessed in standard tasks of false-belief understanding (results that parallel those of Astington & Jenkins, 1995) and at understanding the feelings of those with whom they had close relationships. In the context of playing with a friend, they communicated relatively smoothly, with few failed attempts at conversation and with little conflict; they were responsive to their friends' overtures, and their interactions were characterized by amity. Clearly, conclusions about causal connections between pretend play and friendship cannot be drawn from these correlation (Taylor & Carlson, 1997), but in commonsense terms it seems likely that sharing a fantasy world will foster intimacy and shared enjoyment and that such joint pretend play will flourish when children already like each other and are eager to collaborate in developing a pretend narrative and to resolve conflicts about the course of play smoothly.

Although, in general, engaging in pretend play was associated with smooth communication and lack of conflict between these young friends—supporting the ideas of Gottman (1983, 1986) and Howes et al. (1992)—the findings of this study show how important it is to take into account the themes of the children's fantasies, which differed notably. Some of the children engaged in fantasies about killing, death, physical violence, and arrests, and the first goal was to understand the correlates of this interest in violence, which was significantly more common among the hard-to-manage preschoolers. There were no mean differences between the hard-to-manage group and the control group on the measure of total pretend turns; rather, it was the theme of such pretense that showed the marked difference between the groups. The results showed that the children whose pretend play included a high proportion of violent fantasies were less frequently engaged in pretense than the children whose fantasies were not violent. Furthermore, children's violent fantasizing was correlated—modestly but significantly—with relatively poor skills with regard to understanding others' thoughts, poorer performance on executive function tasks (means-end performance and planning ability), and poorer verbal skills than those of the other children. When the effects of language ability were controlled, the association with understanding others' thoughts was no longer significant; however, the correlation between differences in planning and control—the executive function measures—remained significant. Within the control group, the frequency of violent pretend play was very low; however, the pattern of correlation with the cognitive and behavioral measures, although not significant, was similar, again indicating the potential interest of these particular child characteristics.

Note that this study focused on interaction between friends, as part of a broad research program centered on the nature of and individual differences in friendship. The question of how the children's social skills or interest in fantasy would have differed in the setting of interaction with a "nonfriend" was not addressed here. In general, research indicates that children reveal especially mature understanding of others in the context of interaction with friends as compared with other peers or (disliked) siblings: Interest in resolving conflict, shared positive affect, and sharing of pretend worlds are all higher with friends than nonfriends (e.g., Hartup, 1996). We would therefore not expect such smooth communication or coordination of shared fantasy with a "neutral" or unfamiliar companion.

The children also differed in the frequency with which they engaged in pretend play categorized as "fairytale/magic." The control group children were much more likely to engage in play that involved the stories of Cinderella, Peter Pan and Captain Hook, Sleeping Beauty, and kings and queens, as well as making spells or transforming people into animals. Two points are worth noting about such play. First, the narratives were often quite elaborate; the children were not simply "slavishly" following a Disney story line. The frequency of this category was positively correlated with scores on the vocabulary measure, $r(78) = .32$, $p < .01$ (although not significantly with the social cognition assessments), and negatively with the proportion of violent pretend play for the full sample, $r(80) = -.37$, $p < .05$, and for the two groups considered separately. Sharing the enactment and development of such stories, familiar yet intrinsically exciting to many 4-year-olds, can be plausibly seen as a formative context for friendship development, as Gottman and Paley, among others, have persuasively argued (Paley, 1986, 1988). Second, there were no gender differences in the frequency of this theme, which might have been expected.

The content of the children's pretend play was also related to their emotional regulation and responsiveness. The children who chose to engage in frequent violent pretend play were more frequently angry and less positive in their responses to their friends and engaged in more frequent antisocial acts—bullying, teasing, violence, and rule-breaking—outside the context of their pretend play. The second goal of this study was to investigate the relation of violent pretend play to the quality of children's interactions with their close friends, and here the observations showed the friendships of children who were frequently engaging in violent fantasies to be more conflicted. The children were also less likely to engage in coordinated actions with their friends, and their communication with their friends was relatively poor. Again, to draw causal conclusions about the significance of children's interest in violent pretend play for the development of their friendships would not be warranted. The findings, however, are compatible with the idea that such violent fantasies are particularly evident among children whose goals are more to pursue their own immediate interests than to coordinate harmoniously with those of a friend (Connolly, Doyle, & Reznick, 1988; Garvey, 1990). The preoccupation with violence revealed in these 4-year-olds' fantasies is, these findings suggest, a sign to be taken seriously, because this preoccupation was significantly associated with poor interactions with their friends and with antisocial and aggressive behavior, and thus carried significance for their current and later peer relationships.

The follow-up information on the children's moral sensibility at 6 years of age underlines this point. The children who engaged in a high proportion of violent pretense as 4-year-olds were less likely as 6-year-olds to give empathic explanations of the feelings of those involved as victims of transgressions by others and were more likely to give "hedonistic" or "external" explanations of how the transgressor felt in such incidents. Similarly, their explanations for the emotions of those involved in prosocial incidents were less empathic than those of children who had rarely engaged in violent fantasies as 4-year-olds. It is notable that the violent pretend play measure made a significant unique contribution to the individual differences in later moral understanding, beyond the contribution of group status (hard-to-manage or control), verbal ability, and the other 4-year-old measures considered.

The social experiences that may have influenced the children's interest in violence were not investigated in this study. These restless, inattentive children, both boys and girls, who were easily upset and angry, were choosing aggressive and violent themes in their pretend play when they could have enacted domestic, nurturant themes; fairy-tale stories; narratives of princes and princesses; nursery school hymns; and doctors and nurses—the favorite themes of other children. Clearly, television watching, exposure to violent films and videos, family experiences, and the street and neighborhood lives these children led may all have contributed to their choice of violence in their pretend play. This study of the nature of the identities and narratives that children chose to enact in their pretense provides a window on the interests and preoccupations of preschoolers, but it is only a first step in what is, surprisingly, relatively uncharted territory. Within the category of violent pretend play, the findings indicate that a preoccupation with inflicting injury and pain should be distinguished from dramatic play that primarily involves enacting "conventional" dramas such as doctors and patients or cops and robbers. It was the group of hard-to-manage children—rather than the control children—who were especially likely to engage in fantasies involving pain and violence toward others. An important next step will be to document the social and emotional experiences that foster in such young children the interest in violence that is reflected in their fantasies. The evidence indicates that the focus on the themes of children's pretend play highlights a characteristic of children that is significant for their relationships with peers and for their later moral sensibility, which is relatively easy to measure, and is likely to be of both clinical and developmental significance.

ACKNOWLEDGMENTS

This work was supported by a grant to both authors from the Economic and Social Research Council (R000236432) and a grant to the first author from the National Institute of Child Health and Development (HD23158).

ADDRESSES AND AFFILIATIONS

Corresponding author: Judy Dunn, Social, Genetic and Developmental Psychiatry Research Centre, Institute of Psychiatry, King's College London, 111 Denmark Hill, London SE5 8AF U.K.; e-mail: judy.dunn@ iop.kcl.ac.uk. Claire Hughes was also at King's College London at the time of this study; she is now at the University of Cambridge, Social and Political Sciences Faculty.

REFERENCES

Achenbach, T. (1991). *Manual for the Child Behaviour Checklist/4-18 and 1991 profile.* Burlington: University of Vermont, Department of Psychiatry.

Alessandri, S. (1992). Attention, play and social behavior in ADHD preschoolers. *Journal of Abnormal Child Psychology, 20,* 289–302.

Arsenio, W., & Fleiss, K. (1996). Typical and behaviorally disruptive children's understanding of the emotional consequences of socio-moral events. *British Journal of Developmental Psychology, 14,* 173–186.

Astington, J. W., & Jenkins, J. M. (1995). Theory of mind development and social understanding. *Cognition and Emotion, 9,* 151–165.

Bartsch, K., & Wellman, H. (1989). Young children's attribution of action to beliefs and desires. *Child Development, 60,* 946–964.

Bretherton, I. (1987, April). *Pretense: The form and function of make-believe play.* Paper presented at the biennial meeting of the Society for Research in Child Development, Baltimore, MD.

Bretherton, I. (1995). A communication perspective on attachment relationships and internal working models. *Monographs of the Society for Research in Child Development, 60* (2–3, Serial No. 244).

Bretherton, I., Prentiss, C., & Ridgeway, D. (1990). Family relations as represented in a story completion task at thirty-seven and fifty-four months of age. In I. Bretherton & M. Watson (Eds.), *Children's perspectives on the family* (pp. 85–105). San Francisco: Jossey-Bass.

Bretherton, I., & Watson, M. (1990). *Children's perspectives on the family.* San Francisco: Jossey-Bass.

Bruner, J. (1985). *Actual minds, possible worlds.* Cambridge, MA: Harvard University Press.

Campbell, S. B. (1995). Behavioural problems in preschool children: a review of recent research. *Journal of Child Psychology and Psychiatry and Allied Disciplines, 36,* 113–149.

Campbell, S. B., & Ewing, L. J. (1990). Follow up of hard-to-manage preschoolers: adjustment at age 9 and predictors of continuing symptoms. *Journal of Child Psychology & Psychiatry, 31,* 871–889.

Cassidy, J. C., Parke, R. D., Butkovsky, L., & Braungart, J. M. (1992). Family-peer connections: the roles of emotional expressiveness within the family and children's understanding of emotions. *Child Development, 63,* 603–618.

Connolly, J. A., Doyle, A. B., & Reznick, E. (1988). Social pretend play and social interaction in preschoolers. *Journal of Applied Developmental Psychology, 9,* 301–311.

Cutting, A. L., & Dunn, J. (1999). Theory of mind, emotion understanding, language and family background: individual differences and inter-relations. *Child Development, 70,* 853–865.

Dunn, J., & Brown, J. (1991). Becoming American or English? Talking about the social world in England and the United States. In M. Bornstein (Ed.), *Cross-cultural approaches to parenting* (pp. 155–172). Hillsdale, NJ: Erlbaum.

Dunn, J., & Cutting, A. (1999). Understanding others, and individual differences in friendship interactions in young children. *Social Development, 8,* 201–219.

Dunn, J., Deater-Deckard, K., Pickering, K., O'Connor, T., Golding, J., & the ALSPAC Study Team. (1998). Children's adjustment and pro-social behavior in step-, single-parent and non-step family settings: findings from a community study. *Journal of Child Psychology and Psychiatry, 39,* 1083–1095.

Dunn, J., & Hughes, C. (1998). Young children's understanding of emotions within close relationships. *Cognition and Emotion, 12,* 171–190.

Dunn, L. M., Dunn, L. M., Whetton, C., & Pintillie, D. (1982). *British Picture Vocabulary Scale.* Windsor, U.K.: NFER-Nelson.

Farver, J., & Shin, Y. (1997). Social pretend play in Korean and Anglo-American preschoolers. *Child Development, 68,* 544–556.

Farver, J. A. M., & Howes, C. (1993). Cultural differences in American and Mexican mother–child pretend play. *Merrill Palmer Quarterly, 39,* 344–358.

Garvey, C. (1990). *Play.* Cambridge, MA: Harvard University Press.

Golding, J. (1996). Children of the nineties: a resource for assessing the magnitude of long-term effects of prenatal and perinatal events. *Contemporary Reviews in Obstetrics and Gynecology, 8,* 89–92.

Golomb, C., & Galasso, L. (1995). Make-believe and reality: explorations of the imaginary realm. *Developmental Psychology, 31,* 800–810.

Goodman, R. (1997). The Strengths and Difficulties Questionnaire: a research note. *Journal of Child Psychology and Psychiatry, 38,* 581–586.

Goodman, R., & Scott, S. (1999). Comparing the Strengths and Difficulties Questionnaire and the Child Behaviour Checklist: Is small beautiful? *Journal of Abnormal Child Psychology, 27,* 17–24.

Gottman, J. M. (1983). How children become friends. *Monographs of the Society for Research in Child Development, 48* (3, Serial No. 201).

Gottman, J. M. (1986). The world of coordinated play: same- and cross-sex friendship in young children. In J. M. Gottman & J. G. Parker (Eds.), *Conversations among friends* (pp. 139–191). Cambridge, U.K.: Cambridge University Press.

Gottman, J. M., & Parker, J. G. (1986). *Conversations of friends: Speculations on affective development.* Cambridge, U.K.: Cambridge University Press.

Harris, P. L., Johnson, C., Hutton, D., Andrews, G., & Cooke, T. (1989). Young children's theory of mind and emotion. *Cognition and Emotion, 3,* 379–400.

Hartup, W. W. (1996). The company they keep: friendships and their developmental significance. *Child Development, 67,* 1–13.

Howes, C., & Phillipsen, L. C. (1992). Gender and friendship: relationships within peer groups of young children. *Social Development, 1,* 231–242.

Howes, C., Unger, O., & Mathesen, C. C. (1992). *The social construction of pretend.* Albany: State University of New York Press.

Hughes, C. (1998). Executive function in preschoolers: links with theory of mind and verbal ability. *British Journal of Development Psychology, 16,* 233–253.

Hughes, C., & Dunn, J. (1997). "Pretend you didn't know": preschoolers' talk about mental states in pretend play. *Cognitive Development, 12,* 477–499.

Hughes, C., & Dunn, J. (2000). Hedonism or empathy?. Hard-to-manage children's moral awareness, and links with cognitive and maternal characteristics. *British Journal of Developmental Psychology, 18,* 227–245.

Hughes, C., Dunn, J., & White, A. (1998). Trick or treat?: uneven understanding of mind and emotion and executive function among "hard to manage" preschoolers. *Journal of Child Psychology and Psychiatry, 39,* 981–994.

Hughes, C., & Russell, J. (1993). Autistic children's difficulty with mental disengagement from an object: its implications for theories of autism. *Developmental Psychology, 29,* 498–510.

Hughes, C., White, A., Sharpen, J., & Dunn, J. (2000). Antisocial, angry and unsympathetic: 'hard to manage' preschoolers' peer problems, and possible social and cognitive influences. *Journal of Child Psychology and Psychiatry, 41,* 169–179.

Maguire, M., & Dunn, J. (1997). Friendships in early childhood, and social understanding. *International Journal of Behavioral Development, 21,* 669–686.

Martini, M. (1994). Peer interactions in Polynesia: a view from the Marquesas. In J. Roopnarine, J. Johnson, & F. Hooper (Eds.), *Children's play in diverse cultures.* New York: State University of New York Press.

Moffitt, T. E. (1993). The neuropsychology of conduct disorder. *Development and Psychopathology, 5,* 135–152.

Murray, L., Woolgar, M., Briers, S., & Hipwell, A. I. (1999). Children's social representations in dolls' house play and theory of mind tasks, and their relation to family adversity and child disturbance. *Social Development, 8,* 179–200.

Paley, V. (1986). *Mollie is three: Growing up in school.* Chicago: University of Chicago Press.

Paley, V. (1988). *Bad guys don't have birthdays: fantasy play at four.* Chicago: University of Chicago Press.

Rose, S. L., Rose, S. A., & Feldman, J. R. (1989). Stability of behavior problems in very young children. *Development and Psychopathology, 1,* 5–19.

Rosenberg, D. M. (1983). *The quality and content of preschool fantasy play: correlates in concurrent social-personality functioning and early mother–child attachment relationships.* Unpublished doctoral dissertation, University of Minnesota, Minneapolis.

Rowe, D. C., & Plomin, R. (1977). Temperament in early childhood. *Journal of Personality Assessment, 41,* 150–156.

Samuels, A., & Taylor, M. (1994). Children's ability to distinguish fantasy events from real-life events. *British Journal of Developmental Psychology, 12,* 417–427.

Shallice, T. (1982). Specific impairments in planning. *Philosophical Transactions of the Royal Society of London, B298,* 199–209.

Sodian, B., & Frith, U. (1992). Deception and sabotage in autistic, retarded and normal children. *Journal of Child Psychology and Psychiatry, 33,* 591–605.

Taylor, E., Sandberg, S., Thorley, G., & Giles, S. (1991). *The epidemiology of childhood hyperactivity.* Oxford, U.K.: Oxford University Press.

Taylor, M., & Carlson, S. (1997). The relation between individual differences in fantasy and theory of mind. *Child Development, 68,* 436–455.

Whalen, C. K., & Henker, B. (1992). The social profile of attention-deficit hyperactivity disorder: five fundamental facets. *Child and Adolescent Psychiatric Clinics of North America, 1,* 395–410.

Woolley, J. (1997). Thinking about fantasy: are children fundamentally different thinkers and believers from adults? *Child Development, 68,* 991–1001.

Youngblade, L. M., & Dunn, J. (1995). Individual differences in young children's pretend play with mother and sibling: links to relationships and understanding of other people's feelings and beliefs. *Child Development, 66,* 1472–1492.

5

Ordinary Magic: Resilience Processes in Development

Ann S. Masten

The study of resilience in development has overturned many negative assumptions and deficit-focused models about children growing up under the threat of disadvantage and adversity. The most surprising conclusion emerging from studies of these children is the ordinariness of resilience. An examination of converging findings from variable-focused and person-focused investigations of these phenomena suggests that resilience is common and that it usually arises from the normative functions of human adaptational systems, with the greatest threats to human development being those that compromise these protective systems. The conclusion that resilience is made of ordinary rather than extraordinary processes offers a more positive outlook on human development and adaptation, as well as direction for policy and practice aimed at enhancing the development of children at risk for problems and psychopathology.

During the 1970s a group of pioneering psychologists and psychiatrists began to draw the attention of scientists to the phenomenon of resilience in children at risk for psychopathology and problems in development due to genetic or experiential circumstances. These pioneers argued that research on children who developed well in the context of risk or adversity held the potential to inform theories of etiology in psychopathology and to learn what makes a difference in the lives of children at risk that could guide intervention and policy (Anthony, 1974; Garmezy, 1971, 1974; Murphy, 1974; Murphy & Moriarty, 1976; Rutter, 1979; Werner & Smith, 1982). Their calls to action inspired two decades of investigation that has yielded models, methods, and data about this family of phenomena, as well as controversies, criticisms, and media attention (Luther, Cicchetti, & Becker, 2000; Masten, 1999b; Masten & Coatsworth, 1998).

The recognition and study of resilient children has overturned many negative assumptions and deficit-focused models about the development of children growing up under the threat of disadvantage and adversity. At the same time, the picture emerging from the systematic study of resilience suggests that some of the original assumptions about this class of phenomena were wrong, or at least misleading. Early images of resilience in both scholarly work and mass media implied that there was something remarkable or special about these children, often described by words such as *invulnerable,* or *invincible.* One of the earliest news articles about resilience in American psychology was about "the invulnerables" in the *APA Monitor* (Pines, 1975). Similarly, a headline about this new research field in the *Washington Post* on March 7, 1976, read, "Trouble's a Bubble to Some Kids." The idea of resilient children as remarkable individuals possessing extraordinary strength or inner resiliency has lingered, even in scholarly work. In 1995, "Superkids of the Ghetto" appeared as the title for a book review on resilience in inner-city children published in *Contemporary Psychology* (Buggie, 1995).

The great surprise of resilience research is the ordinariness of the phenomena. Resilience appears to be a common phenomenon that results in most cases from the operation of basic human adaptational systems. If those systems are protected and in good working order, development is robust even in the face of severe adversity; if these major systems are impaired, antecedent or consequent to adversity, then the risk for developmental problems is much greater, particularly if the environmental hazards are prolonged. In this article, I highlight recent evidence accumulating from two major approaches to the study of resilience, one focused on variables and one focused on people. I also discuss the implications of resilience models and findings for research, practice, and policies aimed at understanding and changing the life course of children in developmental jeopardy.

Editor's note. Kennon M. Sheldon and Laura King developed this *Positive Psychology* section.

DEFINING RESILIENCE

Resilience refers to a class of phenomena characterized by *good outcomes in spite of serious threats to adaptation or development.* Research on resilience aims to understand the processes that account for these good outcomes. Resilience is an inferential and contextual construct that requires two major kinds of judgments (Masten, 1999b; Masten & Coatsworth, 1998). The first judgment addresses the threat side of the inference. Individuals are not considered resilient if there has never been a significant threat to their development: there must be current or past hazards judged to have the potential to derail normative development. In other words, there must be demonstrable risk. In many cases, risks are actuarially based predictors of undesirable outcomes drawn from evidence that this status or condition is statistically associated with higher probability of a "bad" outcome in the future (Kraemer et al., 1997; Masten & Garmezy, 1985). Many risk factors, ranging from status variables such as biological child of a parent with schizophrenia or low socioeconomic status to direct measures of exposure to maltreatment or violence, are well-established statistical predictors of subsequent developmental problems, either specific problems or a broad spectrum of difficulties (Masten & Garmezy, 1985; Masten & Wright, 1998).

In studies of resilience, the risk side of the definition has been operationally defined in diverse ways, including socioeconomic status (SES) measures, tabulations of the number of life events that have occurred in recent months or a lifetime, massive community trauma, low birth weight, divorce, and cumulative risk calculations that combine these different kinds of risk factors. The diversity of the risks studied in this literature presents a problem for comparing and interpreting results across studies (Kaufman et al., 1994; Luthar, 1999; Luthar, Cicchetti, & Becker, 2000). On the other hand, convergent findings in the context of such diversity are compelling (Luther Cicchetti, & Becker, 2000).

Investigators quickly realized that risks for specific or general problems in development often co-occur and that cumulation of these risks at one point in time or over time is strongly related to rising risk for poor outcomes on multiple indicators of development, including psychosocial competence, psychopathology, and health (Masten & Wright, 1998; Rutter, 1979, 1990; Seifer & Sameroff, 1987). Such risk gradients are pervasive, and the processes underlying them remain elusive, as evident in recent attempts to understand SES gradients for a wide variety of child and adult criteria of health (broadly defined) and well-being (Keating & Hertzman, 1999). Singular and aggregated risk indices often predict many kinds of undesirable outcomes. The lack of specificity observed in studies of risk (Coie et al., 1993) may reflect in part the tendency for measured and unmeasured risks to co-occur.

Furthermore, most risk gradients can be inverted to create an "asset" or "resource" gradient showing that high levels of assets are associated with better outcomes (Benson et al., 1999; Sameroff, Seifer, & Bartko, 1997). This is because most risk indicators are arbitrarily labeled this way (Kraemer et al., 1997; Masten, 1994; Rutter, 1990; Sameroff, Seifer, & Bartko, 1997; Stouthamer-Leober et al., 1993). Pure risk factors undoubtedly exist (predicting negative outcomes when they occur), such as a car accident, and purely positive assets are conceivable, such as a talent or friend (or a fairy godmother). However, most risk factors actually index continuous, bipolar dimensions that have a positive end associated with positive outcomes (e.g., good parenting vs. poor parenting, high education vs. low education), as well as a negative end associated with negative outcomes. Thus, low risk on a risk gradient indicates high assets in many cases, because of the arbitrary naming of bipolar predictors. However, it is also possible for risks and assets to be inversely related for other reasons, such as a third causal factor, even when they are not opposite ends of the same dimensions (Jessor et al., 1995). Competent parents (causal factor), for example, may produce fewer stressful family life events (risks), choose to live in neighborhoods with low crime rates (risks) and good community resources (assets), and be more likely to hire tutors for their children (assets).

The second judgment involved in an inference about resilience is the criteria by which the quality of adaptation or developmental outcome is assessed or evaluated as "good" or "OK." There is little debate about whether such criteria exist, but much controversy remains about who should define resilience by what standards (Luther et al., 2000; Masten, 1999b). This is a highly complex issue that is only beginning to be addressed empirically.

Many developmental investigators have defined resilience on the basis of an observable track record of meeting the major expectations of a given society or culture in historical context for the behavior of children of that age and situation. These expectations are termed *salient developmental tasks, competence criteria,* or *cultural age expectations* in developmental and life-span theory (Elder, 1998; Masten & Coatsworth, 1995, 1998; Waters & Sroufe, 1983). However, other investigators, particularly in fields concerned with prevention of substance abuse and psychopathology, have focused on the absence of psychopathology or a low level of symptoms and impairment as the criterion for resilience, rather than the presence of academic or social achievements (Conrad & Hammen, 1993; Tiet et al., 1998). Still others include both kinds of criteria (Dubow, Edwards, & Ippolito, 1997; Felner et al., 1995; Greenberg et al., 1999). A related issue is whether to define resilience on the basis of external adaptation criteria (such as academic achievement or the absence of delinquency) or internal criteria (psychological well-being or low levels of distress) or both (Luthar, 1999; Luthar et al., 2000; Masten, 1999b). Clearly, the choices made about the adaptation criteria defining resilience will influence who is included in studies and will reflect cultural norms, whether or not these are articulated in the study. Questions raised by efforts to define "good" development in resilience research warrant their own investigation, which has been rare to date (see Durbrow, 1999; Durbrow et al., in press).

MODELS OF RESILIENCE

Two major approaches have characterized the designs of resilience studies aimed at explaining the variation in outcomes among high-risk children. *Variable-focused* approaches use multivariate statistics to test for linkages among measures of the degree of risk or adversity, outcome, and potential qualities of the individual or environment that may function to compensate for or protect the individual from the negative consequences of risk or adversity. *Person-focused* approaches compare people who have different profiles within or across time on sets of criteria to ascertain what differentiates resilient children from other groups of children. Each approach has advantages and disadvantages, leading some investigators to include both. The variable focus often maximizes statistical power and is well suited to searching for specific and differential links between predictors and outcomes that have implications for intervention. Yet this approach can fail to capture striking patterns in the lives of real people, losing a sense of the whole and overlooking distinctive regularities across dimensions that can indicate who is at greatest risk or needs a particular intervention. The person focus keeps variables assembled in naturally occurring configurations and is well suited to searching for common and uncommon patterns in lives through time that result from multiple processes and constraints on development (Bergman & Magnusson, 1997). On the other hand, person-focused approaches can obscure specific linkages that provide valuable clues to explanatory processes (Shiner, Tellegen, & Masten, in press).

VARIABLE-FOCUSED STUDIES OF RESILIENCE

Main effects in variable-oriented models theoretically reflect the independent contribution of risks or assets or bipolar attributes to the course of the outcome criterion variable, although cansality cannot be determined in these kind of correlational studies (Masten, 1999b). Figure 5.1 shows two common ways to illustrate a main effect found in multivariate, correlational analyses. In Figure 5.1A, regression lines are plotted for two values of an asset variable (representing high vs. low levels of a continuous asset or "present" vs. "absent" conditions for a dichotomous asset). The lines are parallel because the relation of this asset to the criterion of interest does not vary across risk-adversity levels. One is always better off with this asset, although the risk-adversity variable in this picture also has a main effect; scores on the criterion are falling as a function of rising risk. Figure 5.1B uses a path diagram to illustrate the same kind of main effects for an asset variable and a risk-adversity variable, along with the main effect of a bipolar predictor. The path model is more precise in showing the distinction between three kinds of predictors. Such main effect models can be extended through time by predicting positive and negative change in the criterion of interest over time. These prospective, longitudinal models control for the start point on the criterion variable and test for changes (residuals) over time that can be predicted by the asset or risk variables of interest.

Intervention strategies based explicitly or implicitly on such main effect models could focus on adding more assets; theoretically, if enough assets or

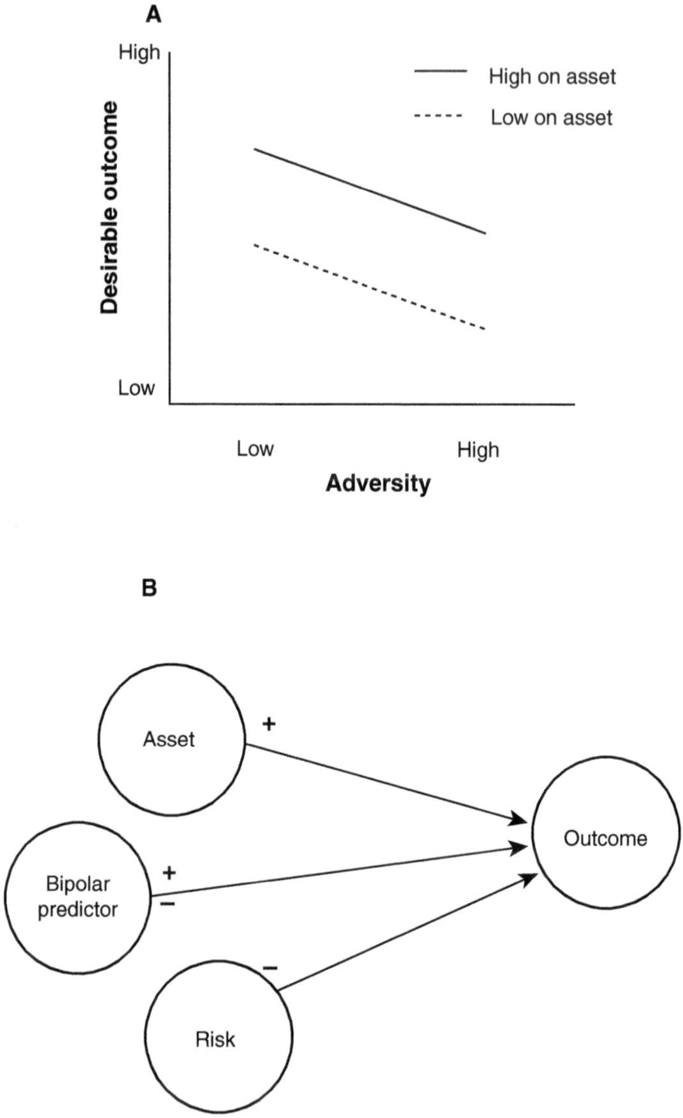

Figure 5.1. Examples of Main Effect Models Based on Multivariate Analyses in Resilience Research.

Note: In A, regression lines are plotted for two values on an asset with a main effect on the criterion; the lines are parallel because this asset is an advantage regardless of adversity or risk level. Adversity also has a main effect in this example so that the criterion falls as adversity increases. B shows a path diagram with the same main effects for an asset variable and an adversity-risk variable, plus an additional bipolar predictor with a main effect on this criterion.

resources were added to a child's life, the outcome variable of interest could be maintained at normative levels, counterbalancing the negative effects of high adversity. The concept of compensatory effects (Garmezy, Masten, & Tellegen, 1984; Masten et al., 1988) refers to the idea that enough positive assets could offset the burden in a child's life from one or many risk influences. Asset-building interventions are based on this assumption.

Interventions could also focus on altering the level of a particular asset or risk in a child's life or in a population. Such strategies reflect models with mediated influence. The focus of intervention could be a mediating attribute within the child, such as when a tutoring program aims to teach a child new academic skills in order to improve the outcome of academic achievement. It is also possible to target asset risk variables in the child's life, such as parenting. Figure 5.2 illustrates a mediation model of how adversity or a positive asset in parents' lives could undermine or enhance the adaptation of a child through their effects on the functioning of the parents. The effects of poverty (McLoyd, 1998) appear to fit this model, in that economic hardship effects on children appear to be at least partially mediated through parenting. This model has been tested by Conger, Elder, and their colleagues in their studies of the farm crisis in the Midwest (Conger, Conger, & Elder, 1997; Conger et al., 1992). Their findings support an indirect pathway whereby the effects of the economic crisis on adolescents are mediated by effects on the mood and interaction of parents that undermine the effectiveness of parenting behavior.

Similar indirect effects suggested by the study of divorce (Hetherington, Bridges, & Glendessa, 1998) led to a randomized experimental prevention

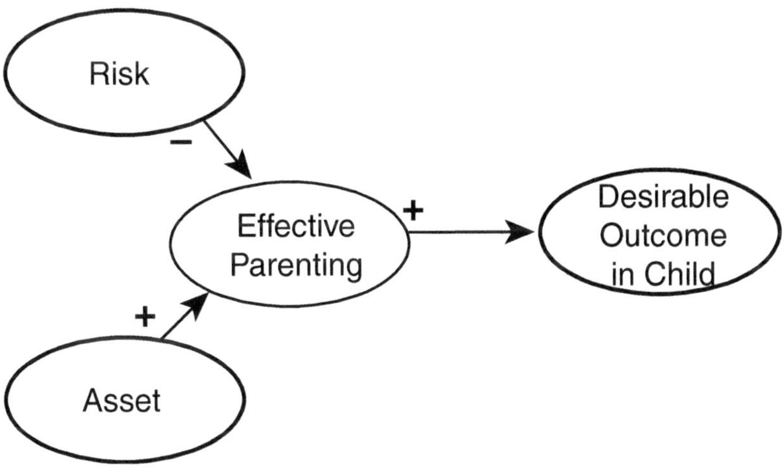

Figure 5.2. Example of an Indirect Model of Risk and Resilience.
Note: Example of an indirect model of risk and resilience where a threat or asset for development works through its effects on a major adaptive system, in this case parenting. Effect of the asset or risk variable in this case is mediated by the parenting variable.

study by Forgatch and DeGarmo (1999). Their study was designed to test the hypothesized protective effect of improving or buffering parenting from the effects of divorce, using an intervention based on coercion theory (Patterson, Reid, & Disbion, 1992). Results supported the effectiveness of the intervention on parenting, which appeared to result in better outcomes among their children. Such intervention trials represent a powerful test of hypothesized protective processes emerging from the resilience literature (Cicchetti & Toth, 1992; Coie et al., 1993; Kellam & Rebok, 1992; Masten & Coatsworth, 1998).

It is also possible to prevent risk factors from occurring altogether, as when universal prenatal care is offered to a population as a preventive intervention for premature birth, a known risk factor for child development. Effective parents probably avert numerous risk factors for their offspring; thus, it is not surprising to find that children with competent parents are exposed to fewer adverse life events (Dubow et al., 1997; Gest et al., 1993; Masten et al., 1999). Total prevention of this kind (the risk factor is averted) could be difficult to detect in studies of naturally occurring resilience, given that one seeks to show something has not occurred. Thus, it is all the more important to develop and test risk-focused models of preventive intervention in randomized experimental designs.

Much also remains to be done to address the transactional dynamics of individual and environmental variables that may contribute to adaptation. Many of these variable-focused models do not accommodate the bidirectional nature of influence in living systems (Masten, 1999b). There is good reason to believe, for example, that children's behavior influences the quality of parenting they receive (Patterson et al., 1992), and that parents influence the development of behavior in children that may be involved in moderating the impact of stress (Gunnar, 2001; Kochanska, 1993). Moreover, some personality characteristics in children and adolescents are associated with more risky behavior that could result in highly damaging life experiences (e.g., Caspi et al., 1997). Rarely examined as yet in resilience research is how the assets, risks, and protective factors in these resilience models may influence each other over time. One study that found parenting to predict child competence, resilience, and change in child competence over time, also found that child competence predicted changes in parenting quality over time (Masten et al., 1999).

Results from variable-focused studies of resilience suggest that parenting qualities, intellectual functioning, SES, and positive self-perceptions have broad and pervasive correlations with multiple domains of adaptive behavior. Substantial main effects are often found for these variables for outcome criteria such as academic achievement, prosocial and antisocial behavior, psychopathology ratings, and peer acceptance (e.g., Cicchetti & Rogosch, 1997; Cicchetti et al., 1993; Conrad & Hammen, 1993; Dubow et al., 1997; Felner et al., 1995; Luthar, 1991; Masten et al., 1988, 1999; Tiet et al., 1998). Main effects for negative life experiences are also found in many of the same studies (e.g., Dubow et al., 1997; Felner et al., 1995; Luthar, 1991; Tiet et al., 1998). However, the explanatory power of negative life experiences is often relatively modest or negligible compared with parenting variables, IQ scores, or SES indicators, particularly when measures of life events exclude events that could be related to the child's behavior and the covariance associated with parenting or SES is controlled (e.g., Cicchetti et al., 1993; Masten et al., 1999).

The possibility that the effects of adversity can be moderated by qualities of the individual or environment is represented and tested by interaction models in variable-focused analyses (Garmezy et al., 1984; Luthar et al., 2000; Masten et al., 1988). Figure 5.3A illustrates an interaction as often portrayed in regression analyses to illustrate the direction of effects after a statistically significant one has been found. Regression lines are plotted for two values of a presumed moderator. In this illustrative case, the contrasting slopes of the two lines suggest that the moderating variable is more important at high levels of adversity; either the individuals high on the variable are protected under high adversity conditions or those disadvantaged on this variable are more vulnerable, or both. It is not clear where the action is in such analyses of covariance.

Path diagram 5.3B illustrates two kinds of interaction with different implications for intervention. One is an enduring attribute unrelated to the risk factor or stressor that alters the impact of risk exposure (e.g., individuals may vary in stress reactivity). The second example is a risk-activated moderator that alters the impact of a hazard, akin to an airbag released in an automobile during a collision that serves to protect the driver (e.g., an adult comforts a child during a hurricane or a 911 call summons crisis intervention).

Interventions based on interaction models could attempt to add risk-activated protections, such as new crisis services. They could also focus on changing the quality of already present moderators, such as efforts to improve emergency social services or parental responses to the needs of children in crisis. Interventions aiming to change the coping behavior of individuals also could be based on such models (Compas, 1998).

Significant interaction effects have not been found very often across the variable-focused resilience literature and results generally have not been consistent, perhaps because of the methodological variability across studies or the general difficulty of detecting interactions or both (Jessor et al., 1995; Luthar et al., 2000). The best evidence for interaction effects in the variable-focused resilience data has accrued for the hypothesis that intellectual functioning moderates the effects of adversity on the development of rule-governed behavior, as indicated by good conduct versus antisocial behavior. Better intellectual skills are generally associated with competence, particularly in school-based domains; however, these capabilities appear to be particularly important protective factors against the development of conduct problems for children growing up in highly disadvantaged circumstances or with high exposure to adverse life events (Kolvin et al., 1988; Masten et al., 1999;

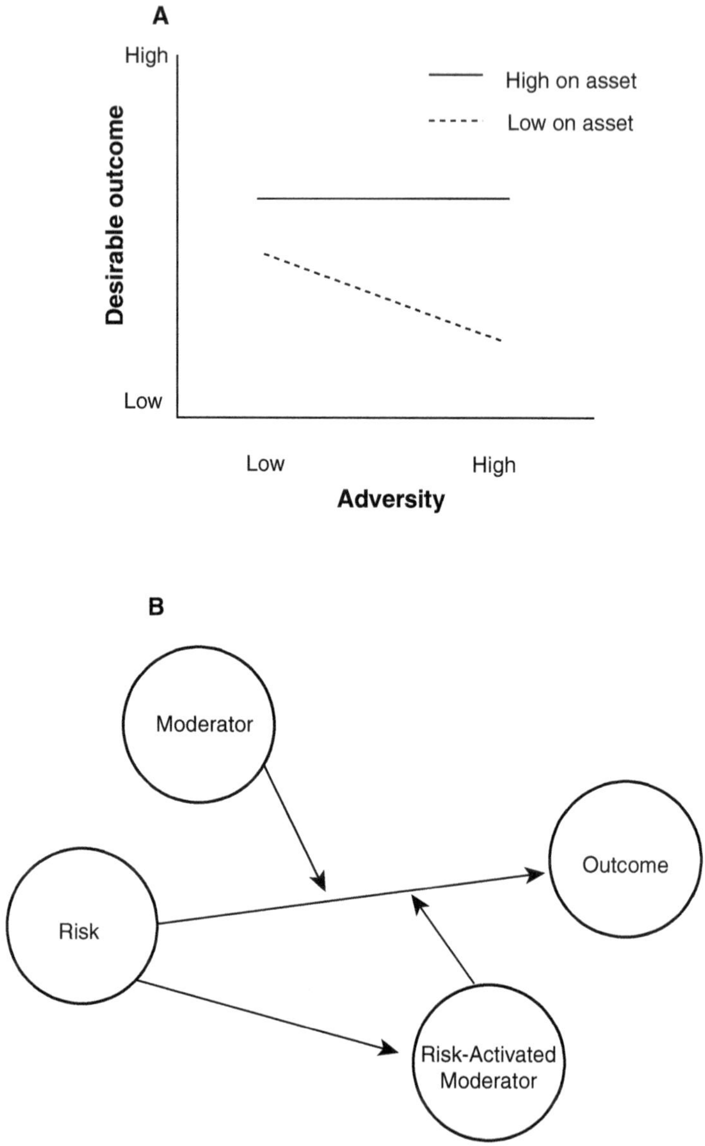

Figure 5.3. Examples of Interaction Models from Resilience Research.
Note: The graph in A illustrates an interaction as typically portrayed in regression analyses in the case where adversity or risk appears to have differential predictive effects on the criterion depending on the level or presence of a protective or vulnerability factor. Path diagram B shows two kinds of moderator effects. One represents an attribute of child or environment that moderates the impact of a risk factor or stressor on the outcome of interest but has no relation to the risk-stressor itself. The other is a risk-activated moderator analogous to an automobile airbag or immune system response.

White, Moffitt, & Silva, 1989). It is not yet clear what exactly it is about intellectual aptitude variables that accounts for this effect. Tests of intellectual functioning are inherently complex and could be markers of motivation as well as a variety of cognitive abilities related to attention, memory, reasoning, and executive functioning.

Effective parenting (e.g., authoritative parenting, monitoring, support) also appears to be protective with respect to antisocial behavior (Dubow et al., 1997; Masten et al., 1999). Again, it is not clear what processes might be involved, including genetic covariance. However, experimental intervention designs that demonstrate a change in child behavior as a function of changes in parenting behavior (e.g., Forgatch & DeGarmo,1999, described above) support the conclusion of resilience investigators that parenting quality has protective power, particularly against antisocial behavior in risky environments.

These findings hint at the possibility of some specificity for cognitive abilities and parenting as moderators of risk for antisocial or disruptive-aggressive behavior when rearing conditions are adverse, although each of these predictors also has extensive links to many other aspects of good and poor developmental outcome, as well as to each other. One might speculate that the development of effective, self-regulation skills are involved in both cases. Clearly, there is empirical and theoretical work to be done before specific protective (or vulnerability) processes are likely to be delineated and adequately tested.

To date, results from variable-focused studies of resilience underscore the importance of well-established individual and family differences for the course of good development. Under conditions of severe adversity, poor cognitive skills and parenting appear to increase the risk of bad outcomes, particularly in the form of antisocial behavior; normative cognition and parenting appear to protect the development of competence under adverse conditions. Parenting appears to play a key mediating role linking major life stressors to child behavior. In low-threat environments, outcomes generally are good, unless the individual has significant handicaps. Very little evidence has emerged from these studies to indicate that severe adversity has major or lasting effects on adaptive behaviors in the environment *unless important adaptive systems, such as cognition and parenting, are compromised prior to or as a result of the adversity.*

PERSON-FOCUSED STUDIES OF RESILIENCE

Resilience studies focused on whole individuals rather than variables corroborate these conclusions. Person-focused approaches attempt to capture the configural patterns of adaptation that naturally occur, in much the same ways that classification systems for mental disorder organize symptoms into patterns that have been observed to occur together. Single case studies of resilience (e.g., Masten & O'Connor, 1989), which are person focused and can be compelling for heuristic purposes, have numerous shortcomings, particularly in terms of generalizability. Most person-focused approaches seek to identify groups of individuals with patterns of good versus poor adaptive functioning (judged on multiple criteria simultaneously) in a life context of high versus low risk or threat, in order to examine what might account for the differences in outcome.

The classic person-focused approach to resilience has been the comparison of two groups drawn from the same high-risk sample who have adaptive and maladaptive outcomes. The Kauai study by Werner and Smith (1982, 1992) has this design, as do the Rochester resilience studies of Cowen, Wyman, and colleagues (Cowen, Lotyczewski, & Weissberg, 1984; Cowen et al., 1997; Cowen, Wyman, Work, & Parker, 1990; Wyman et al., 1999). In the Kauai study, a high-risk group was identified from a birth cohort: the risk group had four or more cumulative risk factors by age 2 (e.g., perinatal problems, low material education, poverty). Then a resilient subgroup was identified on the basis of good competence and few behavior problems at ages 10 and 18. Attributes of these children and their lives were then compared with peers in the high-risk subgroup who developed significant adjustment problems by ages 10 and 18. Many differences were found that favored the resilient group. Resilient individuals had better parenting resources and were more appealing infants. As they grew older, they had better cognitive test scores, more positive self-perceptions, and greater conscientiousness than their maladaptive peers. The competence of the resilient group continued into adulthood, but it is also noteworthy that the investigators have reported a good deal of improvement for the majority of the maladaptive group in the adult years (Werner & Smith, 1992).

Other studies of the classic form base the group categories on a variety of adverse life experiences or conditions. The Rochester investigators formed "stress-affected" and "stress-resilient" groups on the basis of major life stressors (e.g., family violence, death, illness, divorce, poverty) and the pattern of scores on adjustment screening measures indexing behavioral competence and problems (Cowen et al., 1997; Wyman et al., 1999). Richters and Martinez (1993) studied children living in dangerous neighborhoods of Washington, D.C., who were classified as adaptive successes or not on the basis of cutoff scores on the Child Behavior Checklist (total problems fell in the normal range) and teacher ratings of academic progress as average or better. Both of these studies found that parental competence and parenting quality were strongly associated with resilience, although their measures of risk, parenting, and outcome differed. Fergusson and Lynskey (1996) used a cutoff score on a family adversity index based on 39 family risk factors and classified adolescents as resilient on the basis of the absence of externalizing behavior problems, such as drug use, conduct disorders, delinquency, and school problems. The resilient group had significantly lower adversity exposure and higher IQ scores in childhood, as well as less association with deviant peers and less novelty seeking.

What is missing from the classic design are low-risk groups, which could address the question of whether resilient children differ from children who are doing equally well but do not have high-risk profiles. Full classification models of resilience include low-risk groups. Investigators in two of the studies discussed previously with variable-focused analyses also analyzed their data from the person-focused perspective, using cutoff criteria to define four corner groups for analysis (Luthar, 1991; Masten et al., 1999), reflecting cutoff criteria for good versus poor competence as well as high- versus low-adversity-exposure or risk. Once the diagnostic groups were formed, resilient youth (high competence, high adversity) were then compared with both similarly competent peers with low adversity and a group of maladaptive peers who shared a history of high adversity. In both studies, the fourth corner, representing low-risk, maladaptive children (who might be considered highly vulnerable, as in theory they do not fare well even with little adversity) were too few in number for analysis, an empty-cell phenomenon in these school-based samples (see Masten et al., 1999, discussion of the empty cell). Results reported by Masten et al., (1999) revealed that competent, low-adversity, and resilient youth, who shared a profile of average or better competence across three salient domains (academic, conduct, social) had very similar psychosocial resources, including better intellectual functioning and parenting quality and more positive self-concepts. Both competent groups differed markedly from their maladaptive peers on these attributes and resources, even though the resilient and maladaptive groups had similar lifetime histories of severe to catastrophic negative life experiences. Luthar's analysis was designed to assess the possibility that resilient youth suffer internal distress, in contrast to their external competence. Luthar's (1991) results supported this view, although this finding, was not replicated by Masten et al. (1999), who found generally positive well-being among the resilient group.

It is possible to invert the classification in these person-focused studies and group individuals on the basis of adversity and resources, rather than competence. In such cases, children high on a combination of resources represented by scores on variables such as parenting quality, SES, and IQ appear to be well adjusted or competent, even with high-adversity exposure (Cowen et al., 1984; Masten et al., 1999); maladaptive profiles emerge when adversity is high and protective resources are weak.

Discriminant function analysis and cluster analysis also have been used to study resilient persons. Both of these strategies were used by Masten et al. (1999) to corroborate their findings. Maladaptive youth could be readily discriminated from the two competence groups by resources and well-being indicators, whereas the resilient and low-adversity competent groups could not be discriminated from each other. Cluster analysis yielded resilient, maladaptive, and competent groups that were highly comparable with groups defined by cutoff scores, both in terms of who fell into the group and how they compared with each other on other variables.

The most complex person-oriented models of resilience discussed in the literature focus on healthy versus maladaptive pathways of development in lives through time and give special attention to turning points in people's lives (e.g., Bergman & Magnussen, 1997; Cairns & Cairns, 1994; Cicchetti & Rogosch, 1997; Egeland, Carlson, & Sroufe, 1993; Masten, 1994; Rutter, 1990; Sameroff, 1982; Werner & Smith, 1982). The concept of developmental pathways derives from developmental systems theory (Ford & Lerner, 1992), organizational theory (Cicchetti, 1984, 1990; Cicchetti & Schneider-Rosen, 1986; Sroufe, 1979, 1997), and life-course theory (Elder, 1998), all of which assume that patterns of development arise from many interactions of organisms embedded in larger systems and require longitudinal study. Bergman and Magnussen (1997) described this strategy as longitudinal classification analysis.

Most of the resilience investigators of the past decade have assumed that resilience arises from many dynamic interactions within and between organism and environment, but the systematic study of such patterns and pathways is in the nascent stage. To date, much of the discussion of resilient pathways has drawn upon case examples of individuals, often within longitudinal studies (e.g., Cairns & Cairns, 1994; Werner & Smith, 1982). These anecdotes suggest that opportunities and choices at crucial junctures play an important role in the life course of resilient individuals who find mentors, enter the military, find a new or deeper faith, marry healthy partners, leave deviant peer groups, or in other ways take action that has positive consequences for their life course. Resilient youth appear to place themselves in healthier contexts, generating opportunities for success or raising the odds of connecting with prosocial mentors in a manner consistent with the concept of niche seeking (Scar & McCartney, 1983). Such behavior is quite difficult to study in the aggregate because of the variability in timing and situations.

The best recent evidence of resilience in the sense of recovery-to-normal trajectories of development can be found in the follow-up studies of children adopted away from institutional rearing characterized by extreme deprivation. Studies of Romanian adoptees provide dramatic documentation of developmental catch-up in many of the children, both physically and cognitively (Ames, 1997; Rutter & ERA Study Team, 1998); in the words of Rutter et al. "the degree of cognitive catch-up by the age of 4 years was spectacular" (p. 474). As observed in many other situations of extraordinary adversity, the capacity for developmental recovery when normative rearing conditions are restored is amazing (Garnezy, 1985; Masten, Best, & Garmezy, 1990; Wright,

Masten, Northwood, & Hubbard 1997). However, the impressive recovery trajectories of many children following dramatic improvements in rearing conditions do not mean that all children recover well. Significant numbers of children from Romanian orphanages, as well as from other situations of extreme and long-term adversity, have serious and chronic problems that appear to be the residual of their experiences (Ames, 1997; Gunnar, 2001). Nonetheless, the frequency and degree of recovery of these children is compelling evidence of normative restorative processes at work, in response to the provision of good psychological and physical care by an adoptive family.

Pathway models of resilience also offer a conceptual framework for intervention. Several of the most comprehensive efforts to change the life course are conceptualized this way, including Head Start, Fast Track, and the Abecedarian Project (Conduct Problems Prevention Research Group, 1992, 1999; Ramey & Ramey, 1998; Zigler, Taussig, & Black, 1992). Theoretically, such interventions have a developmental systems perspective and they target multiple systems in their intervention. Practical considerations have necessitated simplification of their theoretical models for implementation and evaluation, but in each case, intervention results have been consistent with their models. These models differ, yet they all focus in developmentally sensitive ways on building competence and fostering healthy adaptive systems.

CONCLUSIONS FROM RESEARCH ON RESILIENCE PHENOMENA IN THE LIVES OF CHILDREN

The accumulating data on resilience in development suggest that this class of phenomena is more ordinary than one was led to expect by the extraordinary case histories that often inspired its study. Resilience appears to be a common phenomenon arising from ordinary human adaptive processes. The great threats to human development are those that jeopardize the systems underlying these adaptive processes, including brain development and cognition, caregiver–child relationships, regulation of emotion and behavior, and the motivation for learning and engaging in the environment. This does not mean that in specific instances extraordinary talents or parenting or good fortune may not play a key role for an individual's positive development or recovery; rather, the data suggest that normative processes account for much of the resilience observed across a wide variety of situations. Ironically, expectations that special qualities were required to overcome adversity may have been influenced by prevailing deficit models of psychopathology that the early resilience investigators set out to overturn. In other words, expecting extraordinary qualities in resilient individuals implied that ordinary adaptive resources and systems were not enough.

Evidence from variable-oriented and person-oriented studies of resilience converge on a short list of attributes of child and environment that turn out to be well-established general correlates of competence and psychopathology. Despite all the flaws in the early studies of resilience pointed out by early and later reviewers, recent studies continue to corroborate the importance of a relatively small set of global factors associated with resilience. These include connections to competent and caring adults in the family and community, cognitive and self-regulation skills, positive views of self, and motivation to be effective in the environment (Garmezy, 1985; Luthar et al., 2000; Masten et al., 1990; Masten & Coatsworth, 1998; Masten & Reed, in press; Wyman et al. 2000). Across different situations and research strategies, the consistent support for these resources suggests that basic human adaptational systems are at work, many of which have been studied in some depth under the rubric of constructs such as attachment, authoritative parenting, intelligence, self-regulation, self-efficacy, pleasure-in-mastery, or intrinsic motivation.

Reconceptulizing Intervention Goals, Strategies, Assesment, and Classification

Research on resilience phenomena has changed the nature of the frameworks, goals, assessments, strategies, and evaluations in fields of prevention and treatment (Cicchetti et al. 2000; Cowen, 2000; Luthar et al., 2000; Masten, 1999a; Masten & Coatsworth, 1998; Masten & Reed, in press; Wyman et al., 2000). Goals now incorporate the promotion of competence as well as the prevention or amelioration of symptoms and problems. Strategies include the enhancement of assets as well as the reduction of risks or stressors and the facilitation of protective processes as well as treatment of illness or reduction of harmful processes. Assessments include assets and potential resources as well as problems and risks and competence as well as symptoms and disorder. These changes together reflect a major transformation in the conceptualization of prevention and intervention. This change is evident in reports on interventions, such as one by Hawkins, Catalano, Kosterman, Abbot, and Hill (1999), titled "Preventing Adolescent Health-Risk Behaviors by Strengthening Protection During Childhood." These investigators concluded:

> One explanation for the durability of these effects in contrast to those observed by others is that this intervention focused on increasing school bonding and achievement rather than on developing norms or skills specifically related to avoiding health-risk behaviors. (p. 233)

Similarly, Wyman et al. (2000) proposed the term *cumulative competence promotion and stress protection* to describe how interventions can be conceptualized in terms of resilience. It has also become evident that the classification systems for psychopathology need an overhaul to address more effectively the salient role of competence and adaptive functioning in defining and treating disorder (Masten & Curtis, 2000).

Advancing Research on Adaptive Systems

The roads taken to understand resilience have led investigators toward more integrative studies of adaptive systems in human development, how they work and how these systems develop and respond to variations in the environment. The new frontier for resilience research is understanding these processes at multiple levels, from genes to relationships, and investigating how the individual as a complex living system interacts effectively and ineffectively over time with the systems in which it is embedded. Exciting new work on the linkages among adversity, brain development, and the quality of adaptation in terms of both competence and psychopathology exemplify this frontier (Cicchetti & Cannon, 1999; Maier & Watkins, 1998; Nelson, 1999, 2000).

Research on resilience has underscored the importance of integrating studies of competence and psychopathology, of individual differences and normative patterns in development, and of how developmental processes unfold in normative compared with extremely deviant conditions. These goals are fundamental to the integrative science of developmental psychopathology, which rose to prominence during the same period as resilience (Cicchetti, 1984; Masten & Braswell, 1991; Sroufe & Rutter, 1984). Thus, it is not surprising to find that developmental psychopathologists often have a keen interest in resilience. We are moving toward an integrated science of human adaptation and development (Masten & Curtis, 2000).

Resilience and Positive Psychology

The message from three decades of research on resilience underscores central themes of the positive psychology movement (Seligman & Csikszentmihalyi, 2000; Snyder & Lopez, in press). Psychology has neglected important phenomena in human adaptation and development during periods of focus on risk, problems, pathology, and treatment. Attention to human capabilities and adaptive systems that promote healthy development and functioning have the potential to inform policy and programs that foster competence and human capital and aim to improve the health of communities and nations while also preventing problems. The study of resilience helped to rekindle positive psychology; now the new impetus for research on successful human functioning should serve to illuminate fundamental processes underlying resilience in development (Masten & Reed, in press). In addition, positive psychology poses important questions for resilience investigators about the differentiation of challenging experiences that undermine development versus those that promote development. Concomitantly, the study of resilience raises questions about the nature and development of optimal functioning: whether it arises from an unusual alignment of normative rather than extraordinary processes, what it means under conditions of severe adversity, and how it is scaffolded by the social context over the course of development.

The Power of the Ordinary

What began as a quest to understand the extraordinary has revealed the power of the ordinary. Resilience does not come from rare and special qualities, but from the everyday magic of ordinary, normative human resources in the minds, brains, and bodies of children; in their families and relationships; and in their communities. This has profound implications for promoting competence and human capital in individuals and society. Even the most basic of human adaptational systems are not invulnerable and require nurturance. All too often, children who contend with the greatest adversities do not have the protections afforded by basic resources nor the opportunities and experiences that nurture the development of adaptive systems. If major threats to children are those adversities that undermine basic protective systems for development, it follows that efforts to promote competence and resilience in children at risk should focus on strategies that protect or restore the efficacy of these basic systems. Resilience models and findings also suggest that programs will be most effective when they tap into these basic but powerful systems.

The conclusion that resilience emerges from ordinary processes offers a far more optimistic outlook for action than the idea that rare and extraordinary processes are involved. The task before us now is to delineate how adaptive systems develop; how they operate under diverse conditions; how they work for or against success for a given child in his or her environmental and developmental context; and how they can be protected, restored, facilitated, and nurtured in the lives of children. Fortunately, we know more than we realized about resilience processes because a substantial knowledge base already exists about adaptive processes in human development. Our current knowledge justifies a more positive view of normative, human capabilities; ordinary parents; and the self-righting power of development than either the gloom-and-doom or the rosy-resiliency perspectives could provide.

ACKNOWLEDGMENTS

Author's note. I have had the great fortune of interacting with many resilience researchers over the years who have contributed immeasurably to my thinking about this class of phenomena. Most particularly, I want to thank the following for our illuminating conversations: Norman Garmczy, Suniya Luthar, Michael Rutter, Auke Tellegen, Emmy Werner, and Margaret Wright. Thanks also go to Marie-Gabrielle Reed, Jenifer Powell, John Curtis, Art Sesma, and Robin Mathy for their comments on this article. The writing of this article, as well as my research on resilience, has been facilitated by National Science Foundation Grant NSF/SBR-9729111, the William T. Grant Foundation Gram 97-1845-97, and membership in the Research Network on Psychopathology and Development, funded by the John D. and Catherine T. MacArthur Foundation.

ADDRESS AND AFFILIATIONS

Correspondence concerning this article should be addressed to Ann S. Masten, Institute of Child Development, University of Minnesota, 51 East River Road, Minneapolis, MN 55455-0345. Electronic mail may be sent to amasten@tc.umn.edu.

REFERENCES

Ames, E. W. (1997). *The development of Romanian orphanage children adopted to Canada* (Final report to the National Welfare Grants Program: Human Resources Development Canada). Burnaby, British Columbia, Canada: Simon Fraser University.

Anthony, E. J. (1974). The syndrome of the psychologically invulnerable child. In E. J. Anthony & C. Koupernik (Eds.), *The child in his family: children at psychiatric risk* (pp. 529–545), New York: Wiley.

Benson, P. L., Scales, P. C., Lettert N., & Roehikepartain, E. C. (1999). *A fragile foundation: the state of developmental assets among American youth.* Minneapolis, MN: Search Institute.

Bergman, L. A., & Magnusson, D. (1997). A person-oriented approach in research on developmental psychopathology. *Development and Psychopathology, 9,* 291–319.

Buggie, S. E. (1995). Superkids of the ghetto. *Contemporary Psychology, 40,* 1164–1165.

Cairns, R. B., & Cairns, B. D. (1994). Lifelines and risks: Pathways of youth in our time. New York: Cambridge University Press.

Caspi, A., Begg, D., Dickson, N., Harrington, H., Langley, J., Moffitt, T. E., & Silva, P. A. (1997). Personality differences predict health-risk behaviors in young adulthood: evidence from a longitudinal study. *Journal of Personality and Social Psychology, 73,* 1052–1063.

Cicchetti, D. (1984). The emergence of developmental psychopathology. *Child Development, 55,* 1–7.

Cicchetti, D. (1990). An historical perspective on the discipline of developmental psychopathology. In J. Rolf, A. S. Masten, D. Cicchetti, K. H. Nuechterlein,

& S. Weintraub (Eds.), *Risk and protective factors in the development of psychopathology* (pp. 2–28). New York: Cambridge University Press.
Cicchetti, D., & Cannon, T. D. (Eds.). (1999). Neurodevelopment and psychopathology [Special issue]. *Development and Psychopathology, 11*(3).
Cicchetti, D., Rappaport, J., Sandler, I., & Weissberg, R. P. (Eds.). (2000). *The promotion of wellness in children and adolescents.* Washington, D.C.: Child Welfare League of America Press.
Cicchetti, D., & Rogosch, F. A. (1997). The role of self-organisation in the promotion of resilience in maltreated children. *Development and Psychopathology, 9,* 797–815.
Cicchetti, D., Rogosch, F. A., Lynch, M., & Holt, K. D. (1993). Resilience in maltreated children: processes leading to adaptive outcome. *Development and Psychopathology, 5,* 629–647.
Ciechetti, D., & Schneider-Rosen, K. (1986). An organizational approach to childhood depression. In M. Ratter, C. Izard, & P. Read (Eds.), *Depression in young people: clinical and developmental perspectives* (pp. 71–134). New York: Guilford.
Cicchetti, D., & Toth, S. L. (1992). The role of developmental theory in prevention and intervention. *Development and Psychopathology, 4,* 489–493.
Coie, J. D., Watt, N. F., West, S. G., Hawkins, J. D., Asanow, J. R., Markman, H. J., Ramey, S. L., Shure, M. B., & Long, B. (1993). The science of prevention: a conceptual framework and some directions for a national research program. *American Psychologists, 48,* 1013–1022.
Compas, B. E. (1998). An agenda for coping research and theory: basic and applied developmental issues. *International Journal of Behavioral Development, 22,* 231–237.
Conduct Problems Prevention Research Group. (1992). A developmental and clinical model for the prevention of conduct disorder: the Fast Track program. *Development and Psychopathology, 4,* 509–527.
Conduct Problems Prevention Research Group. (1999). Initial impact of the Fast Track prevention trial for conduct problems: I. The high-risk sample. *Journal of Consulting and Clinical Psychology, 5,* 631–647.
Conger, R. D., Conger. K. J., & Elder, G. H. (1997). Family economic hardship and adolescent academic performance: mediating and moderating processes. In G. Duncan & J. Brooks-Gunn (Eds.), *Consequences of growing up poor* (pp. 288–310). New York: Russell Sage Foundation.
Conger, R. D., Conger, K. J., Elder, G. H., Lorenz, F. O., Simons, R. I., & Whitbeck, L. B., (1992). A family process model of economic hardship and adjustment of early adolescent boys. *Child Development 63,* 526–541.
Conrad, M., & Hammen, C. (1993). Protective and resource factors in high- and low-risk children: a comparison of children with unipolar, bipolar, medically ill, and normal mothers. *Development and Psychopathology, 5*, 593–607.
Cowen, E. L. (2000). Psychological wellness: some hopes for the future. In D. Cicchetti, J. Rappaport, I. Sandler, & R. P. Weissberg (Eds.), *The promotion of wellness in children and adolescents* (pp. 477–503). Washington, D.C.: Child Welfare League of America Press.
Cowen, E. L., Lotyczewski, B. S., & Weissberg, R. P. (1984). Risk and resource indicators and their relationships to young children's school adjustment. *American Journal of Community Psychology, 12,* 353–367.

Cowen, E. L., Wyman, P. A., Work, W. C., Kim, J. Y., Fagen, D. B., & Magnus, B. B. (1997). Follow-up study of young stress-affected and stress resistant urban children. *Development and Psychopathology, 9,* 565–577.

Cowen, E. L., Wyman, P. A., Work, W. C., & Parker, G. R. (1990). The Rochester Child Resilience Project Overview and summary of first year findings. *Development and Psychopathology, 2,* 193–212.

Dubow, E. F., Edwards, S., & Ippolito. M. F. (1997). Life stressors, neighborhood disadvantage, and resources: a focus on inner-city children's adjustment. *Journal of Clinical Child Psychology, 26,* 130–144.

Durbrow, E. H. (1999). Cultural processes in child competence: how rural Caribbean parents evaluate their children. In A. S. Masten (Ed.), *Cultural processes in child development: Vol. 29. Minnesota Symposia on Child Psychology* (pp. 97–121). Mahwah, NJ: Erlbaum.

Durbrow, E. H., Peria, L. F., Masten, A. S., Sesma, A., & Williamson, I. (in press). Mothers' conceptions of child competence in contexts of poverty: the Philippines, St. Vincent, and the United States. *International Journal of Behavioral Development.*

Egeland, B., Carlson, E., & Sroufe, L. A. (1993). Resilience as process. *Development and Psychopathology,* 5, 517–528.

Elder, G. H (1998). The life course as developmental theory. *Child Development, 69,* 1–12.

Felner, R. D., Brand, S., DuBois, D. L., Adm., A. M., Mulhall, P. F., & Evans, E.G., (1995). Socioeconomic disadvantage, proximal environmental experiences, and socioemotional and academic adjustment in early adolescence: investigation of a mediated effects model. *Child Development, 66,* 774–792.

Fergusson, D. M., & Lynskey, M. T. (1996). Adolescent resiliency to family adversity. *Journal of Child Psychology and Psychiatry, 37,* 281–292.

Ford, D. H., & Lerner, R. M. (1992). *Developmental systems theory: an integrative approach.* Newbury Park, CA: Sage.

Forgatch, M. S., & DeGarmo, D. S. (1999). Parenting through change: an effective prevention program for single mothers. *Journal of Consulting and Clinical Psychology, 67,* 711–724.

Garmezy, N. (1971). Vulnerability research and the issue of primary prevention. *American Journal of Orthopsychiatry, 41,* 101–116.

Garamezy, N. (1974). The study of competence in children at risk for severe psychopathology. In E. J. Anthony & C. Koupernik (Eds.), *The child in his family: Vol. 3. Children at psychiatric risk* (pp.77–97). New York: Wiley.

Garmezy, N. (1985). Stress-resistant children: the search for protective factors. In J. E. Stevenson (Ed.), *Recent research in developmental pathopathology* (Journal of Child Psychology and Psychiatry Book suppl. No. 4, pp. 213–233). Oxford, England: Pergamon Press.

Garmezy, N., Masten, A. S., & Tellegen, A. (1984). The study of stress and competence in children: a building block for developmental psychopathology. *Child Development, 55,* 97–111.

Gest, S. D., Neemann, J., Hubbard, J. J., Masten, A. S., & Tellegen, A. (1993). Parenting quality, adversity, and conduct problems in adolescence: testing process-oriented models of resilience. *Development and Psychopathology, 5,* 663–682.

Greenberg, M. T., Lengua, L. J., Coie, J. D., & Pinderhughes, E. E. (1999). Predicting developmental outcomes at school entry using a multiple-risk model: four American communities. *Developmental Psychology, 35,* 403–417.

Gunnar, M. R. (2001). Effects of early deprivation: findings from orphanage-reared infants and children. In C. A. Nelson & M. Luciana (Eds.), *Handbook of developmental cognitive neuroscience* (pp. 617–629). Cambridge, MA: MIT Press.

Hawkins, J. D., Catalano, R. F., Kosterman, R., Abbot, R., & Hill, K. G. (1999). Preventing adolescent health-risk behavior by strengthening protection during childhood. *Archives of Pediatrics and Adolescent Medicine, 153,* 226–234.

Hetherington, E. M., Bridges, M., & Glendessa, M. I. (1998). What matters? What does not? Five perspectives on the association between marital transitions and children's adjustment. *American Psychologist, 53,* 167–184.

Jessor, R., Van Den Bos, J., Vankerryn, J., Costa, F. M., & Turbin, M. S. (1995). Protective factors in adolescent problem behavior: moderator effects and developmental change, *Developmental Psychopathology 31,* 923–933.

Kaufman, J., Cock, A., Amy, L., Jones, B., & Pittinsky, T. (1994). Problems in defining resiliency: illustrations from the study of maltreated children. *Development and Psychopathology, 6,* 215–229.

Keating, D., & Hertzman, C. (Eds.), (1999). *Developmental health* and *the wealth of nations: social, biological and educational dynamics.* New York: Guilford Press.

Kellam, S. G., & Rebok, G. W. (1992). Building developmental and etiological theory through epidemiologically based preventive intervention trials. In J. McCord & R. E. Tremblay (Eds.), *Preventing antisocial behavior: interventions from birth through adolescence* (pp. 162–195). New York: Guilford Press.

Kochanska, G. (1993). Toward a synthesis of parental socialization and child temperament in early development of conscience. *Child Development, 64*, 325–347.

Kolvin, I., Miller, F. J. W., Fleeting, M., & Kolvin, P. A. (1988). Risk/protective factors for offending with particular reference to deprivation. In M. Rutter (Ed.), *Studies of psychosocial risk: the power of longitudinal data* (pp. 77–95). New York: Cambridge University Press.

Kraemer, H. C., Kazdin, A. E., Offord, D. R., Kesler, R C., Jensen, P. S., & Kupfer, D.J. (1997). Coming to term with the terms of risk. *Archives of General Psychiatry, 54,* 337–343.

Luthar, S. S. (1991). Vulnerability and resilience: a study of high-risk adolescents. *Child Development 62,* 600–616.

Luthar, S. S. (1999). Measurement issues in the empirical study of resilience: an overview. In M. Glanz & J. L Johnson (Eds.), *Resilience* and *development: positive life adaptations* (pp. 129–160). New York: Plenum.

Luthar, S. S., Cicchetti, D., & Becker, B. (2000). The construct of resilience: a critical evaluation and guidelines for future work. *Child Development, 71*, 543–562.

Maier, S. F., & Watkins, L. R. (1998). Cytokines for psychologists: implications of bidirectional immune-to-brain communication for understanding behavior, mood, and cognition. *Psychological Review, 105,* 83–107.

Masten, A. S. (1994). Resilience in individual development: successful adaptation despite risk and adversity. In M. Wang & E. Gordon (Eds.), *Risk and resilience* in *inner city America: challenges and prospects* (pp. 3–25). Hillsdale, NJ: Eribaum.

Masten, A. S. (1999a). The promise and perils of resilience research as a guide to preventive interventions: comments on Rolf and Johnson. In M. D. Glantz, J. Johnson, & L. Huffman (Eds.), *Resilience and development: positive life adaptations* (pp. 251–257). New York: Plenum.

Masten, A. S. (1999b). Resilience comes of age: reflections on the past and outlook for the next generation of research. In M. D. Glantz, J. Johnson, & L. Huffman (Eds.), *Resilience and development: positive life adaptations* (pp. 282–296). New York: Plenum.

Masten, A. S., Best. K. M., & Garmezy, N. (1990). Resilience and development: contributions from the study of children who overcome adversity. *Development and Psychopathology, 2,* 425–444.

Masten, A. S., & Braswell, L. (1991). Developmental psychopathology: an integrative framework. In P. R. Martin (Ed.), *Handbook of behavior therapy and psychological science: an integrative oppproach* (pp. 35–56). New York: Pergamon Press.

Masten, A. S., & Coatsworth, J. D., (1995). Competence, resilience, and psychopathology. In D. Cicchetti & D. Cohen (Eds.), *Developmental psychopathology. Vol. 2. Risk, disorder and adaptation* (pp. 715–752). New York: Wiley.

Masten, A. S., & Coatsworth, J. D. (1998). The development of competence in favorable and unfavorable environments: lessons from successful children. *American Psychologist, 53,* 205–220.

Masten, A. S., & Curtis, W. J. (2000). Integrating competence and psychopathology: pathways toward a comprehensive science of adaptation in development. *Development and Psychopathology, 12,* 529–550.

Masten, A. S., & Garmezy, N. (1985). Risk, vulnerability, and protective factors in the developmental psychopathology. In B. B. Lahey & A. E. Kazdin (Eds.), *Advances in clinical child psychology* (Vol. 8. pp. 1–51). New York: Plenum.

Masten, A. S., Garmezy, N., Tellegen, A., Pellegrimi, D. S., Larkin, K., & Larsen, A. (1988). Competence and stress in school children: the moderating effects of individual and family qualities. *Journal* of *Child Psychology and Psychiatry, 29,* 745–764.

Masten, A. S., Hubbard, J. J., Gest, S. D., Tellegen, A., Garmezy., N., & Ramirez, M. (1999). Competence in the context of adversity: pathways to resilience and maladaptation from childhood to late adolescence. *Development and Psychopathology, 11,* 143–169.

Masten, A. S., & O'Connor, M. J. (1989). Vulnerability, stress, and resilience in the early development of a high risk child. *Journal of the American Academy of Child and Adolescent Psychiatry, 28,* 274–278.

Masten, A. S., & Reed, M.G. (in press). Resilience in development. In S. R. Snyder & S. J. Lopez (Eds.), *The handbook of positive psychology.* Oxford, England: Oxford University Press.

Masten. A. S., & Wright, M. O. D. (1998). Cumulative risk and protection models of child maltreatment. In B. B. R. Rossman & M. S. Rosenberg (Eds.), *Multiple victimization of children: conceptual, developmental, research and treatment issues* (pp. 7–30). Binghamton, NY: Haworth.

McLoyd, V. C. (1998). Socioeconomic disadvantage and child development. *American Psychologist,* 53, 185–204.

Murphy, L. B. (1974). Coping, vulnerability, and resilience in childhood. In G. V. Coelho, D. A. Hamburg, & J. E. Adams (Eds.), *Coping and adaptation* (pp. 69–100). New York: Basic Books.

Murphy, L. B., & Moriarty, A. E (1976). *Vulnerability, coping, and growth: from infancy to adolescence.* New Haven, CT: Yale University Press.

Nelson, C. A. (1999). Neural plasticity and human development. *Current Directions in Psychological Science, 8,* 42–45.

Nelson, C. A. (Ed.), (2000). *The effects of adversity on neurobehavioral development: Vol. 31. Minnesota Symposia on Child Psychology.* Mahwah, NJ: Erlbaum.

Patterson, G. R., Reid, J. B., & Disbion, T. J. (1992). *A social learning approach: Vol 4. Antisocial boys.* Eugene, OR: Castaglia.

Pines, M. (1975, December). In praise of "Invulnerables." *APA Monitor,* p. 7.

Ramey, C. T., & Ramey. S. L. (1998). Early intervention and early experience. *American Psychologist, 53,* 109–120.

Richters, J. E., & Martinez, P. E. (1993). Violent communities, family choices, and children's chances: an algorithm for improving the odds. *Development and Psychopathology, 5,* 609–627.

Rutter, M. (1979). Protective factors in children's responses to stress and disadvantage. In M. W. Kent & J. E. Rolf (Eds.), *Primary prevention of psychopathology: Vol 3. Social competence in children* (pp. 49–74). Hanover, NH: University Press of New England.

Rutter, M. (1990). Psychosocial resilience and protective mechanisms. In J. Rolf, A. S. Masten, D. Cicchetti, K. H. Nucchterlein, & S. Weinttaub (Eds.), *Risk and protective factors in the development of psychopathology* (pp. 181–214). New York: Cambridge University Press.

Rutter, M., & the English and Romanian Adoptees (ERA) Study Team (1998). Developmental catch-up and deficit, following adoption after severe global early privation. *Journal of Child Psychology and Psychiatry, 39,* 465–476.

Sameroff, A. J. (1982). Development and the diaelectic: the need for a system approach. In W. A. Collins (Ed.), *The concept of development: Vol. 15. Minnesota Symposia on Child Psychology* (pp. 83–103). Hillsdale, NJ: Erlbaum.

Sameroff, A. J., Seifer, R., & Bartko, W. T. (1997). Environmental perspectives on adaptation during childhood and adolescence. In S. S. Luthar, J. A. Burack, D. Cicchetti, & J. R Weisz (Eds.), *Developmental psychopathology: perspectives on adjustment, risk and disorder* (pp. 507–526). New York: Cambridge University Press.

Scar, S., & McCartney, K. (1983). How people make their own environments: a theory of genotype-environment effects. *Child Development, 54,* 424–435.

Seifer, R., & Samerof, A. J. (1987). Multiple determinants of risk and vulnerability. In E. J. Anthony & B. J. Cohler (Eds.), *The invulnerable child* (pp. 51–69). New York: Guilford.

Seligman, M. E. P., & Csikszentmihalyi, M. (Eds.), (2000). Positive psychology [Special issue]. *American Psychologist, 55*(1).

Shiner, R., Tellegen, A., & Masten, A. S. (in press). Exploring personality across childhood into adulthood: can one describe and predict a moving target? *Psychological Inquiry.*

Snyder, S. R., & Lopez, S. J. (Eds.), (in press). *The handbook of positive psychology.* Oxford, England: Oxford University Press.

Sroufe, L. A. (1979). The coherence of individual development: early care, attachment, and subsequent developmental issues. *American Pschychologist, 34,* 834–841.

Sroufe, L. A. (1997). Psychopathology as an outcome of development. *Development and Psychopathology, 9,* 251–268.

Sroufe, L. A., & Rutter, M. (1984). The domain of developmental psychopathology. *Child Development, 55,* 17–29.

Stouthamer-Loeber, M., Loeber, R., Farrington, D. P., Zhang, Q., van Kammen, W., & Maguin, E. (1993). The double edge of protective and risk factors for delinquency: interrelations and developmental patterns. *Development and Psychopathology, 5,* 683–701.

Tiet, Q. Q., Bird, H. R., Davies, M., Haven, C., Cohen, P., Jense, P. S., & Goodman, S. (1998). Adverse life events and resilience. *Journal of the American Academy of Child and Adolescent Psychiatry, 37,* 1191–1200.

Waters, E. & Sroufe, L. A. (1983). Social competence as a developmental construct. *Developmental Review, 3,* 79–97.

Werner, E. E., & Smith, R. S. (1982). *Vulnerable but invisible: a study of resilient children.* New York: McGraw-Hill.

Werner, E. E., & Smith, R. S. (1992). *Overcoming the odds: high risk children from birth to adulthood.* Ithaca, NY: Cornell University Press.

White, J. L., Moffitt, T. E., & Silva, P. A. (1989). A prospective replication of the protective effects of IQ in subjects at high risk for juvenile delinquency. *Journal of Consulting and Clinical Psychology, 57,* 719–724.

Wright, M O'D., Masten, A. S., Northwood, A., & Hubbard, J. J. (1997). Long-term effects of massive trauma: developmental and psychobiological perspectives. In D. Cicchetti & S. L. Toth (Eds.), *Rochester Symposium on Developmental Psychopathology: Vol. 8. The effect of trauma on the developmental process* (pp. 181–225). Rochester, NY: University of Rochester Press.

Wyman, P. A., Cowes, E. L., Work, W. C., Hoyt-Meyers, L., Magnus, K. B., & Fagen, D. B. (1999). Caregiving and developmental factors differentiating young at-risk urban children showing resilient versus stress-affected outcomes: a replication and extension. *Child Development. 70,* 645–659.

Wyman, P. A., Sandler, I., Wolchik, S., & Nelson, K. (2000). Resilience as cumulative competence promotion and stress protection: theory and intervention. In D. Cicchetti, J. Rappaport, I. Sandler, & R. P. Weissberg (Eds.), *The promotion of wellness* in *children and adolescents* (pp. 133–184), Washington, D.C.: Child Welfare League of America Press.

Zigler, E., Taussig, C., & Black, K. (1992). A promising preventive for juvenile delinquency. *American Psychologist, 47,* 997–1006.

Part II

BIOLOGY AND BEHAVIOR

6

Behavioral Phenotypes of Genetic Syndromes: A Reference Guide for Psychiatrists

Maria Moldavsky, Dorit Lev, and Tally Lerman-Sagie

Objective: *To review the literature on behavioral phenotypes of genetic syndromes, displaying the data as a reference guide for everyday practice.* ***Method:*** *A computerized search was performed for articles published in the past 10 years, and selected papers were surveyed.* ***Results:*** *The behavioral phenotypes of 11 major genetic syndromes were reviewed including the following topics: genetic etiology, genetic counseling, physical features, medical problems, cognitive and behavioral profile, and psychopathology. The speculated correlation between the identified gene and the pathophysiology of the cognitive and behavioral features is discussed.* ***Conclusions:*** *Updated knowledge of behavioral phenotypes will help psychiatrists identify these conditions, refer the patient and his/her family for genetic diagnosis and counseling, make specific treatment recommendations, and contribute to research and syndrome delineation.*

Recently, geneticists have started recognizing not only physical phenotypes and dysmorphology, but also behavioral patterns specific to genetic syndromes. The Society for the Study of Behavioral Phenotypes and a monthly journal, the *American Journal of Medical Genetics (Neuropsychiatric Genetics),* have been instituted.

A behavioral phenotype is defined (Flint, 1998; Flint and Yule, 1994) as the specific and characteristic behavior repertoire exhibited by patients with a genetic or chromosomal disorder. It includes a wide range of developmental and behavioral characteristics including cognitive, language, and social aspects as well as behavioral problems and psychopathology (Finegan, 1998). These patterns of behavior must be consistently associated with the condition (Flint and Yule, 1994) inasmuch as a causal relationship is implied between the genetic lesion and the behavior. It has been proposed, however, that the concept of variability of expression—meaning that individuals with the same syndrome will not express the same abnormality to the same extent (Jones, 1997)—may be applied in the behavioral field as it is widely applied in dysmorphology (Finegan, 1998).

Updated knowledge of behavioral phenotypes is important for every child and adolescent psychiatrist. Some patients will be referred because of their behavioral problems, and the psychiatrist's ability to identify the presenting symptoms as part of a behavioral phenotype will allow referral to a geneticist and an accurate genetic diagnosis. The diagnosis of a genetic syndrome has important implications for parental counseling regarding prognosis and risk in future pregnancies. It will also allow early intervention and specific treatment recommendations

This review describes some well-known behavioral phenotypes and may be used as a reference in everyday practice. Table 6.1 summarizes the cognitive features of genetic syndromes, and Table 6.2 lists their characteristic mental disorders.

DOWN SYNDROME

The frequency of trisomy 21 in the population is 1 in 650 to 1,000 live births (Ensing et al., 1995). Most individuals (95%) with trisomy 21 have three free copies of chromosome 21. In about 5% of patients, one copy is translocated to another acrocentric chromosome. In 2% to 4% of cases with trisomy 21, there is a recognizable mosaicism for a trisomic and a normal cell line.

The risk of having a child with trisomy 21 increases with maternal age. If a parent is a carrier for a structural chromosomal translocation, the recurrence risk is higher.

The syndrome is usually diagnosed at birth because the dysmorphism is distinctive: slanted eyes, epicanthal folds, flat nose. A variety of medical problems may be present: hearing impairment in 60% to 80% of patients, visual problems, short stature, muscular hypotonia, and delayed bone maturation.

The highest development scores are recorded during the infancy years, with progressive slowing as the child gets older (Dykens et al., 1994a). Patients with Down syndrome suffer from moderate to severe mental retardation. A developmental language delay is always present, and usually expressive functions are more affected than receptive ones (Miller et al., 1995). Grammatical abilities are most impaired but the pragmatics of language are good (Fowler, 1990), and in most cases these patients are able to engage in a conversation (Dykens et al., 1994a). Visual processing is usually better than auditory (Pueschel et al., 1987).

Children with Down syndrome have been described as placid and good-tempered (State et al., 1997), but hyperactivity, aggression, and impulsivity

TABLE 6.1
Cognitive Features of Genetic Syndromes

Syndrome/Prevalence	Genetic Locus	Intelligence	Language Rec	Language Exp	Visuospatial Abilities	Memory	Cognitive Strengths	LD
Down 1:650–1,000	Trisomy 21	MR: Mo-Se	↓	↓↓	=	↓ with age	Pragmatics of language	+
Fragile X (M) 1:4,000	X-linked, *FMRI* gene	MR: Mi-Se	↓	↓↓	↓	ST ↓ LT =		+
Fragile X (F)	X-linked, *FMRI* gene	Bord/MR:Mi, in 50%	=	=	=	=		+
Rett 1:10,000-15,000	X-linked, *MECP2* gene	MR: Se	↓↓	↓↓	↓↓	↓↓		+
Prader-Willi 1:16,000–25,000	15q11–13 (paternal)	Bord/MR: Mi	=	=	↑	ST ↓ LT =	Jigsaw puzzles, reading abilities	+M
Angelman 0.08:1,000	15q11–13 (maternal)	MR: Se	↓	None	↓↓	↓↓		+
Isodicentric Chromosome 15	15q duplication	MR	↓	↓	↓	?		+
Williams 1:10,000	17q11.23	Board/MR: Mi-Mo	↓	↑	↓↓	=	Language skills	+
VCF 1:5,000	22q11.2	N/MR: Mi	=	=	=	=	Language skills	+M
Smith-Magenis 1:25,000	17q11.2	MR: Mo	=	↓	↓	LT =	Visual learning	+M
Brunner	*MAOA* gene	Board/MR: Mi	?	?	?	?	?	?
Turner 1:2,500 females	45X	Usually N	=	=	↓	=	Language skills	+M

Note: Rec = receptive; Exp = expressive; LD = learning disabilities; MR = mental retardation; Mi, Mo, Se = mild, moderate, severe; Bord = border line; N = normal; ST, LT = short term, long term; VCF = velocardiofacial; (M) = male; (F) = female ↑ = well-developed ability; (=) = spared, according to intelligence level; ↓ = impaired; ↓↓ = very impaired; + = present; +M = mathematics learning disorder present;? = no information.

TABLE 6.2
Psychopathology in Genetic Syndromes

Syndrome	Anxiety	Depression	Hyperactivity	Aggression	Autistic Features	Psychosis	Additional Behavioral Features
Down	–	In adulthood	+	+	Rarely	Rarely	Placid or subborn
Fragile X(M)	++	–	++	–	++	–	Hypersensitivity to stimuli
Fragile X(F)	++	–	+	–	–	–	Avoidant behavior
Rett	–	–	–	–	+ (mainly in infancy)	–	Loss of purposeful hand movements, stereotypic midline hand movements, eye-pointing
Prader-Willi	+OCD	+	+	+	+	+	Lack of satiety, foraging for food, skin-picking
Angelman	–	–	+	–	+	–	Frequent smiling, outbursts of laughter
Isodicentric chromosome 15	–	–	–	–	++	–	
Williams	+	In adulthood	+	+	+	–	Overfamiliar
VCF	+	+	+	–	–	++	High prevalence of schizophrenia and BSD
Smith-Margenis	–	–	+	+	–	–	Self-injury, self-hug
Brunner	+	–	+	++ (episodic impulsive)	–	–	Sexually aberrant behavior, arson, stereotyped hand movements
Turner	+	+	+	Rarely	Rarely	–	Immature personality, social and self-esteem problems

Note: BSD = bipolar spectrum disorders; (M) = male; (F) = female; OCD = obsessive-compulsive disorder; VCF = velocardiofacial; + = present; ++ = marked; – = not characteristic.

may also be present (Cuskelly and Dadds, 1992). Autistic features are rare but have been described (Ghaziuddin et al., 1992). Early-onset Alzheimer disease is present in a high percentage of persons with Down syndrome (Janicki and Dalton, 2000), but neuropathological changes are more frequent than behavioral manifestations of the disease (Devenny et al., 1996).

FRAGILE X SYNDROME (FRAXA)

Fragile X syndrome is the most common form of inherited mental retardation and must be considered in the differential diagnosis of any child with developmental delay, mental retardation, or learning disability (de Vries et al., 1998). Its prevalence is 1 in 4,000 males. Five folate-sensitive fragile sites have been characterized at the molecular level; three of them (FRAXA, FRAXE, and FRA11B) are associated with clinical problems, and some of the genes (*FMR1* in FRAXA, *FMR2* and *CBL2* in FRAXE) have been identified (Gecz et al., 1996). Fragile X syndrome is caused by a trinucleotide repeat expansion. Affected subjects have expanded CGG repeats (>200) in the first exon of the *FMR1* gene (the full mutation). The pathogenesis of this syndrome is a consequence of absence of the protein product of the *FMR1* gene (FMRP) (Verheij et al., 1993). The premutation in normal carriers expands to a full mutation only when it is transmitted by a female. Females who carry the *FMR1* premutation and full gene mutation may present with learning, cognitive, and/or emotional difficulties, and family members of individuals with fragile X syndrome have ongoing needs and concerns (Staley-Gane et al., 1996).

Prenatal diagnosis of fragile X syndrome using molecular genetic techniques is now a well-established procedure, with the only significant problem being the inability to accurately predict phenotype in female fetuses with full mutations.

Male fragile X patients present with hyperextensible finger joints, double-jointed thumbs, flat feet, arched palate, and velvet-like skin. In adolescence the typical dysmorphism appears: long face, prominent ears, prominent jaw, and macro-orchidism (Hagerman, 1996b). Medical history may include seizures, recurrent infections, hernias, strabismus, and scoliosis (Hagerman, 1996b). Male fragile X patients suffer from sleeping disturbances in the first years of life (Hagerman, 1996a). Family history reveals maternal male relatives with mental retardation or learning disabilities and emotional problems. A history of depression in the mother is frequent (Reiss et al., 1993).

Children with fragile X syndrome suffer from mental retardation in the mild to severe range (Frangiskakis et al., 1991; Merenstein et al., 1996). They have difficulty with abstract thinking, sequential processing, mathematics, short-term memory, and visual-motor coordination (Dykens et al., 1994b). Their language skills increase until they reach an age equivalence of approximately 48 months and then reach a plateau. Fast speech with tangentiality and perseverations is frequently observed. A significant IQ decline is seen in approximately one third of patients in middle to late childhood (Hodapp et al., 1990; Wright-Talamante et al., 1996). This decline is usually not because of regression but a peak in the rate of development relative to chronological age.

Male fragile X patients are hypersensitive to touch, auditory stimuli, and visual stimuli, which is related to their difficulty in establishing eye contact (they turn their head away, cover their eyes with their arm, tightly close their eyes) (Hagerman, 1996b). Hyperactivity, distractibility, and mood lability are very frequent, and 70% of the patients fulfill criteria for attention-deficit/hyperactivity disorder (Hagerman, 1996a).

Some patients show disinterest in social interaction, whereas others present a pattern of approach and withdrawal (Cohen et al., 1989). Stereotypic movements may occur if the patient is overstimulated with excitement or anger (Hagerman, 1996b). Approximately 15% of fragile X syndrome patients fulfill criteria for autism (Reiss and Freund, 1991), and other patients may present with autistic features or schizotypal personality disorder (Kerby and Dawson, 1994). Anxiety disorders are more frequent in fragile X syndrome than in other causes of mental retardation (Baumgardner et al., 1995).

In females with the full mutation, 50% have cognitive deficits with learning disabilities, borderline IQ, or mental retardation, and 50% have normal intellectual functioning (Hagerman et al., 1992). Several studies suggested the presence of molecular-cognitive associations in fragile X females: Abrams and colleagues (1994) found that as activation ratio (the ratio of active normal X chromosome to total normal X chromosome) increased, overall IQ and specific subtest scores increased. Conversely, as mutation amplification size increased, those cognitive measures decreased. Kolehmainen and Karant (1994) documented an approximately linear decrease in mean IQ score as a function of the fraction of cells with the mutation carried on the active X chromosome.

Female fragile X patients show a characteristic behavioral pattern of shyness, poor eye contact, anxiety, social isolation, and odd communication patterns. They may fulfill criteria of social phobia (Hagerman, 1996b) or avoidant personality disorder (Freund et al., 1993). Several cases of selective mutism have been reported (Hagerman et al., 1999). Inattention and distractibility are frequent, and hyperactivity is present in 35% of patients (Hagerman et al., 1992).

A related syndrome due to trinucleotide expansion has been described in association with another folate-sensitive fragile site (FRAXE), causing X-linked mild mental retardation in males (Gecz et al., 1996).

RETT SYNDROME

Rett syndrome is a progressive X-linked dominant encephalopathy which affects almost exclusively females. Its prevalence is estimated at 1 in 10,000 to 15,000 female births (Hagberg et al., 1983). More than 95% of cases are sporadic, but there are rare reports of familial recurrence. Recently, Zoghbi and colleagues (Amir et al., 1999) identified mutations in the *MECP2* gene encoding an X-linked methyl-CpG-binding protein 2 in 50% of cases of Rett syndrome. *MECP2* is thought to mediate transcriptional silencing in the nucleus.

The main features of Rett disorder were summarized by the Rett Syndrome Diagnostic Criteria Work Group (1988) and in the *DSM-IV* (American Psychiatric Association, 1994). The clinical picture is characterized by a progressive course with identifiable stages.

Early development is normal, including a normal head circumference at birth. Between 5 and 48 months of age, deceleration of head growth appears. Loss of previously acquired purposeful hand movements is seen between 6 and 30 months and is temporally associated with communication dysfunction and social withdrawal. The presence of autistic features at this stage of development motivates the inclusion of Rett disorder in the *DSM-IV* category of the pervasive developmental disorders. There are stereotypic midline hand movements, such as hand-wringing, hand-washing, clapping, tapping, and mouthing, with an onset at or after the time when purposeful hand movements are lost. Gait apraxia and truncal apraxia/ataxia appear between 1 and 4 years of age. Severe impairment in the development of expressive and receptive language and severe psychomotor retardation are found. By school age the autistic features are less prominent and development reaches a plateau for some time. Most children remain ambulatory until a final period of motor deterioration.

Because the ability to manipulate objects is lost, gaze is the most important way of interaction with the surroundings. These patients often remain visually attentive to objects and people and show preferences by means of eye-pointing (von Tetzchner et al., 1996).

Additional clinical findings are as follows: EEG abnormalities and seizures, breath-holding spells, periodic hyperventilation, periodic apnea, growth retardation, dystonia, spasticity, scoliosis, and peripheral vasomotor problems.

PRADER-WILLI SYNDROME

The frequency of Prader-Willi syndrome (PWS) is approximately 1 in 16,000 to 25,000, and it is the most common syndromal cause of human obesity. The genetic basis of PWS involves imprinted genes on the proximal long arm of chromosome 15. The basic defect appears to be the absence of function of genes that are normally expressed in a monoallelic fashion only from the paternal chromosome. In 60% to 70% of patients with PWS, the genetic defect is a microdeletion in the area of 15q11-13 on the paternal chromosome. An additional 25% to 30% of patients with PWS do not have paternal deletions, the defect being due to uniparental disomy for maternal chromosome 15 (the presence of two maternally contributed chromosomes 15 and the absence of a paternally contributed chromosome 15). The *SNRPN* (small nuclear ribonucleoprotein-associated polypeptide N) gene has a critical role in the 15q11-13 region, as it is probably part of the putative imprinting center that regulates the expression of several genes in the PWS transcriptional domain. Diagnostic identification by a combination of methods—fluorescence in situ hybridization (FISH) and/or methylation patterns—has become available in recent years, permitting early detection and institution of appropriate management (Cassidy, 1997). PWS usually occurs sporadically. There are only a few reports of familial recurrence.

Hypothalamic dysfunction is presumed to be involved in the pathophysiology of PWS (Swaab, 1997).

The physical phenotype includes a narrow bitemporal diameter, almond-shaped palpebral fissures, and a down-turned mouth with thin upper lip. Additional features are hypopigmentation, short stature, obesity, strabismus, scoliosis, lack of a pubertal growth spurt, and hypogonadism. Personal history is remarkable for prenatal onset of hypotonia with decreased fetal movements. In the neonatal period, the infant with PWS presents with decreased arousal, weak cry, and poor reflexes including a poor suck, which causes feeding problems and often results in failure to thrive. Young children may be placid and show excessive daytime somnolence with or without sleep apnea and depressed motor activity (Dykens and Cassidy, 1996). Older children are stubborn, irritable, impulsive, and aggressive. They present with mood lability and low self-esteem (Dykens and Cassidy, 1995). They may be distractible, but only approximately 5% to 7% of patients meet the criteria for attention-deficit/hyperactivity disorder.

Lack of satiety causing hyperphagia and obesity begins between 1 and 6 years of age. The onset of hyperphagia is often associated with the worsening of behavioral problems (temper tantrums, impulsivity, and aggression). Food-seeking behavior includes hoarding or foraging for food, pica, and stealing food or money to buy food. Obesity complications are frequent, including hypertension, type II diabetes mellitus, and sleep apnea (Dykens and Cassidy, 1996).

Obsessions (preoccupation with food and non-food-related obsessions), compulsions, and repetitive behavior (skin-picking) are characteristic of these patients (Akefeldt and Gillberg, 1999; Dykens and Cassidy, 1995; State et al., 1999). Half of them fulfill the diagnostic criteria for obsessive-compulsive disorder. Depression and anxiety are frequently reported. Psychosis may be associated (Clarke, 1998; Clarke et al., 1998). Some children with PWS present with autistic features (Demb and Papola, 1995).

The average IQ reported in most studies is approximately 70 (Dykens et al., 1992). Mild to moderate mental retardation or borderline intellectual functioning may be found. Adaptively, patients with PWS usually function at a lower level because of the interference of behavioral issues (Dykens and Cassidy, 1996). There is no evidence of IQ decline over time (Dykens et al., 1992).

A remarkable area of cognitive strength in patients with PWS is their visual-spatial integration: they may show unusual skill with jigsaw puzzles (Dykens et al., 1992). They also show good reading decoding and comprehension skills, good long-term memory (Dykens and Cassidy, 1996), and a good expressive vocabulary, but their voice and speech may be peculiar (Akefeldt and Gillberg, 1999). Poor short-term visual and motor memory and arithmetic skills have been found in these patients (Dykens and Cassidy, 1996).

According to Dykens and colleagues (1999), maladaptive behavior ratings are higher in PWS because of paternal deletion than in maternal uniparental disomy, even controlling for the higher IQs of the uniparental disomy group. Another study (Cassidy et al., 1997) compared the phenotype of PWS patients caused by these two different mechanisms and found increased maternal age in the uniparental disomy group. In addition, patients in this group were less likely to have a typical face appearance and to show some of the minor manifestations such as skin-picking, skill with jigsaw puzzles, and high pain threshold.

ANGELMAN SYNDROME

Angelman syndrome results from a lack of maternal contribution from chromosome 15q11-q13, arising from de novo deletion in most cases or from uniparental disomy in rare cases. Rare cases are caused by imprinting mutations. Twenty-five percent of Angelman syndrome cases result from mutations in the *UBE3A* (A ubiquitin-protein ligase) (E6-AP) gene, the product of which functions in protein ubiquitination and may be familial (Kishino et al., 1997). Although Angelman syndrome has an estimated population prevalence of 0.008%, in a recent article at least 1.4% of the moderately to profoundly mentally retarded subjects screened were found to have this syndrome (Jacobsen et al., 1998). The true incidence of Angelman syndrome, especially in adults with severe developmental disabilities, may be underestimated.

Angelman patients present with an unusual facies characterized by a large mandible and open-mouthed expression revealing the tongue. Medical history includes seizures, ataxia with jerky arm movements, and hypotonia. Severe mental retardation is present, and language is severely impaired or absent (Bower and Jeavons, 1967).

A characteristic behavioral pattern is described in these patients: they are cheerful and smiling (Clayton-Smith, 1993) (the syndrome was called happy puppet syndrome). Paroxysmal and excessive laughter may be present (Summers et al., 1995). Nonetheless, noncompliance, hyperactivity, aggression, and temper tantrums have also been found (Summers et al., 1995). Autistic features may be present in these patients (Clayton-Smith, 1993), and they may fulfill the criteria for the diagnosis of autistic disorder (Steffenburg et al., 1996). Repetitive and stereotyped behavior including mouthing of objects is frequent (Summers et al., 1995).

ISODICENTRIC CHROMOSOME 15

The most frequently reported cytogenetic finding in individuals with autistic disorder is maternally derived, de novo, proximal 15q-chromosome anomalies. In two recent reports (Rineer et al., 1998; Wolpert et al., 2000), individuals with autistic disorder and isodicentric 15q anomalies were assessed. Hypotonia, seizures, and speech delay were frequent in these patients. Several candidate genes for an autistic disorder genetic risk factor are being analyzed within this chromosomal region.

WILLIAMS SYNDROME

The frequency of Williams syndrome (WS) is approximately 1 in 10,000. It results from a deletion of 7q11.23 in 90% to 95% of all clinically typical cases. The submicroscopic deletion is detected by FISH. Loss of the LIM-kinase 1 gene may be responsible for the impaired visuospatial constructive cognition characteristic of the syndrome (Frangiskakis et al., 1996). Most cases of WS are sporadic, and the recurrence rate is very low.

Children with WS present with an elfin-like face: stellate irides, epicanthal folds, flat nasal bridge, short up-turned nose with anteverted nostrils, long philtrum, full lips, macrostomia, full lower cheeks, and small, delicate chin (Burn, 1986). Over time, some coarsening of facial features appears (Pober and Dykens, 1996). The dysmorphism may be minor and shows extreme variability.

Medical history includes supravalvular aortic stenosis, other discrete or diffuse arterial stenoses, hypertension, and dental abnormalities (Pober and Dykens, 1996). Growth retardation, hypercalcemia, and hypotonia are frequently found.

Children with WS are typically loquacious and over-friendly and may be willing to follow strangers (Gosch and Pankau, 1997). Some children with WS show autistic-type behavior up to about age 5 years, and a few of them fulfill criteria for autistic disorder (Udwin, 1990). Restlessness, hyperactivity, distractibility, and attention-seeking behavior are present in these children. Hypersensitivity to sounds may also be found (Klein et al., 1990). They are frequently anxious, may obsessively worry about future events, and express somatic concerns (Einfeld et al., 1997; Pober and Dykens, 1996). Adolescents and adults with WS are less over-friendly and may have depressive symptoms (Gosch and Pankau, 1997). The personality profile is so distinct that occasionally the syndrome diagnosis may be ascertained on the basis of the behavioral rather than the physical phenotype.

Mental retardation in the mild-moderate range or low-average intelligence is present (Greer et al., 1997; Pober and Dykens, 1996). Patients with WS make little progress in their educational skills beyond the early teenage years. There is no evidence of cognitive decline over time (Bellugi et al., 1999; Udwin et al., 1996). As adults, they achieve some autonomy (Plissart et al., 1994), but few individuals with WS are able to cope with the demands of employment (Davies et al., 1997). Intelligence tests demonstrate a higher Verbal than Performance IQ (Plissart et al., 1994). Although they may show delay in the earliest stages of language development, once language is acquired it becomes a relative strength in the cognitive profile (Bellugi et al., 1999; Mervis and Klein-Tasman, 2000). Patients with WS tend to use stereotypic adult social phrases (cocktail party talk). Short-term auditory memory for speech sounds is far better than spatial memory, and an increased linguistic affectivity (abundance of prosody and lexical devices used to convey affect) has been described (Bellugi et al., 1999).

The ability to understand complex mental states in other persons (mentalizing ability) (Tager-Flusberg et al., 1998) and face-processing (recognition, classification, memory) are a strength in these individuals (Bellugi et al., 1999). They also display good musical abilities (Lenhoff et al., 1997).

A main area of cognitive weakness is visual-motor integration (Birhle et al., 1989). Lack of cohesion or global organization is typical in the drawings of individuals with WS. Learning disability in all areas is very frequent (Lenhoff et al., 1997).

VELOCARDIOFACIAL SYNDROME

The velocardiofacial syndrome (VCFS) has an estimated prevalence of 1 in 5,000. The majority of cases have a microdeletion of chromosome 22q11.2 (Pike and Super, 1997). It is considered a contiguous gene syndrome. The 22q deletion that causes VCFS is inherited as an autosomal dominant trait, but most cases it occurs sporadically. The diagnosis is made by FISH.

The typical dysmorphism in children with VCFS includes a long face, narrow palpebral fissures, a prominent tubular nose with a bulbous nasal tip, a small open mouth and retrognathia, short stature, and slender hands and digits (Shprintzen et al., 1981).

Medical history is remarkable for cleft palate and velopharyngeal insufficiency (causing feeding difficulties), hypocalcemia, and immunodeficiency (Wang et al., 2000). Cardiac malformations are present: mainly ventricular septal defect or tetralogy of Fallot (Shprintzen et al., 1981; Vantrappen et al., 1999). Hypotonia is present in half of the patients (Wang et al., 2000).

Although language and motor developmental delay and persistent coordination deficits are common (Usiskin et al., 1999; Vantrappen et al., 1999), intelligence is usually in the normal range. Mild mental retardation is less frequent. Verbal IQ is usually higher than Performance IQ (Wang et al., 2000). Learning disabilities in some or all areas (Shprintzen et al., 1981; Vantrappen et al., 1999) are found. The most frequent profile includes poor arithmetic skills but better reading and spelling achievement (Wang et al., 2000). The relative strength in language abilities contrasts with the delay in early language development found in these children. Speech disorder due to the cleft palate is frequent (Shprintzen et al., 1981; Wang et al., 2000). Difficulty with abstract thinking (Shprintzen et al., 1981) and distractibility (Usiskin et al., 1999) may be found.

Children with VCFS are usually withdrawn and have poor social interaction skills (Heineman-de Boer et al., 1999). They show minimal spontaneous facial expression and speak with a nasal, monotonous voice (Usiskin et al., 1999). Blunt or inappropriate affect may be present (Golding-Kushner et al., 1985).

A most remarkable feature in this syndrome is the high frequency of psychiatric illness. Some studies (Papolos et al., 1996) found that VCFS patients suffer mainly from bipolar spectrum disorders including cyclothymia, dysthymia, major depression, and schizoaffective disorder. Other investigators reported paranoid schizophrenia in 30% of VCFS adult patients (Wang et al., 2000). A chronic and disabling course is described in these patients, with poor response to classic neuroleptic drugs and electroconvulsive therapy (Gothelf et al., 1999). Mental illness may have an early age of onset (late childhood or early adolescence) or the usual one (Shprintzen et al., 1992). Psychotic illnesses may be present among relatives (Pulver et al., 1994).

SMITH-MAGENIS SYNDROME

Smith-Magenis syndrome is a multiple congenital anomaly and mental retardation syndrome caused by an interstitial deletion of chromosome 17p11.2 detected by FISH. Its prevalence is estimated as 1 in 25,000. It is probably underdiagnosed because the facial abnormalities are mild and the behavioral problems are dominant, leading to the diagnosis of psychiatric pathology. Smith-Magenis syndrome is considered a contiguous gene syndrome. Genes have been mapped and isolated to the critical region, but their participation in the pathogenesis of the syndrome remains unclear (Elsea et al., 1998). The syndrome occurs sporadically, and the recurrence risk is very low.

The facial dysmorphism in children with Smith-Magenis syndrome includes midface hypoplasia, prominent forehead, up-slanting palpebral fissures, epicanthal folds, broad nasal bridge, and relative prognathism (Greenberg et al., 1991). The shape of the mouth is most characteristic:

a fleshy upper lip with tented appearance. Diagnosis is often difficult in the neonate and infant because the dysmorphism is subtle (Smith et al., 1998). Additional physical and medical features are cardiac defects and renal abnormalities, short stature or failure to thrive, hypotonia, ocular abnormalities (high myopia), a hoarse voice, and hearing loss (Greenberg et al., 1991).

Infants with Smith-Magenis syndrome are sociable and are frequently described as a perfect baby who never cries (Smith et al., 1998). With increasing age, sleep disturbance appears and REM sleep may be reduced or absent (Greenberg et al., 1996; Smith et al., 1998). Children with Smith-Magenis syndrome establish good eye contact, are eager to please, and often have a sense of humor. They constantly seek adult attention (Smith et al., 1998).

Behavior problems include hyperactivity, impulsivity, temper tantrums (mainly in response to changes in routine), and aggression. Self-mutilatory behavior is present in 70% of patients and includes wrist-biting, head-banging, pulling out fingernails and toenails (onychotillomania), and the insertion of foreign bodies in their ears or other body orifices (polyembolokoilamania) (Greenberg et al., 1991; Smith et al., 1998). In some cases, parents have been reported to social services for suspicion of child abuse (Smith et al., 1998).

An additional salient feature is the spasmodic upper-body squeeze or self-hug, which is probably unique to this syndrome. Two types are described: (1) self-hugging and spasmodically tensing the upper body and (2) hand-clasping at chest level or under the chin while squeezing their arms tightly against their chests and sides. These movements appear as an expression of happiness or excitement and they are involuntary, with a tic-like quality (Finucane et al., 1994). People with Smith-Magenis syndrome also hug others (Smith et al., 1998).

Mental retardation—most frequently in the moderate range, but sometimes mild or borderline—is found in individuals with Smith-Magenis syndrome (Greenberg et al., 1996). Speech and language delay is present in most cases. Receptive language skills are generally better than expressive language (Greenberg et al., 1991; Smith et al., 1998). Distractibility is characteristic. The learning abilities are characterized by strength in visual reasoning tasks (they tend to be visual learners) and weakness in sequential processing (counting, mathematical, and multistep tasks). Short-term memory is poor, but long-term memory is a relative strength (Dykens et al., 1997).

BRUNNER SYNDROME

This syndrome is associated with a complete and selective deficiency of enzymatic activity of monoamine oxidase A (MAO-A). Brunner and colleagues (1993a,b) described males with an MAO-A deficiency state resulting from a premature stop codon in the coding region of the *MAOA* gene. This enzyme deficiency is associated with increased levels of MAO-A substrates and reduced amounts of the MAO-A products. In each of five affected males, a point mutation was identified in the eighth exon of the *MAOA* structural gene, which changes a glutamine to a termination codon.

These individuals have no specific dysmorphic signs or congenital abnormalities (Brunner et al., 1993b). Mild mental retardation or borderline intellectual functioning is present (Brunner et al., 1993b). Affected males are described as withdrawn and shy. They show repeated episodes of aggressive or violent behavior (fights, attempted homicide, arson) that tend to cluster in periods of 1 to 3 days, during which the affected male sleeps very little and experiences frequent night terrors (Brunner et al., 1993b). Sexually aberrant behavior may be present, including exhibitionism, voyeurism, grasping or holding of female relatives, and attempted rape. Stereotyped hand movements such as hand-wringing, plucking, or fiddling have been described (Brunner et al., 1993b).

Studies of child psychiatric symptoms consistent with Brunner syndrome have not identified any new cases beyond the described family, thus indicating that MAO-A deficiency states are uncommon (Schuback et al., 1999).

TURNER SYNDROME

The most frequent karyotype in Turner syndrome (TS) is 45,X complete monosomy. Mosaic individuals may be 45,X/46,XX. In addition, structural abnormalities of the X chromosome (for example, a ring chromosome) may produce partial monosomy. TS occurs sporadically.

Considerable phenotypic variation has been described among affected persons. The full phenotype consists of short stature, webbing of the neck, low hairline on the back of the neck, cubitus valgus, a broad chest with broad-spaced nipples, coarctation of the aorta, gonadal dysgenesis, renal anomalies, and hemangiomas. There is decreased ovarian estrogen production, which results in absent breast development, amenorrhea, and infertility (Hall and Gilchrist, 1990).

Intelligence is usually normal (Siegel et al., 1998). Mental retardation is found in only 5% of girls with a classic TS karyotype and in 30% of those with rare TS karyotype anomalies (Swillen et al., 1993). The Performance IQ is typically lower than the Verbal IQ, because of the relative weakness of visuospatial subtests. Poor visual-motor skills have also been demonstrated. Verbal and language abilities are normal (Ross et al., 1995; Swillen et al., 1993). Learning disabilities, mainly difficulty in mathematics, are typical (Siegel et al., 1998). The ability to discriminate facial affect (McCauley et al., 1987) and prosody affect (Ross et al., 1995) were identified as additional areas of cognitive weakness, which may underlie the social relationship problems found in these girls as a result of their difficulty in processing affective cues in social situations. The clinical picture may be described as a nonverbal learning disability which is related to a right hemisphere dysfunction (Ross et al. 1995; Siegel et al., 1998). Additional areas of difficulty are attention, short-term memory (Siegel et al., 1998), and executive function including verbal fluency, planning skills, and flexibility (Rovet, 1994).

Emotional disturbance and social adjustment problems are found in girls with TS. McCauley and colleagues (1994) described changes in the behavioral profile according to age. Younger girls are more immature, hyperactive, and anxious while older ones report anxiety, depression, and unsatisfactory social relationships. Around the age of normal puberty, a tendency to hypoactivity is described (Swillen et al., 1993). Severe psychopathology is infrequent in girls with TS (Siegel et al., 1998).

A correlation has been found between structural abnormalities of the X chromosome and the severity of behavior problems (Rovet and Ireland, 1994). The behavioral phenotype of TS patients with a ring X chromosome has been studied by El-Abd et al. (1999) and includes mental retardation, autistic features, attentional problems, impulsiveness, aggression toward self and others, and obsessive-compulsive symptoms.

A study on phenotypic variability as a result of systematic differences in the parental origin of the single X chromosome in TS (Skuse et al., 1999) showed that quality of life of patients with a maternal X chromosome is poorer than that of girls with a paternal one.

Girls with TS have a feminine gender identity. There is no evidence that they have less feminine attitudes than their normal age-matched peers (El-Abd et al., 1995), although less independence from parents and less frequency of living with a partner and marrying has been described (Nielsen et al., 1977).

DISCUSSION

Technological advances arising from the Human Genome Project have stimulated renewed interest in research focused on the behavioral phenotypes of genetic syndromes. The hope is that further description of such phenotypes will enable identification of genes important for human cognitive and behavioral disorders. At present, the correlation between the identified gene and the pathophysiology of the behavioral phenotype is speculated in only a few syndromes.

The poor visual-spatial constructive ability in WS may be related to a deletion in the LIM-kinase 1 gene which encodes for a novel protein kinase which is strongly expressed in the brain (Frangiskakis et al., 1996). However, the common WS deletion region has not been completely characterized, and genes for additional features, including mental retardation and the unique personality profile, are yet to be discovered (Meng et al., 1998).

The description of syndromes due to genes involved in the metabolism of neurotransmitters or their receptors enables an understanding of the effect of these substances on specific behavior. An example is the discovery of a deficiency of MAO-A in patients with Brunner syndrome who exhibit impulsive and aggressive behavior (Brunner et al., 1993a,b). Patients with a deficiency of MAO-B do not exhibit the same behavioral phenotype (Lenders et al., 1996). Animal models (MAO-A and MAO-B knock-out mice) exist that provide a further opportunity to study the biology of aggression (Shih and Chen, 1999). Mice with MAO-A knock-out manifest aggression and have elevated levels of norepinephrine, dopamine, and serotonin, whereas mice with MAO-B knock-out are not aggressive and have elevated phenylethylamine only.

Patients with VCFS may present with psychiatric manifestations. The explanation for these symptoms may be involvement of the catechol-*O*-methyltransferase (*COMT*) gene within the deleted area on 22q11. Lachman and colleagues (1996) described an association between an additional low-activity allele on the nondeleted chromosome and the development of bipolar spectrum disorder. Individuals with low *COMT* activity would be expected to have higher levels of transynaptic catecholamines due to a reduced degradation of norepinephrine and dopamine.

Hyposensitivity of a subset of γ-aminobutyric acid (GABA) receptors is suggested in patients with Prader-Willi and Angelman syndromes (Ebert et al., 1997), inasmuch as three genes for subsets of GABA receptors are contained within the distal part of the imprinted region (the GABA type A receptor subunits 3 [*GABRB3*], a 5 [*GABRA5*], and 3 [*GABRG3*]). These genes are involved in inhibitory synaptic transmission in the brain (Lalande et al., 1999). The modified sensitivity of the receptors may explain not only the epileptic trait in Angelman syndrome but also some of the behavioral abnormalities in both syndromes (DeLorey and Olsen, 1999).

Abnormalities of hormone secretion, due to genetic aberrations, during critical periods of brain development may also influence cognitive processes. In Turner syndrome, the absence of estrogen at a critical stage of puberty seems to be related to an immature pattern of response in event-related brain potentials (Johnson et al., 1993) and to low scores on visuospatial tasks (Swillen et al., 1993).

Skuse and colleagues (1999) found a different social-cognitive outcome in girls with Turner syndrome based on which parent's X chromosome is present. When the single X chromosome is of maternal origin, psychiatric and cognitive impairments are more severe, suggesting that an imprinted X-linked locus influences social-cognitive skills and behavior. This finding may have implications for the overrepresentation of males (whose X chromosome is of maternal origin) in prepubertal psychiatric disorders.

Behavioral phenotypes may also be caused by mutations or rearrangements in genes involved in the normal development of the central nervous system. Different neuroimaging techniques are used to identify specific structural brain abnormalities in genetic syndromes. Jakala and colleagues (1997) found minor abnormalities in temporal lobe structures in adult fragile X subjects with full mutations. Mostofsky and colleagues (1998) found that posterior vermis size is significantly decreased in fragile X, more so in males than in females. In females with fragile X, posterior vermis size predicted performance on selected cognitive measures (Mostofsky et al., 1998). FMRP, the deficient protein in fragile X, is synthesized in postsynaptic dendritic terminals. It is suggested that synthesis of FMRP may be essential for activity-based synapse maturation and elimination, a key process in normal brain development (Weiler and Greenough, 1999). This could be an explanation for the structural abnormalities found in this syndrome.

CONCLUSION

Updated knowledge of behavioral phenotypes will help psychiatrists identify these conditions, refer the patient and his/her family for genetic diagnosis and counseling, make specific treatment recommendations, and contribute to research and syndrome delineation.

ACKNOWLEDGMENTS

REFERENCES

Abrams MT, Reiss AL, Freund LS, Baumgardner TL, Chase GA, Denckla MB (1994), Molecular-neurobehavioral associations in females with the fragile X full mutation. *Am J Med Genet* 51: 317–327.

Akefeldt A, Gillberg C (1999), Behavior and personality characteristics of children and young adults with Prader-Willi syndrome: a controlled study. *J Am Acad Child Adolesc Psychiatry* 38: 761–769.

American Psychiatric Association (1994), *Diagnostic and Statistical Manual of Mental Disorders, 4th edition (DSM-IV).* Washington, D.C.: American Psychiatric Association.

Amir RE, Van den Veyver IB, Wan M, Tran CQ, Francke U, Zoghbi HY (1999), Rett syndrome is caused by mutations in X-linked MECP2, encoding methyl-CpG-binding protein 2. *Nat Genet* 23: 185–188.

Baumgardner TL, Reiss AL, Freund LS (1995), Specification of the neurobehavioral phenotype in males with fragile X syndrome. Pediatrics 95: 744–752.

*Bellugi U, Lichtenberger L, Mills D, Galaburda A, Korenberg JR (1999), Bridging cognition, the brain and molecular genetics: evidence from Williams syndrome. *Trends Neurosci* 22: 197–207.

Birhle AM, Bellugi U, Delis D et al., (1989), Seeing either the forest or the trees: dissociation in visuospatial processing. *Brain Cogn* 11: 37–49.

Bower BD, Jeavons PM (1967), The happy puppet syndrome. *Arch Dis Child* 42: 298–301.

Brunner HG, Nelen M, Breakefield XO, Ropers HH, van Oost BA (1993a), Abnormal behavior associated with a point mutation in the structural gene for monoamine oxidase A. Science 262: 578–580.

Brunner HG, Nelen MR, van Zandvoort P et al., (1993b), X-linked borderline mental retardation with prominent behavioral disturbance: phenotype, genetic localization and evidence for disturbed monoamine metabolism. *Am J Hum Genet* 52: 1032–1039.

Burn J (1986), Williams syndrome. *J Med Genet* 23: 389–395.

Cassidy SB (1997), Prader-Willi syndrome. *J Med Genet* 34: 917–923.

Cassidy SB, Forsythe M, Heeger S et al., (1997), Comparison of phenotype between patients with Prader-Willi syndrome due to deletion 15q and uniparental disomy 15. *Am J Med Genet* 68: 433–440.

Clarke D (1998), Prader-Willi syndrome and psychotic symptoms, 2: a preliminary study of prevalence using the Psychopathology Assessment Schedule for Adults With Developmental Disability Checklist. *J Intellect Disabil Res* 42: 451–454.

Clarke D, Boer H, Webb T et al., (1998), Prader-Willi syndrome and psychotic symptoms, 1: case descriptions and genetic studies. *J Intellect Disabil Res* 42: 440–450.

Clayton-Smith J (1993), Clinical research on Angelman syndrome in the United Kingdom: observations on 82 affected individuals. *Am J Med Genet* 46: 12–15.

Cohen IL, Vietze PM, Sudhalter V (1989), Parent-child dyadic gaze patterns in fragile X males and in non-fragile X males with autistic disorder. *J Child Psychol Psychiatry* 30: 845–856.

Cuskelly M, Dadds M (1992), Behavioral problems in children with Down syndrome and their siblings. *J Child Psychol Psychiatry* 33: 749–761.

Davies M, Howlin P, Udwin O (1997), Independence and adaptive behavior in adults with Williams syndrome. *Am J Med Genet* 70: 188–195.

de Vries BB, Halley DJ, Oostra BA, Neirmeijer MF (1998), The fragile X syndrome. *J Med Genet* 35: 579–589.

DeLorey TM, Olsen RW (1999), GABA and epileptogenesis: comparing GABRB3 gene deficient mice with Angelman syndrome in man. *Epilepsy Res* 36: 123–132.

Demb HB, Papola P (1995), PDD and Prader-Willi syndrome. *J Am Acad Child Adolesc Psychiatry* 34: 539–540.

Devenny DA, Silverman WP, Hill AL, Jenkins E, Sersen EA, Wisniewski KE (1996), Normal aging in adults with Down's syndrome: a longitudinal study. *J Intellect Disabil Res* 40: 208–221.

Dykens EM, Cassidy SB (1995), Correlates of maladaptive behavior in children and adults with Prader-Willi syndrome. *Am J Med Genet* 60: 546–549.

*Dykens EM, Cassidy SB (1996), Prader-Willi syndrome: genetic, behavioral, and treatment issues. *Child Adolesc Psychiatr Clin N Am* 5: 913–927.

Dykens EM, Cassidy SB, King BH (1999), Maladaptive behavior differences in Prader-Willi syndrome due to paternal deletion versus maternal uniparental disomy. *Am J Ment Retard* 104: 67–77.

Dykens E, Finucane B, Gayley C (1997), Cognitive and behavioral profiles in persons with Smith-Magenis syndrome. *J Autism Dev Disord* 27: 203–211.

Dykens EM, Hodapp RM, Evans DW (1994a), Profiles and development of adaptive behavior in children with Down syndrome. *Am J Ment Retard* 98: 580–587.

Dykens EM, Hodapp RM, Leckman JF (1994b), *Behavior and Development in Fragile X Syndrome*. Thousand Oaks, CA: Sage.

Dykens EM, Hodapp RM, Walsh K, Nash LJ (1992), Profiles, correlates and trajectories of intelligence in individuals with Prader-Willi syndrome. *J Am Acad Child Adolesc Psychiatry* 31: 1125–1130.

Ebert MH, Schmidt DE, Thompson T, Butler MG (1997), Elevated plasma gamma-aminobutyric acid (GABA) levels in individuals with either Prader-Willi syndrome or Angelman syndrome. *J Neuropsychiatry Clin Neurosci* 9: 75–80.

Einfeld SL, Tonge BJ, Florio T (1997), Behavioral and emotional disturbance in individuals with Williams syndrome. *Am J Ment Retard* 102: 45–53.

El-Abd S, Patton MA, Turk J, Hoey H, Howlin P (1999), Social, communicational and behavioral deficits associated with ring X Turner syndrome. *Am J Med Genet* 88: 510–516.

El-Abd S, Turk J, Hill P (1995), Psychological characteristics of Turner syndrome. *J Child Psychol Psychiatry* 36: 1109–1125.

Elsea SH, Fritz E, Schoener-Scott R, Meyn MS, Patel PI (1998), Gene for topoisomerase III maps within the Smith-Magenis syndrome critical region: analysis of cell-cycle distribution and radiation sensitivity. *Am J Med Genet* 75: 104–108.

Ensing GJ, Everett LA, Green ED et al., (1995), Down syndrome, trisomy 21. In: *Metabolic Basis of Inherited Disease,* Scriver CR, Beaudet AL, Sly WS, Valle D, eds. New York: McGraw-Hill, pp. 749–794.

*Finegan JA (1998), Study of behavioral phenotypes: goals and methodological considerations. *Am J Med Genet* 81: 148–155.

Finucane BM, Konar D, Haas-Givler B, Kurtz MB, Scott Jr CI (1994), The spasmodic upper-body squeeze: a characteristic behavior in Smith-Magenis syndrome. *Dev Med Child Neurol* 36: 78–83.

*Flint J (1998), Behavioral phenotypes: conceptual and methodological issues. *Am J Med Genet* 81: 235–240.

Flint J, Yule W (1994), Behavioral phenotypes. In: *Child and Adolescent Psychiatry,* Rutter M, Taylor E, Hersov L, eds. Oxford, England: Blackwell Scientific Publications, pp. 666–687.

Fowler A (1990), Language abilities in children with Down syndrome. In: *Children With Down Syndrome: A Developmental Perspective,* Cicchetti D, Beeghly M, eds. New York: Cambridge University Press, pp. 302–328.

Frangiskakis JM, Ewart AK, Morris CA et al., (1991), Cognitive profiles associated with the fra(X) syndrome in males and females. *Am J Med Genet* 38: 542–547.

Frangiskakis JM, Ewart AK, Morris CA et al., (1996), LIM-kinase 1 hemizygosity implicated in impaired visuospatial constructive cognition. *Cell* 86: 59–69.

Freund LS, Reiss AL, Abrams M (1993), Psychiatric disorders associated with fragile X in the young female. *Pediatrics* 91: 321–329.

Gecz J, Gedeon AK, Sutherland GR, Mulley JC (1996), Identification of the gene FMR2, associated with FRAXE mental retardation. *Nat Genet* 13: 105–108.

Ghaziuddin M, Tsail Y, Ghaziuddin N (1992), Autism in Down's syndrome: presentation and diagnosis. *J Intellect Disabil Res* 36: 449–456.

Golding-Kushner KJ, Weller G, Shprintzen RJ (1985), Velo-cardio-facial syndrome: language and psychological profiles. *J Craniofac Genet Dev Biol* 51: 259–266.

Gosch A, Pankau R (1997), Personality characteristics and behaviour problems in individuals of different ages with Williams syndrome. *Dev Med Child Neurol* 39: 527–533.

Gothelf D, Frisch A, Munitz H et al., (1999), Clinical characteristics of schizophrenia associated with velo-cardio-facial syndrome. *Schizophr Res* 35: 105–112.

Greenberg F, Guzzetta V, Montes de Oca-Luna R et al., (1991), Molecular analysis of the Smith-Magenis syndrome: a possible contiguous-gene syndrome associated with del(17)(p11.2). *Am J Hum Genet* 49: 1207–1218.

Greenberg F, Lewis RA, Potocki L et al., (1996), Multi-disciplinary clinical study of Smith-Magenis syndrome (deletion 17p11.2). *Am J Med Genet* 62: 247–254.

Greer MK, Brown 3rd FR, Pai GS, Choudry SH, Klein AJ (1997), Cognitive, adaptive, and behavioral characteristics of Williams syndrome. *Am J Med Genet* 74: 521–525.

Hagberg B, Aicardi J, Dias K, Ramos O (1983), A progressive syndrome of autism, dementia, ataxia and loss of purposeful hand use in girls: Rett's syndrome: report of 35 cases. *Ann Neurol* 14: 471–479.

*Hagerman RJ (1996a), Fragile X syndrome. *Child Adolesc Psychiatr Clin N Am* 5: 895–911

Hagerman RJ (1996b), Physical and behavioral features. In: *Fragile X Syndrome: Diagnosis, Treatment and Research,* 2nd ed, Hagerman RJ, Cronister AC, eds. Baltimore: Johns Hopkins University Press, pp. 83–87.

Hagerman RJ, Hills J, Scharfenaker S, Lewis H (1999), Fragile X syndrome and selective mutism. *Am J Med Genet* 83: 313–317.

Hagerman RJ, Jackson C, Amiri K, Silverman AC, O'Connor R, Sobesky W (1992), Girls with fragile X syndrome: physical and neurocognitive status and outcome. *Pediatrics* 89: 395–400.

Hall JD, Gilchrist DM (1990), Turner syndrome: its variants. *Pediatr Clin North Am* 37: 1421–1440.

Heineman-de Boer JA, Van Haelst MJ, Cordia-de Haan M, Beemer FA (1999), Behavior problems and personality aspects of 40 children with velo-cardio-facial syndrome. *Genet Couns* 10: 89–93.

Hodapp RM, Dykens EM, Hagerman RJ, Schreiner R, Lachiewicz AM, Leckman JF (1990), Developmental implications of changing trajectories of IQ in males with fragile X syndrome. *J Am Acad Child Adolesc Psychiatry* 29: 214–219.

Jacobsen J, King BH, Leventhal BL, Christian SL, Ledbetter DH, Cook Jr EH (1998), Molecular screening for proximal 15q abnormalities in a mentally retarded population. *J Med Genet* 35: 534–538.

Jakala P, Hanninen T, Ryynanen M et al., (1997), Fragile-X: neuropsychological test performance, CGG triplet repeat lengths, and hippocampal volumes. *J Clin Invest* 100: 331–338.

Janicki MP, Dalton AJ (2000), Prevalence of dementia and impact on intellectual disability services. *Ment Retard* 38: 276–288.

Johnson Jr R, Rohbaugh JW, Ross JL (1993), Altered brain development in Turner's syndrome: an event-related potential study. *Neurology* 43: 803–808.

Jones KL (1997), *Smith's Recognizable Patterns of Human Malformation*. Philadelphia: Saunders.

Kerby DS, Dawson BL (1994), Autistic features, personality, and adaptive behavior in males with the fragile X syndrome and no autism. *Am J Ment Retard* 98: 455–462.

Kishino T, Lalande M, Wagstaff J (1997), UBE3A/E6-AP mutations cause Angelman syndrome. *Nat Genet* 15: 70–73.

Klein AJ, Armstrong BL, Greer MK et al., (1990), Hyperacusis and otitis media in individuals with Williams syndrome. *J Speech Hear Disord* 55: 339–344.

Kolehmainen K, Karant Y (1994), Modeling methylation and IQ scores in fragile X females and mosaic males. *Am J Med Genet* 51: 328–338.

Lachman HM, Morrow B, Shprintzen R et al., (1996), Association of codon 108/158 catechol-*O*-methyltransferase gene polymorphism with the psychiatric manifestations of velo-cardio-facial syndrome. *Am J Med Genet* 67: 468–472.

Lalande M, Minassian BA, DeLorey TM, Olsen RW (1999), Parental imprinting and Angelman syndrome. *Adv Neurol* 79: 421–429.

Lenders JW, Eisenhofer G, Abeling NG et al., (1996), Specific genetic deficiencies of the A and B isoenzymes of monoamine oxidase are characterized by distinct neurochemical and clinical phenotypes. *J Clin Invest* 97: 1010–1019.

Lenhoff HM, Wang PP, Greenberg F, Bellugi U (1997), Williams syndrome and the brain. *Sci Am* 277: 68–73.

McCauley E, Kay T, Ito J, Treder R (1987), The Turner syndrome: cognitive deficits, affective discrimination, and behavior problems. *Child Dev* 58: 464–473.

McCauley E, Ross J, Sybert V (1994), Self-concept and behavioral profiles in females with Turner syndrome. In: *Growth, Stature and Adaptation,* Stabler B, Underwood LE, eds. Chapel Hill: University of North Carolina, pp. 181–194.

Meng X, Lu X, Li Z et al., (1998), Complete physical map of the common deletion region in Williams syndrome and identification and characterization of three novel genes. *Hum Genet* 103: 590–599.

Merenstein SA, Sobesky WE, Taylor AK, Riddle JE, Tran HX, Hagerman RJ (1996), Molecular-clinical correlations in males with an expanded FMR1 mutation. *Am J Med Genet* 66: 388–394.

Mervis CB, Klein-Tasman BP (2000), Williams syndrome: cognition, personality, and adaptive behavior. *Ment Retard Dev Disabil Res Rev* 6: 148–158.

Miller JF, Leddy M, Miolo G, Sedey A (1995), The development of early language skills in children with Down syndrome. In: *Down Syndrome: Living and Learning in the Community,* Nadel L, Rosenthal D, eds. New York: Wiley, pp. 115–120.

Mostofsky SH, Mazzocco MM, Aakalu G, Warsofsky IS, Denckla MB, Reiss AL (1998), Decreased cerebellar posterior vermis size in fragile X syndrome: correlation with neurocognitive performance. *Neurology* 50: 121–130.

Nielsen NJ, Nyborg H, Dahl G (1977), Turner's syndrome: a psychiatric psychological study of 45 women with Turner's syndrome. *Acta Jutlandica* 45: 1–190.

Papolos DF, Faedda GL, Veit S et al., (1996), Bipolar spectrum disorders in patients diagnosed with velo-cardio-facial syndrome: does a hemizygous deletion of chromosome 22q11 result in bipolar affective disorder? *Am J Psychiatry* 153: 1541–1547.

Pike AC, Super M (1997), Velocardiofacial syndrome. *Postgrad Med J* 73: 771–775.

Plissart L, Borghgraef M, Volcke P, Van den Berghe H, Fryns JP (1994), Adults with Williams-Beuren syndrome: evaluation of the medical, psychological and behavioral aspects. *Clin Genet* 46: 161–167.

Pober BR, Dykens EM (1996), Williams syndrome: an overview of medical, cognitive and behavioral features. *Child Adolesc Psychiatr Clin N Am* 5: 929–943.

Pueschel SM, Gallagher PL, Zartler AS, Pezzulo JC (1987), Cognitive and learning process in children with Down syndrome. *Res Dev Disabil* 8: 21–37.

Pulver AE, Nestadt G, Goldberg R et al., (1994), Psychotic illness in patients diagnosed with velo-cardio-facial syndrome and their relatives. *J Nerv Ment Dis* 182: 476–478.

Reiss AL, Freund L (1991), Behavioral phenotype of fragile X syndrome: *DSM-III-R* autistic behavior in male children. *Am J Med Genet* 43: 35–46.

Reiss AL, Freund L, Abrams M, Boehm C, Kazazian H (1993), Neurobehavioral effect of the fragile X premutation in adult women: a controlled study. *Am J Hum Genet* 52: 884–894.

Rett Syndrome Diagnostic Criteria Work Group (1988), Diagnostic criteria for Rett syndrome. *Ann Neurol* 23:425–428.

Rineer S, Finucane B, Simon EW (1998), Autistic symptoms among children and young adults with isodicentric chromosome 15. *Am J Med Genet* 81: 428–433.

Ross JL, Stefanatos G, Roeltgen D, Kushner H, Cutler Jr GB (1995), Ullrich-Turner syndrome: neurodevelopmental changes from childhood through adolescence. *Am J Med Genet* 58: 74–82.

Rovet J, Ireland L (1994), Behavioral phenotype in children with Turner syndrome. *J Pediatr Psychol* 19: 779–790.

Rovet JF (1994), School outcome in Turner syndrome. In: *Growth, Stature and Adaptation,* Stabler B, Underwood LE, eds. Chapel Hill: University of North Carolina, pp. 165–180.

Schuback DE, Mulligan EL, Sims KB et al., (1999), Screen for MAOA mutations in target human groups. *Am J Med Genet* 88: 25–28.

Shih JC, Chen K (1999), MAO-A and -B gene knock-out mice exhibit distinctly different behavior. *Neurobiology* (Bp) 7: 235–246.

Shprintzen RJ, Goldberg R, Golding-Kushner KJ, Marion R (1992), Late-onset psychosis in the velo-cardio-facial syndrome. *Am J Med Genet* 42: 141–142.

Shprintzen RJ, Goldberg RB, Young D, Wolford L (1981), The velo-cardio-facial syndrome: a clinical and genetic analysis. *Pediatrics* 67: 167–172.

Siegel PT, Clopper R, Stabler B (1998), The psychological consequences of Turner syndrome and review of the National Cooperative Growth Study psychological substudy. *Pediatrics* 102: 488–491.

Skuse D, Elgar K, Morris E (1999), Quality of life in Turner syndrome is related to chromosomal constitution: implications for genetic counselling and management. *Acta Paediatr Suppl* 428: 110–113.

*Smith ACM, Dykens E, Greenberg F (1998), Behavioral phenotype of Smith-Magenis syndrome (del 17p11.2). *Am J Med Genet* 81: 179–185.

Staley-Gane L, Flynn L, Neitzel K, Cronister A, Hagerman RJ (1996), Expanding the role of the genetic counselor. *Am J Med Genet* 64: 382–387.

State MW, Dykens EM, Rosner B, Martin A, King BH (1999), Obsessive-compulsive symptoms in Prader-Willi and Prader-Willi-like patients. *J Am Acad Child Adolesc Psychiatry* 38: 329–334.

State MW, King BH, Dykens E (1997), Mental retardation: a review of the past 10 years. Part II. *J Am Acad Child Adolesc Psychiatry* 36: 1664–1671.

Steffenburg S, Gillberg CL, Steffenburg U, Kyllerman M (1996), Autism in Angelman syndrome: a population-based study. *Pediatr Neurol* 14: 131–136.

Summers JA, Allison DB, Lynch PS, Sandler L (1995), Behaviour problems in Angelman syndrome. *J Intellect Disabil Res* 39: 97–106.

Swaab DF (1997), Prader-Willi syndrome and the hypothalamus. *Acta Paediatr Suppl* 423: 50–54.

Swillen A, Fryns JP, Kleczkowska A, Massa G, Vanderschueren-Lodeweyckx M, Vanden- Berghe H (1993), Intelligence, behaviour and psychosocial development in Turner syndrome: a cross-sectional study of 50 pre-adolescent and adolescent girls (4-20 years). *Genet Couns* 4: 7–18.

Tager-Flusberg H, Boshart J, Baron-Cohen S (1998), Reading the windows of the soul: evidence of domain-specific sparing in Williams syndrome. *J Cogn Neurosci* 10: 631–639.

Udwin O (1990), A survey of adults with Williams syndrome and idiopathic infantile hypercalcemia. *Dev Med Child Neurol* 32: 129–141.

Udwin O, Davies M, Howlin P (1996), A longitudinal study of cognitive abilities and educational attainment in Williams syndrome. *Dev Med Child Neurol* 38: 1020–1029.

Usiskin SI, Nicolson R, Krasnewich DM et al., (1999), Velo-cardio-facial syndrome in childhood-onset schizophrenia. *J Am Acad Child Adolesc Psychiatry* 38: 1536–1543.

Vantrappen G, Devriendt K, Swillen A et al., (1999), Presenting symptoms and clinical features in 130 patients with the velo-cardio-facial syndrome: the Leuven experience. *Genet Couns* 10: 3–9.

Verheij C, Bakker CE, de Graaff E et al., (1993), Characterization and localization of the FMR-1 gene product associated with fragile X syndrome. *Nature* 363: 722–724.

von Tetzchner S, Jacobsen KH, Smith L, Skjeldal OH, Heiberg A, Fagan JF (1996), Vision, cognition and developmental characteristics of girls and women with Rett syndrome. *Dev Med Child Neurol* 38: 212–226.

Wang PP, Woodin MF, Kreps-Falk R, Moss EM (2000), Research on behavioral phenotypes: velocardiofacial syndrome (deletion 22q11.2). *Dev Med Child Neurol* 42: 422–427.

Weiler IJ, Greenough WT (1999), Synaptic synthesis of the fragile X protein: possible involvement in synapse maturation and elimination. *Am J Med Genet* 83: 248–252.

Wolpert CM, Menold MM, Bass MP et al., (2000), Three probands with autistic disorder and isodicentric chromosome 15. *Am J Med Genet* 96: 365–372.

Wright-Talamante C, Cheema A, Riddle JE, Luckey DW, Taylor AK, Hagerman RJ (1996), A controlled study of longitudinal IQ changes in females and males with fragile X syndrome. *Am J Med Genet* 64: 350–355.

7

Approaches to Gene Mapping in Complex Disorders and Their Application in Child Psychiatry and Psychology

Philip J. Asherson and Sarah Curran

Background: *Twin studies demonstrate the importance of genes and environment in the etiology of childhood psychiatric and neurodevelopmental disorders. Advances in molecular genetics enable the identification of genes involved in complex disorders and enable the study of molecular mechanisms and gene–environment interactions.* ***Aims:*** *To review the role of molecular genetics studies in childhood behavioral and developmental traits.* ***Method:*** *Molecular approaches to complex disorders are reviewed, with examples from autism, reading disability, and attention-deficit hyperactivity disorder (ADHD).* ***Results:*** *The most robust finding in ADHD is the association of a variable number tandem repeat polymorphism in exon 3 of the DRD4 gene. Other replicated associations with ADHD are outlined in the text. In autism, there is a replicated linkage finding on chromosome 7. Linkage studies in reading disability have confirmed a locus on chromosome 6 and strongly suggest one on chromosome 15.* ***Conclusions:*** *In the next 5 to 10 years susceptibility genes for these disorders will be established. Describing their relationship to biological and behavior behavioral function will be a far greater challenge.*

INTRODUCTION

The classic genetic approaches of family, twin, and adoption studies have provided considerable evidence that genetic influences play an important role in the development of child behavior and cognition. There have also been remarkable advances in the application of molecular methods in medicine, together with technological progress in mapping and sequencing the human genome. As a result, many are now persuaded that the time is right to focus on the identification of genes that may give rise to childhood psychiatric and behavioral disorders. Expectations aroused by work in this area are high, so that molecular genetic strategies now have a pivotal role in research aimed at elucidating both the biological basis (nature) and environmental basis (nurture) of childhood behavioral and neurodevelopmental disorders, with the hope of major developments in prevention and treatment. In this review we focus on contemporary approaches to gene discovery in complex disorders and describe how they have been applied in child psychiatry and psychology.

COMBINING QUANTITATIVE GENETIC AND MOLECULAR GENETIC APPROACHES

Molecular genetic research in the field of child development and psychopathology is comparatively new. In part, this is because of difficulties in defining childhood disorders and the scarcity of sufficiently detailed family, twin, and adoption studies demonstrating familial resemblance between close family members and the relative contribution of genes and environment. In many clinical areas the question of familial risk is only now starting to be addressed using more rigorous protocols. Indeed, the relative ease with which molecular genetic studies can be performed has in many cases led to molecular approaches being pursued in advance of good phenotypic definition. As a result many groups are developing both quantitative and molecular approaches side by side, since they are complementary in the investigation of complex behavioral disorders (for general reviews see McGuffin et al., 1994; Plomin et al., 1994, 2000; Rutter et al., 1999b).

One of the key issues for those engaged in molecular genetic studies is the identification of heritable phenotypes. Traditional diagnostic categories are useful in practice, but their validity in terms of their underlying etiology is uncertain. Nevertheless, the general approach so far has been to use categorical criteria based on definitions such as those in *DSM-IV* (American Psychiatric Association, 1994) or *ICD-10* (World Health Organization, 1992).

Alternative approaches aimed at identifying quantitative trait loci (QTLs) can be applied whenever a behavioral or developmental trait is continuously distributed throughout the population. These approaches may be particularly applicable to child psychopathology, since with few exceptions, behavioral disorders of childhood can be conceptualized as extremes on continuously distributed dimensions. Many of the conditions encountered in childhood seem to have close parallels in normal variations in human behavior. Questions therefore arise about the relationship between quantitative dimensions of behavior and extreme diagnostic categories, and whether genes that exert an influence across a normal range of behavior also exert their influence at the pathological extremes.

Quantitative genetic studies using twin samples have approached this issue by considering the relationship between diagnostic categories or cutoffs on dimensional scores in twin probands and quantitative scores in their twin partners (DeFries & Fulker, 1985, 1988). A simple multiple regression procedure is used to test the hypothesis that quantitative trait scores of twin partners (co-twins) should be more similar to those of the probands for identical co twins compared with nonidentical co-twins. Using this approach, mild learning difficulties (Plomin et al., 1991), hyperactivity, and spelling disability (Stevenson et al., 1993) appear to represent extremes of continuously distributed traits, whereas severe learning difficulties (Plomin et al., 1991) and early language delay (Dale et al., 1998) appear to be distinct disorders.

STRATEGIES FOR MOLECULAR GENETIC RESEARCH

Molecular genetic research has had a dramatic impact on the study of simple genetic disorders with Mendelian patterns of inheritance. Over 100 genes that are the sole or main cause of such disorders have been identified using a variety of positional cloning and targeted candidate gene strategies (see the Online Mendelian Inheritance in Man [OMIM] database at http://www3.ncbi.nlm.nih.gov/Omim). In most cases this has laid the foundation for further functional studies resulting in considerable insights into the molecular and biochemical basis of these disorders. One of the most exciting aspects of this work has been the ability to discover genes involved in disease processes in the absence of *a priori* hypotheses, by first identifying chromosomal regions containing disease genes and then screening genes within the region for functional mutations. Conditions such as autism, attention-deficit hyperactivity disorder (ADHD), reading disability, and mild mental impairment, however, are said to show complex inheritance. They do not conform to Mendelian patterns of segregation and are thought to result from the combined effects of several genes (oligogenic) or perhaps many genes (polygenic), each of which, on its own, has only a small effect. In these cases, variations of single genes are neither sufficient nor necessary to cause the disorder, but such genes act as susceptibility genes, increasing risk for the disorder. Mapping and identifying the genes responsible for such complex disorders represents a greater challenge than that posed by rarer Mendelian diseases, but one that is becoming rapidly more tractable.

Linkage analysis using multiply affected families

Early genetic studies of common behavioral disorders such as schizophrenia and bipolar disorder were based on the assumption of single-gene inheritance. Large, multiply affected families were identified, and this appeared to show Mendelian inheritance. In some cases results using this approach suggested the identification of rare familial forms segregating single genes of major effect.

For example, there are three independent reports of linkage between markers on chromosome 4p near to the dopamine D5 receptor gene, and bipolar and schizoaffective disorder (Blackwood et al., 1996; Asherson et al., 1998; Ewald et al., 1998).

However, analyses of such families using traditional linkage approaches have in general been unsuccessful and are unlikely to identify genetic risk factors for common forms of these disorders. As a result, more recent linkage studies of behavioral phenotypes have focused on using sibling pairs and small nuclear families rather than multiplex pedigrees (reviewed by Craddock & Owen, 1996; Risch, 2000).

Linkage analysis using affected sibling pairs

Pairs of siblings affected with the same disorder are presumed to share susceptibility genes inherited from the same parent. This hypothesis can be tested by ascertaining a series of affected sibling pairs and genotyping the sample with markers spread evenly throughout the genome. Where affected siblings share parental alleles more often than by chance alone, this indicates linkage between a susceptibility gene and the marker alleles. These studies can be robust in the sense that diagnostic criteria can be specified in an attempt to reduce genetic and aetiological heterogeneity, and no assumptions are required about the underlying mode of inheritance. The major limitation is the power of the technique, so that large numbers of affected pairs are needed to detect genes of moderate to small effect.

A measure frequently used to evaluate the power of affected sibling pair linkage is the ratio of the risk to the sibling of an affected proband and population prevalence, a parameter known as λ_s. Low λ_s values may be due to a variety of factors such as polygenic transmission, genetic heterogeneity, phenocopies, and low penetrance, which may require unfeasibly large sample sizes to overcome. Disorders such as autism may be more amenable to this approach since the estimated λ_s is very large (100 to 200), well within the theoretical resolution of linkage strategies. On the other hand, disorders such as ADHD have an estimated λ_s somewhere between 2 and 5 (Biederman et al., 1990, 1992). Indeed, if more than one gene causes ADHD, then the λvalue for any single gene (the gene-specific λ or λ_g) must be very low.

Association strategies

Association studies compare the frequencies of marker alleles in a group of affected individuals with those in a sample of control subjects without the disorder or drawn from the general population. A statistically significant difference suggests either tight linkage, resulting in linkage disequilibrium between a marker allele and the susceptibility locus, or that the marker allele itself confers susceptibility to disorder. Linkage disequilibrium (LD) describes the phenomenon where two loci are so close together on a chromosome that they are not separated by recombination events over many generations. Loci linked together in such a way reflect fragments of ancestral chromosomes that remain intact despite many meiotic events over multiple generations and therefore appear to be associated even in individuals from different families.

The power of association to detect genes of small effect is well known. Risch and Merikangas (1996), using stringent criteria that took into account the large number of loci required to screen the entire genome, estimated that a sample of 340 unrelated cases would detect association with a susceptibility gene with a frequency of 0.5 and gene-specific λ of 2.0. In comparison, 2,498 affected sibling pairs would be required to detect the same gene by linkage analysis. Despite this, the usefulness of the approach has been limited by the fact that thousands of markers are required to perform a whole genome search. For this reason association approaches are still in their infancy and in most cases have only been applied to the analysis of a few candidate genes. Fortunately, the development of a new-generation high-density marker map and the technology to screen these in large numbers is under way, so that LD mapping strategies are fast becoming the focus of current interest in the study of complex disorders (Chakravati, 1999; Kruglyak & Nickerson, 2001).

Association studies in behavioral disorders have unfortunately thrown up a number of contradictory results (for example, see O'Donovan & Owen, 1999). This has been in part because of the problems of diagnosis and comparability of patient populations from different centers, and inadequate sample sizes in many studies. A confounding factor in case–control studies is the selection of control subjects, which can result in stratification effects. The solution to this problem is to sample both parents of affected probands and use the nontransmitted parental alleles as control genotypes (haplotype relative risk analysis) (Falk & Rubinstein, 1987), or look for increased transmission of a specific allele from heterozygote parents (transmission disequilibrium test) (Spielman & Ewens, 1996).

Quantitative trait loci mapping

An alternative approach to mapping genes for disorders using categorical criteria is the analysis of traits that are continuously distributed in the population (Plomin et al., 1994, 2000). Such quantitative traits are influenced by the action and co-action of multiple genes or QTLs. Developmental traits such as general cognitive ability (*g*) and reading ability, and behavioral traits such as hyperactivity, may be better perceived in this way. In QTL linkage, the difference in trait values, measured on a dimensional scale for pairs of siblings, is squared and examined as a function of the number of shared parental alleles (Haseman & Elston, 1972; Kruglyak & Lander, 1995). An alternative approach selects one sibling from the top few percent (diagnosed cases) and regresses the phenotypic score of the other sibling onto the number of shared parental alleles (Fulker et al., 1995; Fulker & Cherney, 1996). Considerable additional power can be gained by the use of phenotypically discordant as well concordant sibling pairs and the selection of siblings within the top and bottom deciles (Risch & Zhang, 1995; Purcell et al., 2001). Furthermore, both concordant and discordant siblings provide a powerful resource for QTL association mapping as well as linkage, using variance component approaches (Fulker et al., 1999).

Genetic maps and high-throughput genotyping

Investigators working before DNA markers became readily accessible were restricted to the use of 'classic' genetic markers such as red blood cell antigens (ABO, MNS, and Rh) and the human leucocyte antigens (HLA). The use of DNA markers began with the discovery of techniques for measuring variation within genomic DNA. Modern maps were introduced following the discovery that within noncoding regions of genomic DNA there are simple sequence repeats (SSRs) of short (two to four) nucleotide sequences (Weber & May, 1990). The usefulness of these markers lies in the ease with which they can be typed, following introduction of the polymerase chain reaction (PCR) and the use of efficient gel electrophoresis systems that allow multiple SSRs to be analyzed together. Newer machines using capillaries instead of conventional slab gels enable the processing of 6,000 to 18,000 individual genotypes on one machine in a day. This rate of production is adequate for genome-wide linkage, but for association mapping a much closer grid of markers is required, so that even more rapid methods are needed.

New approaches to very rapid genotyping

New approaches that are expected to have far-reaching consequences for mapping genes in complex disorders depend upon the detection of single-nucleotide polymorphisms (Anon., 1999; Craig et al., 2000). Single-nucleotide polymorphisms (SNPs) consist mainly of single-base substitutions and are the most frequent type of variation in the human genome. The SNP Consortium and International Human Genome Sequencing Consortium have identified and mapped 1.42 million SNPs, which are distributed throughout the human genome at an average density of one SNP every 1,900 base pairs (International SNP Map Working Group, 2001). Further developments aim at screening gene sequences directly, so that instead of searching for associations with anonymous markers, genome scans will be able to focus on variation within genes that affects protein sequence and expression, or lies very close to such functional variants. So far 60,000 of the identified SNPs fall within protein coding sequences and 85% of coding regions are within 5,000 base pairs of the nearest SNP. It has been estimated that a systematic approach to cataloging all the variation that may be relevant to human behavior would involve around 10,000 genes, an achievable goal within the next few years. Such polymorphisms will then be available for use in behavioral genetics association studies.

In parallel with the identification of SNPs, methods are under development for efficient SNP genotyping (see Landegren et al., 1998, for review). The approaches which have gained widest publicity are the development of DNA micro-arrays, commonly referred to as DNA chips (Lander, 1999), and, more recently, matrix-assisted laser desorption/ionization time-of-flight mass spectrometry (MALDITOF) (Griffin et al., 1999). The impact of these technologies on gene mapping is likely to be profound, since it will be possible to screen very large samples for linkage and association with extremely dense marker maps, greatly increasing the power to detect genes of small effect in complex disorders.

MOLECULAR GENETIC STUDIES OF CHILDHOOD BEHAVIORAL AND DEVELOPMENTAL TRAITS

The search for genetic variations that exert an influence on child behavior and development has only just begun. Nevertheless, there has been considerable progress in the study of autism, ADHD, and reading disability. Here we will review the most prominent of these findings, which will also serve to illustrate the range of gene mapping strategies being applied.

Molecular studies of autism

Autism is a pervasive developmental disorder with onset by 3 years of age and is defined by the presence of a triad of social and communication impairments with restricted, repetitive, or stereotyped behaviors. The disorder is interesting from a genetic perspective because, unlike most complex disorders, it is relatively rare and has a high degree of familiality. Nevertheless, it shows a complex mode of inheritance best explained by the action of several genes. Familial clustering is high, with an estimated λ_s of about 100, calculated from a population prevalence of around 2 to 4 per 10,000 and a risk to siblings of around 3%. Such clustering may be the result of shared environmental factors, but findings from twin studies provide overwhelming evidence for the importance of genetic influences: monozygotic (MZ) concordance rates are 60 to 90%, compared with less than 5% in dizygotic (DZ) twins, giving an estimated broad heritability of over 90% (reviewed by Rutter et al., 1999a,b). Twin studies also suggest that traditional diagnostic boundaries are far too restricted, since a higher MZ:DZ concordance ratio is found using a broad autistic phenotype, consisting of a combination of cognitive and social deficits similar to autism but in milder form (Bailey et al., 1998).

In the light of these findings it is not surprising that there has been a concerted effort to pursue genetic linkage studies using affected sibling pairs. This was first achieved by the International Molecular Genetic Study of Autism Consortium, which brought together groups from across Europe and the united states. In large collaborative projects the reliability of clinical assessments and subsequent diagnosis across multiple groups is always a key issue, especially with behavioral phenotypes, which are difficult to measure accurately and are generally quantitative rather than qualitative. However, this was facilitated by the adoption by all participating groups of the same assessment instruments: the Autism Diagnostic Interview (ADI) (Le Couteur et al., 1989) and the Autism Diagnostic Observation Schedule (ADOS) (Lord et al., 1989). A public information resource and DNA databank known as the Autism Genetic Resource Exchange has been established (http://www.agre.org).

The first report of a full genome linkage screen for autism identified three chromosomal regions showing evidence suggestive of linkage. The most significant of these was on the long arm of chromosome 7, which gave rise to a gene-specific λ of 5.0 (International Molecular Genetic Study of Autism Consortium, 1998). Consistent evidence for the chromosome 7 locus and another locus on chromosome 2 has come from several published and unpublished data-sets (Barrett et al., 1999; Phillipe et al., 1999; Risch et al., 1999; Auranen et al., 2000; reviewed by Lamb et al., 2000). If the identified genetic loci acted in a simple additive fashion they would contribute less than 10% to the overall λ_s value of around 100, suggesting that there must be multiple genes of very small effect or—perhaps more likely—important gene–gene and gene–environment interactions. The next step is to identify the genes themselves, by genotyping dense maps of SSR and SNP markers to refine the linkage regions and search for associations with particular genes and functional variants.

Molecular studies of reading disability

Familial transmission of reading disability has been recognized for a long time and twin studies demonstrate a substantial heritable component, estimated to be between 50% and 70% (DeFries et al., 1987; Gillis et al., 1992; Alarcon et al., 1998). Furthermore, twin studies suggest that the QTL perspective, which views genetic factors involved in reading disability as the same as those contributing to the quantitative dimension of the disability, is valid and should inform the design of molecular genetic studies. In fact, molecular studies of reading disability began in 1983 using traditional linkage approaches, giving suggestive but inconclusive results on chromosomes 6 and 15 (Smith et al., 1983; Bisgaard et al., 1987; Gross-Glenn et al., 1991; Rabin et al., 1993).

Cardon et al. (1994) were the first to apply a QTL approach to linkage mapping. This was achieved by deriving a continuous measure of reading ability from a battery of psychometric tests used to test the siblings of probands with reading disability. They found considerable evidence for a gene in the chromosome 6 region implicated earlier, with a moderate to strong influence on reading ability. Further evidence for the chromosome 6 and chromosome 15 loci came from an analysis of six large families (Grigorenko et al., 1997), which found that these loci were linked to two distinct reading-related phenotypes: phonological awareness with chromosome 6, and single-word reading with chromosome 15. Final confirmation for the chromosome 6 locus has come from two linkage studies (Fisher et al., 1999; Gayan et al., 1999). Since then, association mapping with simple sequence repeat markers has been used to screen the chromosome 6 and 15 linkage regions. Association was detected with chromosome 15 markers in two series of probands giving an overall significance value of $P = 0.00000008$ (Morris et al., 2000). Current work is focused on identifying the specific genes involved.

Molecular studies of ADHD

Attention-deficit hyperactivity disorder is characterized by a persistent pattern of overactivity, inattention, and impulsivity that is pervasive across social situations and accompanied by substantial social impairments. The disorder is common, occurring in 2% to 5% of children, affecting boys two to three times more frequently than girls, and is one of the major causes of childhood behavioral problems (Taylor et al., 1996). Hyperactivity is known to aggregate within families (Cantwell, 1972; Biederman et al., 1990, 1992) and twin studies have consistently shown it to be among the most highly heritable behaviors in childhood (reviewed in Thapar et al., 1999). Although ADHD is diagnosed using operational criteria to define diagnostic categories, measures of hyperactivity are continuously distributed in the general population. Recent twin studies have used dimensional rating scales, with clinical cutoffs applied when diagnostic categories were required. These studies all show high heritabilities regardless of where these cutoffs had been made and regardless of whether diagnostic or continuous criteria had been applied. This suggests strongly that a dimensional perspective on hyperactivity is a valid and powerful approach to the identification of QTLs and should be considered complementary to the study of defined clinical types. Despite this, most studies to date have applied categorical definitions based on current DSM definitions of ADHD.

Molecular genetic studies in ADHD began by focusing on candidate genes within the dopamine system, based on *a priori* hypotheses from neurochemical and neuropharmacological research. Replicated associations have been reported with variations in genes for the dopamine receptors 4 (*DRD4*) and 5 (*DRD5*) and the dopamine transporter (*DAT1*) (Collier et al., 2000). The most robust of these findings is the association between ADHD and the 7-repeat of a 48 bp sequence within the coding region of *DRD4*, which is commonly repeated two, three, four, or seven times (reviewed by Mill et al., 2001). A recent meta-analysis of seven case–control and fourteen within-family studies of this association, including both published and unpublished data, supports this finding, with odds ratios of 1.8, $P = 4 \times 10^{-8}$ and 1.3, $P = 2 \times 10^{-2}$, respectively (Faraone et al., 2001).

An interesting feature of the *DRD4* data is the wide range of sampling procedures giving rise to positive findings. Swanson et al. (1998) used a highly selected group of children who all responded to methylphenidate and had the combined subtype of ADHD without significant comorbidity. This contrasts greatly with the studies by Rowe et al. (1998), who assessed children attending a behavioral clinic and applied diagnostic criteria following completion of *DSM-IV* rating scales, and Smalley et al. (1998), who applied broader *DSM-III-R* and *DSM-IV* criteria following diagnostic interview. An alternative approach adopted by Curran et al. (2001a) was to take a QTL perspective in which ADHD was conceptualized as the extreme of a normally distributed trait. In this study, they examined the relationship of the *DRD4* polymorphism in a sample of children selected from the general population on the basis of high and low scores on five ADHD items of the Strengths and Difficulties Questionnaire as rated by the parents, and found a significant association with high-scoring individuals ($\chi^2 = 8.63$, $P = 0.003$; odds ratio 2.09).

The *DAT1* findings are of particular interest since stimulant drugs interact directly with the transporter protein. To date, there have been nine published association studies of ADHD with a 480 bp allele of a variable number tandem repeat (VNTR) polymorphism in the 3'-untranslated region of the gene: five support an association and four do not (summarized by Curran et al., 2001b). Meta-analysis of these data is consistent with a very small main effect for the 480 bp allele and is not yet convincing ($\chi^2 = 3.45$, $P = 0.06$, OR $= 1.15$). However, there is significant evidence of heterogeneity between the combined data-sets ($\chi^2 = 22.64$, d.f. $= 8$, $P = 0.004$), suggesting that the studies may divide into two groups: those in which the associated *DAT1* allele has a main effect and those in which the allele does not. In this case, failure to replicate the association in some studies may result from variation in the strength of the genetic influence in different populations. The cause of such heterogeneity remains unknown and requires further investigation.

Finally, association and linkage to a marker near to *DRD5* has been reported by several groups (Daly et al., 1999; Barr et al., 2000; Tahir et al., 2000)

THE FUTURE

The identification of susceptibility genes is only an initial step. Describing the molecular mechanisms involved and their relationship to biological and behavioral function will be a far greater challenge. Bridges will need to be built between structure and function, between molecular mechanisms and behavior, and between social, genetic, and developmental psychiatry. This area of functional genomics will be the real challenge in the post-genomic era if we are to see tangible benefits from current progress in mapping out the genetic and environmental influences on child behavioral and neurodevelopmental disorder.

CLINICAL IMPLICATIONS AND LIMITATIONS

Clinical Implications

Both genes and environment are implicated in many child psychiatric conditions and psychological traits.
Molecular genetic studies aim to identify common genetic risk factors.
Long-term benefits are expected from an improved understanding of the genetic and environmental mechanisms involved.

Limitations

Very large samples are required to reliably detect genes for such complex human traits.
Further advances are required in the rate of genetic marker data.
Bridging the gap between gene structure and function in relation to behavioral outcomes remains a major challenge.

ACKNOWLEDGMENTS

The authors thank the U.K. Medical Research Council for their support of this research. Dr. Sarah Curran is a Wellcome Trust Training Fellow.

ADDRESSES AND AFFILIATIONS

Social, Genetic and Developmental Psychiatry Research Centre, Institute of Psychiatry, London, United Kingdom. Correspondence: Philip J. Asherson, Social, Genetic and Developmental Psychiatry Research Centre, Institute of Psychiatry, De Crespigny Park, Denmark Hill, London SE5 8AF, United Kingdom.

REFERENCES

Alarcon, M., Plomin, R., Fulker, D. W., et al. (1998). Multivariate path analysis of specific cognitive abilities data at 12 years of age in the Colorado adoption project. *Behavior Genetics*, *28*, 255–264.

American Psychiatric Association (1994). *Diagnostic and Statistical Manual of Mental Disorders* (4th ed.) (DSM-IV). Washington, D.C.: APA.

Anon. (1999). SNP attacks on complex traits (editorial). *Nature Genetics*, *20*, 3. [CrossRef]

Asherson, P., Mant, R., Williams, N., et al. (1998). A study of chromosome 4p markers and dopamine D5 receptor gene in schizophrenia and bipolar disorder. *Molecular Psychiatry*, *3*, 310–320. [CrossRef] [Medline]

Auranen, M., Nieminen, T., Majuri, S., et al. (2000). Analysis of autism susceptibility gene loci on chromosomes 1p, 4p, 6q, 7q, 13q, 15q, 16p, 17q, 19q and 22q in Finnish multiplex families. *Molecular Psychiatry*, *5*, 320–322.

Bailey, A., Palferman, S., Heavey, L., et al. (1998). Autism: the phenotype in relatives. *Journal of Autism and Developmental Disorders*, *28*, 369–392.

Barr, C. L., Wigg, K. G., Feng, Y., et al. (2000). Attention-deficit hyperactivity disorder and the gene for the dopamine D5 receptor. *Molecular Psychiatry*, *5*, 548–551.

Barrett, S., Beck, J. C., Bernier, R., et al. (1999). An autosomal genomic screen for autism. Collaborative linkage study of autism. *American Journal of Medical Genetics*, *88*, 609–615.

Biederman, J., Faraone, S. V., Keenan, K., et al. (1990). Family-genetic and psychosocial risk factors in DSM-III attention deficit disorder. *Journal of the American Academy of Child and Adolescent Psychiatry*, *29*, 526–533.

Biederman, J., Faraone, S. V., Keenan, K., et al. (1992). Further evidence for family-genetic risk factors in attention deficit hyperactivity disorder: patterns of comorbidity in probands and relatives in psychiatrically and pediatrically referred samples. *Archives of General Psychiatry*, *49*, 728–738.

Bisgaard, M. L., Eiberg, H. & Moller, N. (1987). Dyslexia and chromosome 15 heteromorphism: negative lod score in a Danish material. *Clinical Genetics*, *32*, 118–119. [Medline]

Blackwood, D. H. R., He, L., Morris, S. W., et al. (1996). A locus for bipolar affective disorder on chromosome 4p. *Nature Genetics*, *12*, 427–430. [Medline]

Cantwell, D. P. (1972). Psychiatric illness in families of hyperactive children. *Archives of General Psychiatry*, *27*, 728–738.

Cardon, L. R., Smith, S. D., Fulker, D. W., et al. (1994). Quantitative trait locus for reading disability on chromosome 6. *Science*, *266*, 276–279. [Medline]

Chakravati, A. (1999). Population genetics: making sense out of sequence. *Nature Genetics*, *21*, 56–60. [CrossRef] [Medline]

Collier, D. A., Curran, S. & Asherson, P. (2000). Mission: not impossible? Candidate gene studies in child psychiatric disorders. *Molecular Psychiatry*, *5*, 457–460. [CrossRef] [Medline]

Craddock, N. & Owen, M. J. (1996). Modern molecular genetic approaches to psychiatric disease. *British Medical Bulletin*, *52*, 434–452. [Abstract]

Craig, I. W., McClay, J., Plomin, R., et al. (2000). Chasing behavior genes into the next millenium. *Tibtech*, *18*, 22–26.

Curran, S., Mill. J., Sham, P., et al. (2001a). QTL association analysis of the DRD4 exon 3 VNTR polymorphism in a population sample of children screened with a parent rating scale for ADHD symptoms. *American Journal of Medical Genetics*, in press.

Curran, S., Mill. J., Tahir, E., et al. (2001b). Association study of a dopamine transporter polymorphism and attention deficit hyperactivity disorder in UK and Turkish samples. *Molecular Psychiatry*, in press.

Dale, P. S., Simonoff, E., Bishop, D. V. M., et al. (1998). Genetic influence on language delay in two-year-old children. *Nature America*, *1–4*, 324–328.

Daly, G., Hawi, Z., Fitzgerald, M., et al. (1999). Mapping susceptibility loci in attention deficit hyperactivity disorder: preferential transmission of parental alleles at DATI, DBH and DRD5 to affected children. *Molecular Psychiatry*, *4*, 192–196.

Daniels, J., Holmans, P., Williams, N., et al. (1998). A simple method for analyzing microsatellite allele image patterns generated from DNA pools and its application to allelic association studies. *American Journal of Human Genetics*, *62*, 1189–1197.

DeFries, J. C. & Fulker, D. W. (1985). Multiple regression analysis of twin data. *Behavior Genetics*, *15*, 467–473.

DeFries, J. C. & Fulker, D. W. (1988). Multiple regression analysis of twin data: etiology of deviant scores versus individual differences. *Acta Geneticae Medicae et Gemellologiae*, *37*, 205–216.

DeFries, J. C., & Fulker, D. W. & LaBuda, M. C. (1987). Evidence for a genetic aetiology in reading disability of twins. *Nature*, *329*, 537–539.

Ewald, H., Degn, B., Mors, O., et al. (1998). Support for the possible locus on chromosome 4p16 for bipolar affective disorder. *Molecular Psychiatry*, 3, 442–448.

Falk, C. T. & Rubinstein, P. (1987). Haplotype relative risks: an easy reliable way to construct a proper control sample for risk calculations. *Annals of Human Genetics*, *51*, 227–233.

Faraone, S. V., Doyle, A. E., Mick, E., et al. (2001). Meta-analysis of the association between the dopamine D4 gene 7-repeat allele and attention deficit hyperactivity disorder. *American Journal of Medical Genetics*, in press.

Fisher, S. E., Marlow, A. J., Lamb, J., et al. (1999). A quantitative-trait locus on chromosome 6p influences different aspects of developmental dyslexia. *American Journal of Human Genetics*, *64*, 146–156.

Fulker, D. W. & Cherny, S. S. (1996). An improved multipoint sib-pair analysis of quantitative traits. *Behavior Genetics*, *26*, 527–532.

Fulker, D. W. & Cherny, S. S. & Cardon, L. R. (1995). Multipoint interval mapping of quantitative trait loci, using sib pairs. *American Journal of Human Genetics*, *56*, 1224–1233.

Fulker, D. W. & Cherny, S. S., Sham, P. C., et al. (1999). Combined linkage and association sib-pair analysis for quantitative traits. *American Journal of Human Genetics*, *64*, 259–267.

Gayan, J., Smith, S. D., Cherney, S. S., et al. (1999). Quantitative-trait locus for specific language and reading deficits on chromosome 6p. *American Journal of Human Genetics, 64*, 157–164.

Gillis, J. J., Gilger, J. W., Pennington, B. F., et al. (1992). Attention deficit disorder in reading-disabled twins: evidence for a genetic aetiology. *Journal of Abnormal Child Psychology*, *20*, 303–315.

Griffin, T. J., Hall, J. G., Prudent, J. R., et al. (1999). Direct genetic analysis by matrix-assisted laser desorption/ionization mass spectrometry. *Proceedings of the National Academy of Sciences of the USA*, *96*, 6301–6306.

Grigorenko, E. L., Wood, F. B., Meyer, M. S., et al. (1997). Susceptibility loci for distinct components of developmental dyslexia on chromosomes 6 and 15. *American Journal of Human Genetics*, *60*, 27–39.

Gross-Glenn, K., Duara, R., Barker, W. W., et al. (1991). Positron-emission tomographic studies during serial word-reading by normal and dyslexic adults. *Journal of Clinical and Experimental Neuropsychology*, *13*, 531–544.

Haseman, J. K. & Elston, R. (1972). The investigation of linkage between a quantitative trait and a marker locus. *Behavior Genetics*, *2*, 3–19.

International Molecular Genetic Study of Autism Consortium (1998). A full genome screen for autism with evidence for linkage to a region on chromosome 7q. *Human Molecular Genetics*, *7*, 571–578.

International SNP Map Working Group (2001). A map of human genome sequence variation containing 1.42 million single nucleotide polymorphisms. *Nature*, *409*, 928–932.

Kruglyak, L. & Lander, E. S. (1995). Complete multipoint sib-pair analysis of qualitative and quantitative traits. *American Journal of Human Genetics*, *57*, 439–454.

Kruglyak, L. & Nickerson, D. A. (2001). Variation is the spice of life. *Nature Genetics*, *27*, 234–236.

Lamb, J. A., Moore, J., Bailey, A., et al. (2000). Autism: recent molecular genetic advances. *Human Molecular Genetics*, *9*, 861–868.

Landegren, U., Nilsson, M. & Kwok, P. Y. (1998). Reading bits of genetic information: methods for single-nucleotide polymorphism analysis. *Genome Research*, *8*, 769–776.

Lander, E. (1999). Array of hope. *Nature Genetics*, *21* (suppl.), 3–4.

Lander, E. & Kruglyak, L. (1995). Genetic dissection of complex traits: guidelines for interpreting and reporting linkage results. *Nature Genetics*, *11*, 241–247.

Le Couteur, A., Rutter, M., Lord, C., et al. (1989). Autism diagnostic interview: a standardized investigator-based instrument. *Journal of Autism Developmental Disorders*, *19*, 363–387.

Lord, C., Rutter, M., Goode, S., et al. (1989). Autism diagnostic observation schedule: a standardized observation of communicative and social behavior. *Journal of Autism and Developmental Disorders*, *19*, 185–212.

Maestrini, E., Marlow, A. J., Weeks, D. E., et al. (1998). Molecular genetic investigations of autism. *Journal of Autism and Developmental Disorders*, *28*, 427–437.

McGuffin, P., Owen, M. J., O'Donovan, M. C., et al. (1994). *Seminars in Psychiatric Genetics*. London: Gaskell.

Mill, J., Curran, S., Kent, L., et al. (2001). Attention deficit hyperactivity disorder (ADHD) and the dopamine D4 receptor gene: evidence of association but no linkage in a UK sample. *Molecular Psychiatry*, in press.

Morris, D. W., Robinson, L., Turic, D., et al. (2000). Family-based association mapping provides evidence for a gene for reading disability on chromosome 15q. *Human Molecular Genetics*, *9*, 843–848. [Abstract/Free Full Text]

O'Donovan, M. C. & Owen, M. J. (1999). Candidate-gene association studies of schizophrenia. *American Journal of Human Genetics*, *65*, 587–592. [CrossRef] [Medline]

Phillipe, A., Martinez, M., Guilloud-Bataille, M., et al. (1999). Genome-wide scan for autism susceptibility genes. Paris Autism Research International Sibpair Study. *Human Molecular Genetics*, *8*, 805–812. [Abstract/Free Full Text]

Plomin, R., McClearn, G. E. & Gora-Maslak, G. (1991). Quantitative trait loci and psychopharmacology. *Journal of Psychopharmacology*, *5*, 1–9.

Plomin, R., Owen, M. J. & McGuffin, P. (1994). The genetic basis of complex human behaviors. *Science*, *264*, 1733–1739.

Plomin, R., DeFries, J. C., McClearn, G. E., et al. (2000). *Behavioral Genetics* (4th ed.). New York: Worth Freeman.

Purcell, S., Cherney, S. S., Hewitt, J. K., et al. (2001) Optimal sibship selection for genotyping in QTL Linkage Analysis. *Human Heridity*, in press.

Rabin, M., Wen, X. L., Hepburn, M., et al. (1993). Suggestive linkage of developmental dyslexia to chromosome I p34–p36. *Lancet*, *342*, 178.

Risch, N. (2000) Searching for genetic determinants in the new millennium. *Nature*, *405*, 847–856.

Risch, N. & Merikangas, K. (1996). The future of genetic studies of complex human diseases. *Science*, *273*, 1516–1517.

Risch, N. & Zhang, H. (1995). Extreme discordant sib pairs for mapping quantitative trait loci in humans. *Science*, *268*, 1584–1589.

Risch, N., Spiker, D., Lotspeich, L., et al. (1999). A genomic screen of autism: evidence for a multilocus etiology. *American Journal of Human Genetics*, *65*, 493–507.

Rowe, D. C., Stever, C., Giedinghagen, L. N., et al. (1998). Dopamine DRD4 receptor polymorphism and attention deficit hyperactivity disorder. *Molecular Psychiatry*, *3*, 419–426.

Rutter, M., Silberg, J., O'Connor, T., et al. (1999a). Genetics and child psychiatry: I. Advances in quantitative and molecular genetics. *Journal of Child Psychology and Psychiatry and Allied Disciplines*, *40*, 3–18.

Rutter, M., Silberg, J., O'Connor, T., et al. (1999b). Genetics and child psychiatry: II. Empirical research findings. *Journal of Child Psychology and Psychiatry and Allied Disciplines*, *40*, 19–55.

Smalley, S. L., Bailey, J. N., Palmer, C. G., et al. (1998). Evidence that the dopamine D4 receptor is a susceptibility gene in attention deficit hyperactivity disorder. *Molecular Psychiatry*, *3*, 427–430.

Smith, S. D., Kimberling, W. J., Pennington, B. F., et al. (1983). Specific reading disability: identification of an inherited form through linkage analysis. *Science*, *219*, 4590, 1345–1347.

Spielman, R. S. & Ewens, W. J. (1996). The TDT and other family-based tests for linkage disequilibrium and association. *American Journal of Human Genetics*, *59*, 983–989.

Stevenson, J., Pennington, B. F., Gilger, J. W., et al. (1993). Hyperactivity and spelling disability: testing for shared genetic aetiology. *Journal of Child Psychology and Psychiatry and Allied Disciplines*, *34*, 1137–1152.

Sunohara, G. A., Roberts, W. Malone, M., et al. (2000). Linkage of the dopamine D4 receptor gene and attention-deficit/hyperactivity disorder. *Journal of the American Academy of Child and Adolescent Psychiatry*, *39*, 537–542.

Swanson, J. M., Sunohara, G. A., Kennedy, J. L., et al. (1998). Association of the dopamine receptor D4 (DRD4) gene with a refined phenotype of attention deficit hyperactivity disorder (ADHD): a family-based approach. *Molecular Psychiatry*, *3*, 38–41. [CrossRef] [Medline]

Tahir, E., Yazgan, Y., Cirakoglu, B., et al. (2000). Association and linkage of DRD4 and DRD5 with attention deficit hyperactivity disorder (ADHD) in a sample of Turkish children. *Molecular Psychiatry*, *5*, 396–404. [CrossRef] [Medline]

Taylor, E., Chadwick, O., Heptinstall, E., et al. (1996). Hyperactivity and conduct problems as risk factors for adolescent development. *Journal of the American Academy of Child and Adolescent Psychiatry*, *35*, 1213–1226. [Medline]

Thapar, A., Holmes, J., Poulton, K., et al. (1999). Genetic basis of attention deficit and hyperactivity. *British Journal of Psychiatry*, *174*, 105–111. [Abstract]

Weber, J. L. & May, P. E. (1990). Dinucleotide repeat polymorphism at the D22S156 locus. *Nucleic Acids Research*, *18*, 6465.

World Health Organization (1992). *Tenth Revision of the International Classification of Diseases and Related Health Problems* (ICD-10). Geneva: WHO.

8

Functional Neuroanatomy of Visuospatial Working Memory in Fragile X Syndrome: Relation to Behavioral and Molecular Measures

Hower Kwon, Vinod Menon, Stephan Eliez, Ilana S. Warsofsky, Christopher D. White, Jennifer Dyer-Friedman, Annette K. Taylor, Gary H. Glover, and Allan L. Reiss

Objective: *Fragile X syndrome is a neurogenetic disorder that is the most common known heritable cause of neurodevelopmental disability. This study examined the neural substrates of working memory in female subjects with fragile X syndrome. Possible correlations among behavioral measures, brain activation, and the FMR1 gene product (FMRP expression), as well as between IQ and behavioral measures, were investigated.* ***Method:*** *Functional magnetic resonance imaging was used to examine visuospatial working memory in 10 female subjects with fragile X syndrome and 15 typically developing female subjects (ages 10 to 23 years). Subjects performed standard 1-back and 2-back visuospatial working memory tasks. Brain activation was examined in four regions of the cortex known to play a critical role in visuospatial working memory. Correlations between behavioral, neuroimaging, and molecular measures were examined.* ***Results:*** *Relative to the comparison group, subjects with fragile X syndrome performed significantly worse on the 2-back task but not on the 1-back task. In a region-of-interest analysis focused on the inferior frontal gyrus, middle frontal gyrus, superior parietal lobule, and supramarginal gyrus, comparison subjects showed significantly increased brain activation between the 1-back and 2-back tasks, but subjects with fragile X syndrome showed no change in activation between the two tasks. Significant correlations were found in comparison subjects between activation in the frontal and parietal regions and the rate of correct responses on the 2-back task, but not on the 1-back task. In subjects with fragile*

X syndrome, significant correlations were found during the 2-back task between FMRP expression and activation in the right inferior and bilateral middle frontal gyri and the bilateral supramarginal gyri. ***Conclusions:*** *Subjects with fragile X syndrome are unable to modulate activation in the prefrontal and parietal cortex in response to an increasing working memory load, and these deficits are related to a lower level of FMRP expression in fragile X syndrome subjects than in normal comparison subjects. The observed correlations between biological markers and brain activation provide new evidence for links between gene expression and cognition.*

INTRODUCTION

Fragile X syndrome is the most common inherited cause of neurodevelopmental disability, occurring at a frequency of approximately one in every 2,000 to 4,000 live births.[1] The syndrome arises from disruption in expression of the FMR1 gene, which is most commonly caused by expansion of a CGG repeat stretch in the gene, with resultant methylation and silencing of expression. The absence of the FMR1 gene product (FMRP) in neurons is associated with abnormal morphology of dendritic spines and a reduction in the length of synapses in the cortex.[2,3] The neuropsychological profile of fragile X syndrome is notable for mental retardation, as well as difficulties in visual memory and perception, mental manipulation of visuospatial relationships among objects, visual-motor coordination, processing of sequential information, and executive function.[4–6] In this study, we used a working memory task to investigate deficits in higher-order cognition in subjects with fragile X syndrome. Impairment in visuospatial working memory may be an important contributing factor to the behavioral profile of people with fragile X syndrome. For example, impairment in the processing and retention of information in social situations, an area of cognition known to be heavily dependent on nonverbal skills, may be implicated in difficulties known to occur in subjects with fragile X syndrome, such as poor social relatedness, avoidance, and anxiety.[7–9]

Working memory is the ability to hold and manipulate information online in the brain.[10–12] The component processes involved in working memory —encoding, rehearsal, storage, and executive processes on the contents of stored memory—represent key cognitive operations of the human brain. Neurophysiological studies have suggested that the prefrontal cortex plays a critical role in working memory,[13–16] although other brain regions, notably the parietal cortex, also play an important role.[17,18] Positron emission tomography (PET) and functional magnetic resonance imaging (fMRI) studies have investigated the neural substrates of visuospatial working memory and its components, and most studies have shown significant prefrontal cortex as well as parietal cortex involvement.[19–23]

Although there are a few behavioral and functional neuroimaging studies involving subjects with fragile X syndrome,[24–26] we are aware of no studies that have specifically examined working memory in this population, even by using behavioral measures. In this study, we investigated the neural substrates of working memory in female subjects with fragile X syndrome. Given that subjects with fragile X syndrome show significant deficits in visuospatial cognition as well as in executive function, we hypothesized that they would show significant impairment in performance on visuospatial 1-back and 2-back working memory tasks. We also hypothesized that they would show significant deficits in activation in brain regions known to be involved in working memory—particularly, the inferior and middle frontal gyri, the dorsolateral prefrontal cortex, and the parietal cortex. Whole-brain voxel-by-voxel analyses were utilized to investigate differences in areas outside the regions of interest. We then examined possible correlations among behavioral measures, brain activation, and FMRP expression, as well as between IQ and behavioral measures.

METHOD

Subjects, Diagnosis, and Molecular Measures

Ten female subjects with a diagnosis of fragile X syndrome (mean age = 17.2 years, *SD* = 4.5, range = 10 to 23) were recruited from throughout the United States (Table 8.1). Subjects were recruited through advertisements in national newsletters for fragile X syndrome patients and their caregivers, through prior clinical contacts, and through contact at national conferences. After complete description of the study to the subjects and caregivers, written informed consent was obtained. Fifteen female comparison subjects also participated (mean age = 15.1 years, *SD* = 4.6, range = 8 to 22). The diagnosis of fragile X syndrome (presence of an FMR1 full mutation) was confirmed by DNA analysis. Standard Southern blot and polymerase chain reaction analyses were performed, followed by FMR1-specific probe hybridization.[27] The CGG repeat number was calculated from the Southern blot autoradiogram images. A PhosphorImager (Molecular Dynamics, Inc., Sunnyvale, Calif.) was used to quantitate the radioactive intensity of the normal methylated and unmethylated bands of each sample on the Southern blot. The FMR1 gene activation ratio, the intensity of the normal unmethylated band divided by the sum of the intensities of both the normal unmethylated and methylated bands, was calculated.[28] The FMR1 gene activation ratio represents the proportion of

TABLE 8.1
Demographic and Neuropsychological Characteristics of Female Subjects with Fragile X Syndrome and Healthy Comparision Subjects in a Study of Visuopatial Working Memory

	Subjects With Fragile X Syndrome (N = 10)			Comparison Subjects (N = 15)			Analysis		
Characteristics	Mean	SD	Range	Mean	SD	Range	t	df	p
Age (years)	17.23	4.49	10.2–22.7	15.05	4.58	7.66–21.6	1.17	23	0.25
IQ									
Full-scale	84	12	65–108	117	13	93–137	6.46	23	<0.001
Verbal	86	13	66–111	115	12	94–134	5.67	23	<0.001
Performance	85	13	62–104	117	13	93–132	6.09	23	<0.001
Judgment of Line Orientation score	11.1	9.6	0.0–24.0	25.3	4.0	18.0–30.0	4.23	22	<0.001
Woodcock-Johnson spatial reasoning test score	41.0	7.7	31.0–53.0	61.9	7.3	50.0–75.0	6.37	20	<0.001

the normal (nonmutant) FMR1 gene that is on the active X chromosome and reflects the proportion of cells that can express FMRP. FMRP expression was ascertained by calculating the percentage of peripheral lymphocytes containing FMRP by using immunostaining techniques.[29]

Neuropsychological Assessment

IQ was determined by using the Wechsler intelligence scales. The WISC-III[30] was administered to those under age 17 years, and the WAIS-III[31] was administered to those over age 17 years. Spatial reasoning and recognition were assessed by using the Woodcock-Johnson spatial reasoning test[32] and the Judgment of Line Orientation test.[33]

Experimental Design

The visuospatial 1-back and 2-back working memory tasks consisted of rest, experimental (E), and control (C) epochs in the following order: rest-E-C-E-C-E-C-rest-E-C-E-C-E-C-rest. Thus, there were three rest epochs, six experimental epochs, and six control epochs in each task. Each rest epoch was 30 seconds long, during which subjects passively viewed a blank screen. Experimental epochs began with a 4-second display of the instructions, "Push for 1 Back," in the 1-back task, and "Push for 2 Back," in the 2-back task. Control epochs began with a 4-second display of the instructions, "Push for Center." Each control and experimental epoch consisted of 16 stimuli presented for 500 millisecond(msec) each, with a 1,500-millisecond interstimulus interval. The stimulus was the letter "O" presented in one of nine distinct visuospatial locations in a 3 × 3 matrix. In the 1-back task, the subject was instructed to respond if the stimulus was in the same location as in the previous trial. In the 2-back task, the subject was instructed to respond if the stimulus was in the same location as in two trials back. In the control task, the subject was instructed to respond if the stimulus was in the center position.

Behavioral Data Analysis

The rate of correct responses refers to the percentage of stimulus trials in which the subject responded correctly, either with an appropriate button push or an appropriate inhibition. The miss rate is the percentage of trials in which the subject failed to respond appropriately. The false alarm rate is the percentage of stimuli to which the subject responded with a button push when no response was needed. Subjects' reaction times also were measured.

fMRI Acquisition

Images were acquired on a 1.5-T GE Signa scanner with Echospeed gradients (General Electric Medical Systems, Milwaukee) by using a custom-built whole-head coil that provides a 50% advantage in signal-to-noise ratio over that provided by the standard GE coil.[34] Eighteen axial slices (6 mm thick, 1 mm skip) parallel to the anterior and posterior commissures covering the whole brain were imaged with a temporal resolution of 2 seconds by using a T_{2*}-weighted, gradient echo, spiral pulse sequence (TR = 2000 msec, TE = 40 msec, flip angle = 89° and 1 interleave).[35] The field of view was 240 mm, and the effective in-plane spatial resolution was 4.35 mm. To aid in localization of functional data, a high-resolution T_1-weighted, spoiled gradient recalled echo acquisition in the steady state, three-dimensional MRI sequence with the following parameters was used: TR = 35 msec, TE = 6 msec, flip angle = 45°, 24 cm field of view, 124 slices in coronal plane, 256 × 192 matrix, acquired resolution = 1.5 × 0.9 × 1.2 mm. On several scans of subjects with fragile X syndrome, a faster protocol was utilized to decrease time of acquisition of the spoiled gradient recalled echo acquisition in the steady state image, with TR = 11 msec, TE = 2 msec, and flip angle = 15°. The images were reconstructed as a 124 × 256 × 256 matrix with a 1.5 × 0.9 × 0.9 mm spatial resolution.

The task was programmed by using PsyScope[36] on a Macintosh (Sunnyvale, Calif.) computer. The initiation of the scan and the task was synchronized by using a TTL (transistor–transistor logic) pulse delivered to the scanner timing microprocessor board from a "CMU Button Box" microprocessor (http://psyscope.psy.cmu.edu) connected to the Macintosh computer. The stimuli were presented visually at the center of a screen by using a custom-built, magnet-compatible projection system (Resonance Technology, Los Angeles).

Image Preprocessing

The images were reconstructed, by using inverse Fourier transform, for each of the 261 time points into 64 × 64 × 18 image matrices (voxel size: 3.75 × 3.75 × 7 mm). The fMRI data were preprocessed by using statistical parametric mapping (SPM 99) software (Wellcome Department of Cognitive Neurology, Institute of Neurology, University College, London). The images were corrected for movement by using least-square minimization without higher-order corrections for spin history and were normalized to stereotaxic Talairach coordinates.[37] The images were then resampled every 2 mm by using sinc interpolation and smoothed with a 4-mm Gaussian kernel to decrease spatial noise.

Statistical Analysis

Statistical analysis was performed on individual and group data by using the general linear model and the theory of Gaussian random fields as implemented in SPM 99. This method takes advantage of multivariate regression analysis and corrects for temporal and spatial autocorrelations in the fMRI data.[38]

In the first step, a within-subject procedure was used to model all the effects of interest, covariates, and nuisance variables for each subject. The individual subject models were identical across subjects (i.e., a balanced design was used). Confounding effects of fluctuations in global mean were removed by proportional scaling where, for each time point, each voxel was scaled by the global mean at that time point. Low-frequency noise was removed with a high-pass filter (0.5 cycles/minute) applied to the fMRI time series at each voxel. A temporal smoothing function (Gaussian kernel corresponding to dispersion of 8 seconds) was applied to the fMRI time series to enhance the temporal signal-to-noise ratio. We then defined the effects of interest for each subject with the relevant contrasts of the parameter estimates. For each of these contrasts, a corresponding contrast image was also generated. Voxel-wise t statistics were normalized to z scores to provide a statistical measure of activation that is independent of size of the study group. Finally, to determine the presence of significant clusters of activation, the joint expected probability distribution of the height and extent of the z scores (39), with height ($z > 2.33$, $p < 0.01$, with corrected p values) and extent ($p < 0.05$) thresholds, was used to correct for spatial correlations in the data.

Whole brain analysis

The aim of this analysis was to determine which brain regions showed significant activation for each main effect and interaction of interest. The group analysis was performed by using a random-effects model with a two-stage hierarchical procedure. This model estimates the error variance for each condition of interest across subjects, rather than across scans,[40] and therefore provides a stronger generalization to the population. This analysis consisted of two steps. In the first step, contrast images for each subject and each effect of interest were generated, as described above. In the second step, these contrast images were compared by using a general linear model analysis to determine appropriate t statistics. Thus, for example, with one contrast image per subject, reflecting activation during the 2-back experimental condition contrasted with the control condition, a one-way t test was used to determine group activation for that contrast. Finally, the t statistics were normalized to z scores, and significant clusters of activation were determined by using the joint expected probability distribution of height and extent of z scores, with height ($z > 2.33$, $p < 0.01$) and extent ($p < 0.05$) thresholds.

Region-of-interest analysis

The aim of this analysis was to investigate the profile of regional task-related differences in activation. The group analysis was conducted by using z scores derived from the individual subject analysis, as described above. The percentage of voxels, in each region of interest, with $z > 2.33$ ($p < 0.01$) was determined for each relevant contrast and entered into an analysis of variance (ANOVA). A four-way repeated measures ANOVA with the factors region of interest (inferior frontal gyrus, middle frontal gyrus, superior parietal lobule, supramarginal gyrus), hemisphere (left, right), task (1-back, 2-back), and condition (experimental, control) was done. A standard analysis framework[41] was used to interpret interactions, simple effects, and main effects. An alpha level for significance of $p < 0.05$ (two-tailed) was used.

Regions of Interest

Regions of interest were demarcated separately in the left and right hemispheres from the average T_1-weighted Talairach normalized images.

Inferior frontal gyrus. By using a surface rendering of the average brain, the anterior border was identified by the junction of the lateral orbital sulcus and inferior frontal sulcus. The posterior border was defined by the precentral sulcus. The superior border was defined by the inferior frontal sulcus. The inferior border was defined by the lateral orbital sulcus until it could no longer be visualized. For the most posterior part of the inferior frontal gyrus, the inferior border was the horizontal ramus of the lateral fissure. Medially, the border was defined by a straight line joining the deepest point of the inferior frontal sulci and the deepest point of the lateral orbital sulci. These definitions closely followed surface sulci demarcated by Duvernoy[42] and Ono et al.[43]

Middle frontal gyrus. The superior frontal sulcus defined the medial boundary for this region. The frontomarginal sulcus and the inferior frontal sulcus defined the lateral boundary. At more posterior slices where the inferior frontal sulcus disappears, the superior precentral sulcus was used as the lateral boundary. The posterior boundary for this region was the precentral gyrus.

Parietal cortex. Information from triplanar views was used to delineate the parietal lobe and parcel the lobe into the superior parietal lobule, supramarginal gyrus, and angular gyrus. The parietal lobe was delineated by first marking the postcentral sulcus as its anterior border. The inferior border was the sylvian fissure until it was no longer identifiable in the coronal section progressing in the anterior to posterior direction. At this point, the inferior and medial borders were defined by the parallel sulcus and the interhemispheric fissure, respectively. Next, in the midsagittal view, a line parallel to the parieto-occipital fissure was identified and linearly interpolated to the parieto-occipital notch on the lateral surface. This defined the posterior border of the parietal lobe. The parietal lobe was then parceled by using neuroanatomical landmarks identified in the axial plane. The intraparietal sulcus was used to demarcate the superior parietal lobule from the supramarginal gyrus and angular gyrus. The intraparietal sulcus and the ascending posterior segment of the parallel sulcus were then used to separate the supramarginal gyrus and angular gyrus.

Data Analysis

IQ data and results on the Woodcock-Johnson spatial reasoning test and the Judgment of Line Orientation test were compared between groups by using t tests and an alpha level of 0.05. Correct and incorrect response rates and reaction times on the visuospatial working memory tasks were compared by using a two-by-two factorial analysis of covariance (ANCOVA) with the factors diagnosis, task (1-back versus 2-back), and condition (experimental versus control); an alpha level of 0.05; and full-scale IQ as a nuisance covariate. Pearson product-moment correlation was used to analyze the relationship between performance on the working memory tasks and functional brain activation. Spearman correlations were also performed when data were suspected of being nonnormalized.

RESULTS

Neuropsychological Measures

The mean full-scale IQ was 84 for the fragile X syndrome group and 117 for the comparison group, a significant difference (Table 8.1). Group differences on verbal IQ and performance IQ were also significant (Table 8.1). Significant group differences of similar magnitude were also observed on the Woodcock-Johnson spatial reasoning test and the Judgment of Line Orientation test (Table 8.1).

Behavioral Task Analysis

Because comparison and fragile X syndrome groups differed significantly in IQ, full-scale IQ was used as a covariate in all behavioral analyses described below. There was a statistically significant correlation between full-scale IQ and performance on the experimental condition of the 2-back task for the combined groups ($r = 0.78$, $df = 21$, $p < 0.001$) (Figure 8.1). When data for

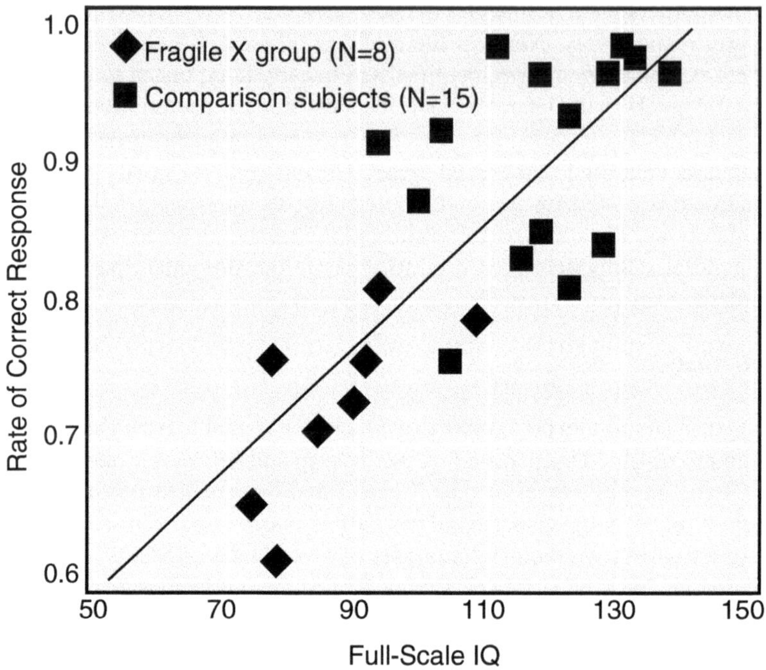

Figure 8.1. Correlation Betewen Full-Scale IQ and Accuracy in the Experimental Condition of a 2-Back Visuospatial Working Memory Task[a] of Female Subjects with Fragile X Syndrome and Healthy Comparison Subjects.

[a] Subjects were presented with a series of 3 × 3 matrices with nine distinct visuospatial locations. Subjects were instructed to respond if the stimulus was in the same location as two trials back.

each group were examined separately, no significant correlation was seen in either the fragile X syndrome group ($r = 0.70$, $df = 7$, $p = 0.051$) or the comparison group ($r = 0.35$, $df = 14$, $p = 0.19$), although the former correlation approached significance. Experimental behavioral data were successfully collected from all comparison subjects and from 8 of the 10 subjects with fragile X syndrome

The percentages of correct responses on the visuospatial working memory tasks in the two groups were compared by using ANCOVA (Table 8.2). Main effects of task ($F = 26.5$, $df = 1, 21$, $p < 0.0001$) and condition ($F = 106.4$, $df = 1, 21$, $p < 0.0001$) were observed, but a main effect of diagnosis was not ($F = 0.6$, $df = 1, 20$, $p = 0.44$). There was a significant interaction of diagnosis, task, and condition ($F = 8.9$, $df = 1, 21$, $p < 0.008$). A separate two-way ANCOVA examining the interaction of diagnosis and task was not significant for the control condition ($F = 0.2$, $df = 1, 21$, $p < 0.70$) but was significant for the experimental condition (Figure 8.2). Planned comparisons of this two-way

TABLE 8.2

Performance on 1-Back and 2-Back Visuospatial Working Memory Tasks of Female Subjects with Fragile X Syndrome and Healthy Comparison Subjects

	Subjects With Fragile X Syndrome (N = 8)								Comparison Subjects (N = 15)							
	% Correct[b]		% Missed[c]		% False Alarms[d]		Reaction Time (msec)		% Correct[b]		% Missed[c]		% False Alarms[d]		Reaction Time (msec)	
Task and Condition[a]	Mean	SD	Mean	SD	Mean	SD	Mean	SD	Mean	SD	Mean	SD	Mean	SD	Mean	SD
1-back task																
Control condition	98	2	2	2	1	1	630	177	98	2	1	1	1	2	654	147
Experimental condition	86	11	6	5	8	8	714	195	95	4	4	3	2	3	684	150
2-back task																
Control condition	97	3	2	2	1	1	642	179	98	2	1	2	0	1	629	113
Experimental condition	73	7	15	3	13	8	727	190	91	7	6	5	3	5	725	215

[a]Subjects were presented with a series of 3 x 3 matrices with nine distinct visuospatial locations. In the experimental condition, subjects were instructed to respond if the stimulus was in the same location as in the previous trial for the 1-back task or in two trials back for the 2-back task. In the control condition, subjects were instructed to respond if the stimulus was in the center location.

[b]Percentage of stimulus trials in which the subject responded or inhibited response appropriately.

[c]Percentage of stimulus trials in which the subject failed to respond appropriately.

[d]Percentage of stimulus trials in which the subject responded when response should have been inhibited.

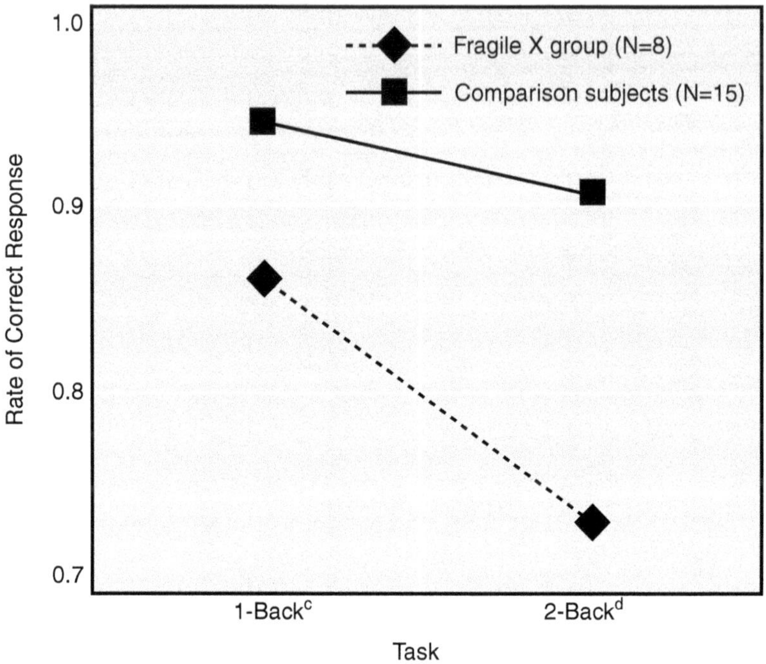

Figure 8.2. Accuracy in Experimental Conditions of 1-Back and 2-Back Visuospatial Working Memory Tasks[a] of Female Subjects with Fragile X Syndrome and Healthy Comparison Subjects.[b]

[a] Subjects were presented with a series of 3 x 3 matrices with nine distinct visuospatial locations. Subjects were instructed to respond if the stimulus was in the same location as in the previous trial for the 1-back task or in two trials back for the 2-back task.

[b] Significant interaction of diagnosis and task, covaried by full-scale IQ (F = 9.8, df = 1, 21, p < 0.005).

[c] Significant difference between groups (F = 6.9, df = 1, 21, $p < 0.02$).

[d] Significant difference between groups (F = 32.7, df = 1, 21, $p < 0.0001$).

interaction showed that comparison subjects did not differ significantly in performance on the 2-back versus the 1-back task (91% correct responses on 2-back task vs. 95% on the 1-back task) ($F = 4.2$, $df = 1, 21$, $p = 0.052$), whereas subjects with fragile X syndrome performed significantly worse on the 2-back task than on the 1-back task (73% correct responses on 2-back task versus 86% on the 1-back task) ($F = 28.9$, $df = 1, 21$, $p < 0.0001$). Moreover, subjects with fragile X syndrome performed worse than comparison group subjects on the experimental conditions of both tasks, with the difference statistically significant on both tasks (Figure 8.2).

Analysis of false alarms showed main effects of task ($F = 24.5$, $df = 1, 21$, $p < 0.0001$) and condition ($F = 26.2$, $df = 1, 21$, $p < 0.0001$) but not of diagnosis ($F < 0.1$, $df = 1, 20$, $p = 0.92$). The two-way interaction of diagnosis and task was significant ($F = 10.9$, $df = 1, 21$, $p < 0.004$). Subjects with fragile X syndrome had significantly higher false alarm rates ($F = 26.1$, $df = 1, 21$, $p < 0.0001$) in the 2-back versus the 1-back task. The comparison subjects showed no difference ($F = 1.9$, $df = 1, 21$, $p = 0.18$) in false alarms between the tasks. No significant three-way interaction (diagnosis-by-task-by-condition) was observed ($F = 4.2$, $df = 1, 21$, $p = 0.053$). For reaction time, there were no significant interactions of diagnosis with any of the factors. There was no main effect of diagnosis ($F = 0.4$, $df = 1, 20$, $p = 0.56$). A main effect of condition was observed ($F = 18.6$, $df = 1, 21$, $p < 0.0003$).

Brain Activation: Whole Brain Analysis

Comparison subjects. In the 1-back experimental condition compared to the control condition, comparison subjects showed significant activation in the right middle frontal gyrus and superior frontal gyrus and in the left middle frontal gyrus and superior frontal gyrus (Table 8.3, Figure 8.3). In the 2-back experimental condition compared to the control condition, comparison subjects showed significant activation in the left pre-supplemental motor area, right middle frontal gyrus, right inferior frontal gyrus, right precuneus, right angular gyrus, right superior parietal lobule, right inferior parietal lobule, right supramarginal gyrus, left superior parietal lobule, left inferior parietal lobule, left middle frontal gyrus/precentral gyrus, and the right superior cerebellum bordering on the fusiform gyrus (Table 8.3, Figure 8.3). When the 1-back and 2-back tasks were directly compared, comparison group subjects showed significantly greater activation in the 2-back task in the pre-supplemental motor area, left inferior parietal lobule, left supramarginal gyrus, intraparietal sulcus, and right superior parietal lobule.

Subjects with fragile X syndrome. In the 1-back condition compared to the control condition, significant activation in subjects with fragile X syndrome was found in the right middle frontal gyrus, right superior frontal gyrus, right inferior frontal gyrus, right inferior parietal lobule, right insula, pre-supplemental motor area, left middle frontal gyrus, left superior parietal lobule, left precuneus, left inferior parietal lobule, and left angular gyrus (Table 8.3, Figure 8.3). In the 2-back condition compared to the control condition, subjects with fragile X syndrome activated the pre-supplemental motor area, right middle frontal gyrus, right inferior frontal gyrus, left superior frontal gyrus, left middle frontal gyrus, right inferior parietal lobule, right superior parietal lobule, and right supramarginal gyrus (Table 8.3, Figure 8.3). When the 1-back and 2-back tasks were directly compared, subjects with fragile X syndrome showed significantly greater activation in the 2-back task in the right superior frontal gyrus and left inferior frontal gyrus bordering on the left superior temporal gyrus.

TABLE 8.3

Brain Regions with Significant Activation During 1-Back and 2-Back Visuospatial Working Memory Tasks. Relative to a Control Condition,[a] in Healthy Comparison Subjects and Female Subjects With Fragile X Syndrome

Subject Group, Task, and Activated Regions	Number of Voxels	z Score (maximum)	p (corrected for height and extent of z score)	Talairach Coordinates of Location of Peak Activation		
				x	y	z
Comparison group (N=15)						
1-back task						
Right middle frontal gyrus (Brodmann's areas 6 and 9)	1,507	4.49	<0.001	42	6	38
Right superior frontal gyrus (Brodmann's area 6)	774	4.41	<0.001	2	22	54
Left middle frontal gyrus, superior frontal gyrus (Brodmann's areas 6 and 45)	665	3.78	<0.001	−54	24	38
2-back task						
Pre-supplemental motor area, right middle frontal gyrus (Brodmann's area 6)	4,787	4.93	<0.001	−2	32	50
Right inteior frontal gyrus and middle frontal gyrus (Brodmann's area 47)	498	4.85	0.001	36	24	−6
Right precuneus, inferior parietal lobule, angular gyrus, superior parietal lobule, supramarginal gyrus (Brodmann's areas 7 and 19): left superior parietal lobule, inferior parietal lobule (Brodmann's area 40)	6,004	4.83	<0.001	2	−64	56
Left middle frontal gyrus, precentral gyrus (Brodmann's area 6)	2,679	4.75	<0.001	−26	2	60
Right fusiform/cerebellum (Brodmann's area 40)	272	3.73	<0.04	18	−58	−12

Fragile X syndrome group (N=10)						
1-back task						
Right inferior parietal lobule (Brodmann's area 40)	324	4.92	0.002	52	-42	46
Right superior frontal gyrus, middle frontal gyrus (Brodmann's areas 10 and 8)	1,444	4.70	<0.001	28	56	4
Left superior parietal lobule, precuneus (Brodmann's area 7)	224	4.22	<0.03	−6	−66	62
Right middle frontal gyrus, superior frontal gyrus (Brodmann's area 6)	265	3.95	0.007	28	8	56
Left superior parietal lobule, interior parietal lobule, angular gyrus (Brodmann's areas 7 and 30)	241	3.85	<0.02	−42	−62	52
Right insula, middle frontal gyrus, inferior frontal gyrus (Brodmann's areas 45 and 47)	261	3.77	0.008	36	26	−2
Pre-supplemental motor area (Brodmann's area 8)	303	3.47	0.003	4	36	54
Left middle frontal gyrus – dorsolateral prefrontal cortex (Brodmann's areas 9 and 45)	295	3.40	0.003	−48	30	34
2-back task						
Pre-supplemental motor area (Brodmann's area 8)	751	5.30	0.001	0	40	40
Left middle frontal gyrus, superior frontal gyrus (Brodmann's area 6)	226	4.12	<0.04	−24	8	60
Right Inferior parietal lobule, superior parietal lobule (Brodmann's area 7)	438	4.05	<0.001	32	−62	44
Right supramarginal gyrus (Brodmann's area 40)	469	3.92	<0.001	54	−16	32
Right middle frontal gyrus (Brodmann's areas 8 and 9)	428	3.72	<0.001	30	36	42
Right middle frontal gyrus, inferior gyrus (Brodmann's areas 8 and 44)	263	3.51	0.02	34	8	30

[a]Subjects were presented with a series of 3 x 3 matrices with nine distinct visuospatial locations. In the experimental condition, subjects were instructed to respond if the stimulus was in the same location as in the previous trial for the 1-back task or in two trials back for the 2-back task. In the condition, subjects were instructed to respond if the stimulue was in the counter location.

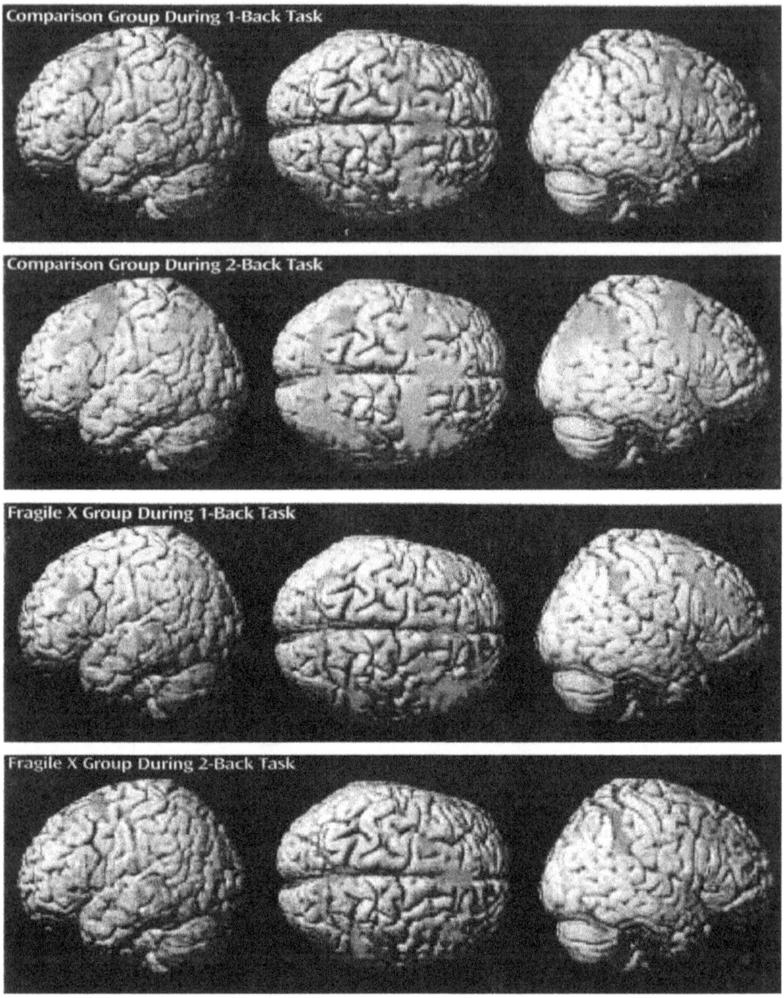

Figure 8.3. Whole-Brain Activation During 1-Back and 2-Back Working Memory Tasks, Relative to a Control Condition,[a] in Female Subjects with Fragile X Syndrome (N = 10) and Healthy Comparison Subjects (N = 15).[b]

[a] Subjects were presented with a series of 3 × 3 matrices with nine distinct visuospatial locations in each task. In the experimental condition, subjects were instructed to respond if the stimulus was in the same location as in the previous trial for the 1-back task or in two trials back for the 2-back task. In the control condition, subjects were instructed to respond if the stimulus was in the center location.

[b] Areas of significant activation for subjects groups determined by using a general linear model to yield images of group activation for each contrast.

Brain Activation: Region-of-Interest Analysis

Regional differences in activation were investigated by using a four-way ANCOVA, with one between-group factor, diagnosis (comparison group vs. fragile X syndrome group), and three within group factors (region of interest, task, and hemisphere), with full-scale IQ as a covariate.

Statistically significant main effects were observed for region of interest (middle frontal gyrus > inferior frontal gyrus > superior parietal lobule > supramarginal gyrus; $F = 9.8$, $df = 3, 69$, $p < 0.0001$), hemisphere (right > left; $F = 8.4$, $df = 1, 23$, $p = 0.008$), and task (2-back > 1-back; $F = 8.1$, $df = 1, 23$, $p = 0.009$). There was no main effect of diagnosis ($F = 0.2$, $df = 1, 22$, $p = 0.65$). However, a significant diagnosis-by-task interaction was observed ($F = 10.8$, $df = 1, 23$, $p = 0.003$). The comparison subjects showed a significant increase in activation between the 1-back and 2-back tasks ($F = 23.6$, $df = 1, 23$, $p < 0.0001$), but subjects with fragile X syndrome showed no difference between the two tasks ($F = 0.1$, $df = 1, 23$, $p = 0.78$). When each task was examined separately, the comparison subjects and subjects with fragile X syndrome did not differ significantly on the 1-back ($F = 0.4$, $df = 1, 22$, $p = 0.51$) or 2-back ($F = 0.1$, $df = 1, 22$, $p = 0.79$) tasks. Therefore, the diagnosis-by-task interaction was driven almost entirely by the working memory load-specific increases in activation shown by the comparison subjects together with the absence of any such increase in subjects with fragile X syndrome. Furthermore, no regional differences in activation were observed as indicated by the lack of an interaction of region of interest, diagnosis, and task. Other higher-order interactions were nonsignificant.

The pattern for each region of interest was that of a significant increase in activation between the 1-back and 2-back tasks for comparison group subjects and a generally flat response for subjects with fragile X syndrome (Figure 8.4). All four regions of interest showed significant diagnosis-by-task interactions in activation. In the inferior frontal gyrus, comparison subjects showed significant increase in activation from the 1-back to the 2-back task ($F = 6.1$, $df = 1, 23$, $p = 0.02$), whereas subjects with fragile X syndrome showed a nonsignificant decrease ($F = 1.7$, $df = 1, 23$, $p = 0.20$). Similarly, the comparison subjects showed significant increases in the middle frontal gyrus ($F = 10.7$, $df = 1, 23$, $p = 0.003$), superior parietal lobule ($F = 44.3$, $df = 1, 23$, $p < 0.001$), and supramarginal gyrus ($F = 34.6$, $df = 1, 23$, $p < 0.001$), while subjects with fragile X syndrome did not show such increases ($p > 0.20$).

Brain Activation and Performance

As a corollary to the analysis that showed an association between performance on the visuospatial working memory tasks and full-scale IQ

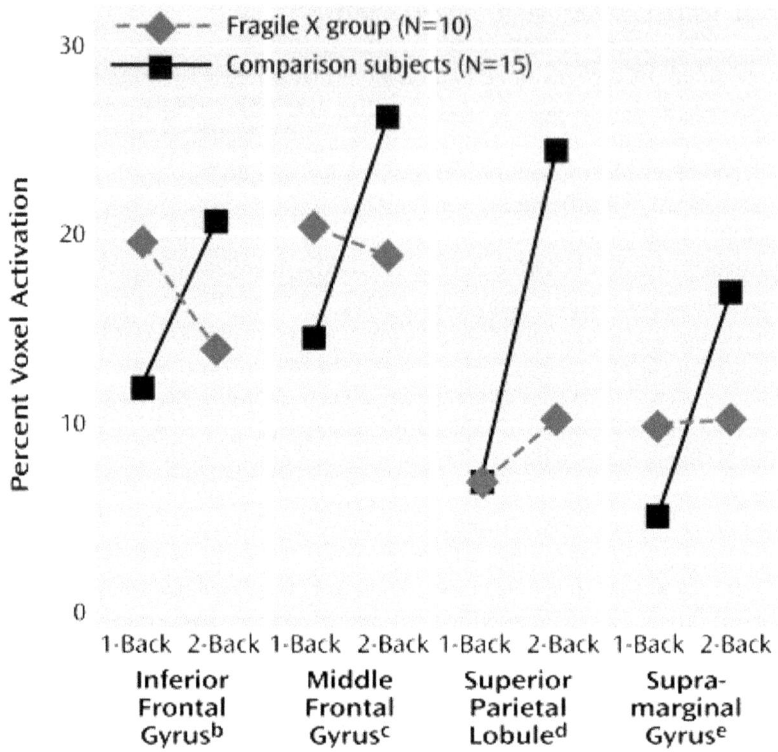

Figure 8.4. Brain Activation in Regions of Interest During 1-Back and 2-Back Working Memory Tasks, Relative to a Control Condition,[a] in Female Subjects with Fragile X Syndrome and Healthy Comparison Subjects.

[a] Subjects were presented with a series of 3 × 3 matrices with nine distinct visuospatial locations in each task. In the experimental condition, subjects were instructed to respond if the stimulus was in the same location as in the previous trial for the 1-back task or in two trials back for the 2-back task. In the control condition, subjects were instructed to respond if the stimulus was in the center location.

[b] Significant interaction of diagnosis and task ($F = 6.7$, $df = 1, 23$, $p = 0.02$).

[c] Significant interaction fo diagnosis and task ($F = 5.4$, $df = 1, 23$, $p = 0.03$).

[d] Significant interaction of diagnosis and task ($F = 11.8$, $df = 1, 23$, $p = 0.02$).

[e] Significant interaction of diagnosis and task ($F = 12.8$, $df = 1, 23$, $p = 0.002$).

(Figure 8.1), the relationship between brain activation and full-scale IQ was examined. When the two subject groups were combined ($N = 25$), Pearson product-moment correlation analysis showed a significant correlation between full-scale IQ and activation during the 2-back task in the left inferior frontal gyrus ($r = 0.42$, $df = 23$, $p < 0.04$), left superior parietal lobule ($r = 0.41$,

$df = 23, p < 0.05$), left supramarginal gyrus ($r = 0.50$, $df = 23$, $p = 0.01$), and right supramarginal gyrus ($r = 0.42$, $df = 23$, $p < 0.04$). No significant correlations between full-scale IQ and activation were observed in the 1-back task. However, when the groups were examined separately, neither group showed significant correlations between full-scale IQ and brain activation during the 2-back task, suggesting that the average group differences in full-scale IQ and activation were driving the correlation observed when the groups were combined. Nonparametric Spearman analysis also showed no significant correlation between full-scale IQ and brain activation, either within or across groups.

In the comparison subjects, response accuracy on the 2-back task was correlated with activation in the left inferior frontal gyrus, right inferior frontal gyrus, left middle frontal gyrus, right middle frontal gyrus, left superior parietal lobule, right superior parietal lobule, left supramarginal gyrus, and right supramarginal gyrus (Table 8.4). No such correlations were found in the subjects with fragile X syndrome. In the subjects with fragile X syndrome, reaction time on the 2-back task was significantly inversely correlated with activation in both frontal lobe regions of interest bilaterally (left inferior frontal gyrus, right inferior frontal gyrus, left middle frontal gyrus, and right middle frontal gyrus) (Table 8.4). The comparison subjects showed no such correlations on the 2-back task.

In the 1-back task, significant correlations were seen for reaction time but not for accuracy. Reaction time correlated positively in the comparison group ($N = 15$) with activation in the right inferior frontal gyrus ($r = 0.56$, $df = 13$, $p < 0.03$) and negatively in the fragile X syndrome group ($N = 8$) with activation in the right inferior frontal gyrus ($r = -0.80$, $df = 6$, $p < 0.02$) and right superior parietal lobule ($r = -0.78$, $df = 6$, $p < 0.03$).

Brain Activation, FMRP Expression, and FMR1 Gene Activation Ratio

In the subjects with fragile X syndrome, brain activation during the 1-back task in the left middle frontal gyrus was significantly correlated with both the FMR1 gene activation ratio and FMRP expression (Table 8.5). In the 2-back task, the FMR1 gene activation ratio was significantly correlated with activity in the right inferior frontal gyrus, left middle frontal gyrus, and right middle frontal gyrus, while FMRP expression was significantly correlated with activity in the right inferior frontal gyrus, left middle frontal gyrus, right middle frontal gyrus, left supramarginal gyrus, and right supramarginal gyrus (Table 8.5).

No significant correlations were seen between the FMR1 gene activation ratio or FMRP expression and any of the behavioral measures on either task.

TABLE 8.4

Correlation Between Two Measures of Performance on a 2-Back Visuospatial Working Memory Task[a] and Activation in Brain Regions of Interest in Healthy Comparison Subjects and Female Subjects With Fragile X Syndrome

	Comparison Group (N = 15)				Fragile x Syndrome Group (N=8)			
	Correct Response Rate		Reaction Time		Correct Response Rate		Reaction Time	
Region of Interest	r	p	r	p	r	p	r	p
Left inferior frontal gyrus	0.72	0.002	–0.01	0.97	0.13	0.76	–0.85	0.008
Right interior frontal gyrus	0.59	<0.03	0.12	0.67	–0.16	0.70	–0.89	0.003
Left middle frontal gyrus	0.59	<0.03	–0.09	0.74	0.19	0.66	–0.79	<0.02
Right middle frontal gyrus	0.55	<0.04	–0.05	0.86	0.11	0.80	–0.90	0.003
Left superior parietal lobule	0.66	0.008	–0.22	0.42	0.24	0.57	0.19	0.66
Right superior parietal lobule	0.61	<0.02	0.04	0.90	0.22	0.60	–0.26	0.53
Left supramarginal gyrus	0.54	0.04	–0.44	0.10	0.41	0.31	–0.19	0.65
Right supramarginal gyrus	0.61	<0.02	–0.04	0.90	0.51	0.20	–0.67	0.07

[a]Subjects were presented with a series of 3 x 3 matrices with nine distinct visuospatial locations. In the experimental condition, subjects were instructed to respond if the stimulus was in the same location as two trials back. In the control condition, subjects were instructed to respond if the stimulus was in the center location.

TABLE 8.5

Correlation of FMR1 Gene Activation Ratio and FMR1 Gene Product (FMRP) Expression with Brain Activation in Regions of Interest During 1-Back Visuospatial Working Memory Tasks[a] in Female Subjects with Fragile X Syndrome (N = 10)

	1-Back Task				2-Back Task			
	FMR1 Gene Activation Ratio[b]		FMRP Expression[c]		FMR1 Gene Activation Ratio[b]		FMRP Expression[c]	
Region of Interest	r	p	r	p	r	p	r	p
Left inferior frontal gyrus	0.53	0.12	0.53	0.12	0.55	0.10	0.62	0.055
Right interior frontal gyrus	0.59	0.07	0.48	0.17	0.70	<0.03	0.69	<0.03
Left middle frontal gyrus	0.67	<0.04	0.70	<0.03	0.77	0.009	0.81	0.004
Right middle frontal gyrus	0.57	0.09	0.56	0.09	0.66	<0.04	0.71	<0.03
Left superior parietal lobule	–0.18	0.62	–0.15	0.68	0.34	0.33	0.39	0.26
Right superior parietal lobule	–0.20	0.58	–0.19	0.59	0.39	0.27	0.43	0.22
Left supramarginal gyrus	0.15	0.68	0.19	0.59	0.61	0.06	0.70	<0.03
Right supramarginal gyrus	0.11	0.77	0.15	0.69	0.61	0.06	0.70	<0.03

[a] Subjects were presented with a series of 3 x 3 matrices with nine distinct visuospatial locations. In the experimental condition, subjects were instructed to respond if the stimulus was in the same location as in the previous trial for the 1-back task or in two trials back for the 2-back task. In the control condition, subjects were instructed to respond if the stimulus was in the center location.

[b] Represents the proportion of the normal (nonmutant) FMR1 gene on the active X chromosome, which reflects the proportion of cells that can express FMRP.

[c] Ascertained by calculating the percentage of lymphocytes containing FMRP.

DISCUSSION

To our knowledge, this report presents the first study to examine the neural substrates of working memory in individuals with fragile X syndrome. Behaviorally, we found significant visuospatial working memory deficits in the subjects with fragile X syndrome, even after accounting for differences in IQ. Relative to the comparison subjects, the subjects with fragile X syndrome also showed significant differences in brain activation. Significant correlations were found between brain activation and both FMRP expression and performance in the 2-back task. Significant correlations also were seen on the 1-back task for both subject groups, but they were more limited in degree and extent.

Behavioral Results

Behavioral deficits in the fragile X syndrome group were observed after covarying for IQ, suggesting that even after accounting for overall cognitive level, subjects with fragile X syndrome may be especially deficient in working memory skills. Subjects with fragile X syndrome showed good performance on the control condition of the working memory tasks, suggesting intact attention and impulse control when working memory load is relatively low. Performance on the 2-back task was significantly worse than on the 1-back task for both subject groups. However, subjects with fragile X syndrome experienced a significantly greater decrease in accuracy (13% for the fragile X syndrome subjects vs. 4% for the comparison subjects) with increased memory load. In addition to experiencing lower overall accuracy, subjects with fragile X syndrome had higher rates of errors of omission and commission. These findings may be related to clinical descriptions of greater difficulties with attention and impulsivity in this population.[8,44]

Our results agree with prior neuropsychological studies showing that visuospatial perception and short-term memory, attention, and manipulation of visuospatial relationships are impaired in the fragile X syndrome population.[4,6] Prior data also have suggested that subjects with fragile X syndrome are particularly weak in visual short-term memory and sequential processing relative to other cognitive domains.[4] However, unlike these prior neuropsychological studies, which involved several cognitive processes in addition to working memory, the study reported here used a task that better operationalized working memory and provided direct evidence for specific deficits in working memory in subjects with fragile X syndrome. These deficits were observed even after differences in IQ were taken into account, implying that the ability to maintain and manipulate information in memory is specifically affected in fragile X syndrome.

Neuroimaging Findings

In conjunction with these behavioral deficits, differences in patterns of brain activation between comparison subjects and subjects with fragile X syndrome were found. The activation patterns seen in the comparison group, namely involvement of bilateral prefrontal and parietal cortices, are in good agreement with previous findings that these regions play critical roles in working memory. For example, electrophysiological[14,17] and lesion[45,46] studies have consistently indicated that the prefrontal cortex is essential in successful working memory performance. Other fMRI studies have found bilateral dorsolateral prefrontal cortex involvement in visuospatial working memory processing.[47,48] Furthermore, several PET and fMRI studies have shown a correlation between activation increases in the dorsolateral prefrontal cortex and increased memory load.[49,50] A previous study using an n-back task similar to the task in our study reported robust activation in the middle frontal gyrus only during the 2-back task.[48] Prior imaging studies have reported consistent activation of the parietal lobe during both verbal and visuospatial working memory tasks.[51] Imaging studies also have suggested that the ventral aspects of the parietal cortex are involved in the short-term storage and retrieval of object-related material, while the dorsal aspects of the parietal areas are involved in the storage and retrieval of visuospatially encoded information.[11] On the basis of prior findings of frontal and parietal lobe involvement in the storage, retrieval, and executive manipulations of the contents of working memory, we selected these regions as regions of interest for the current study.

The subjects with fragile X syndrome showed significant activation in bilateral frontal and parietal areas in both the 1-back and 2-back tasks. As such, they showed little change in the pattern of activation in a comparison between the tasks of differing working memory load. On the other hand, the comparison subjects had significantly greater activation in bilateral areas of the parietal cortex in the 2-back task compared to the 1-back task. To further clarify group differences, we proceeded to a region-of-interest analysis.

The statistical significance of a two-way ANCOVA of diagnosis and task across all regions of interest (Figure 8.4) confirmed our hypothesis that the subjects with fragile X syndrome had different patterns of brain activation than the comparison subjects. The level of activity seen in the subjects with fragile X syndrome in the experimental conditions may represent nonspecific, generalized activation that is not modulated in response to increasing demands. It is also possible that activation reaches a ceiling in subjects with fragile X syndrome during the 1-back task. In contrast, Callicott et al.[52] reported the presence in normally developing adults of a threshold in performance and recruitment of neural resources by a 3-back visuospatial working memory task.

Taken together, the behavioral and neuroimaging analyses reveal significant deficits in working memory systems in subjects with fragile X syndrome. These differences in brain activation may arise from synaptic and dendritic abnormalities known to be present in subjects with fragile X syndrome.[2,3] This, in turn, may lead to dysregulation of neural processes critical to working memory performance.

Relationship between Brain Activation and Performance

In contrast to correlations between activation and accuracy on the 1-back or 2-back tasks in the comparison subjects, no correlation was found in subjects with fragile X syndrome. This finding supports the hypothesis of generalized nonspecific activation in subjects with fragile X syndrome. However, an inverse correlation was seen between reaction time on the 2-back task and brain activation for subjects with fragile X syndrome bilaterally in the inferior frontal gyrus and the middle frontal gyrus. This correlation was not observed in the comparison subjects. This finding suggests that despite a relative impairment of working memory function, subjects with fragile X syndrome show an association between activation in these frontal areas and the speed of working memory processing.

Effects of FMRP Expression on Neural Activation

The subjects with fragile X syndrome showed robust patterns of activation during the 1-back task in the bilateral prefrontal cortex and parietal cortices but showed a correlation between FMRP expression and brain activation during the 1-back task only in the left middle frontal gyrus. In contrast, significant correlations were seen in the 2-back task in the right inferior frontal gyrus, bilateral middle frontal gyrus, and bilateral supramarginal gyrus. These findings may be explained by a ceiling effect. The subjects with fragile X syndrome may have recruited all of their neural resources needed for working memory in the 1-back task, resulting in an absence of any correlation between brain activation and FMRP. In the 2-back task, the fragile X syndrome group experienced significant deterioration in performance along with the lack of coherent recruitment in areas subserving working memory. The degree to which subjects can recruit areas adequately appears to be related to FMRP expression. These results indicate that FMRP may play a dynamic role in modulating brain activation in response to working memory load.

Some studies have begun to elucidate the role of FMRP in neurons. These studies point to the function of FMRP as an RNA-binding protein, possibly involved in the transport and/or stabilization of RNA from the nucleus to the dendrites.[53,54] Levels of a rat homologue of FMRP have been shown to increase rapidly (on the order of minutes) in response to neuronal stimulation,[54] indicating a possible role of FMRP in the regulation of protein synthesis in response to increased synaptic input. Furthermore, low levels of FMRP in subjects with fragile X syndrome have been associated with abnormal morphology of dendritic spines and a reduction in the length of synapses in the cortex,[2,3] although the precise mechanism by which this occurs is not known.

On the basis of these findings, we hypothesize that intracellular FMRP levels increase rapidly in normally developing individuals in response to a working memory task. In light of the role of FMRP in transporting and/or stabilizing mRNA, increased FMRP may act as a precursor to increased protein synthesis in dendritic processes. In the fragile X syndrome population, in which the level of FMRP is lower, the degree of dendritic protein synthesis may be limited by the ability of the neuron to synthesize FMRP for its role in modulating protein translation. The resulting limit in protein translation may lead to impairments in synaptic maturation or plasticity. These dynamic impairments in translation would occur in addition to the baseline abnormalities in neural activation likely to result from synaptic and dendritic dysmorphology.

This study is the first we are aware of to examine the relationship between brain activation and a molecular marker of genetic dysfunction in the context of working memory load. We plan future studies that will compare IQ-matched populations and will involve subjects with a more limited age range to avoid the confounding effects of development and age. Differences in neural architecture and functioning may exist between prepubertal and adolescent subjects, although a recent developmental study of spatial working memory reported similar areas of activation in frontal and parietal regions.[23]

In conclusion, this study shows that subjects with fragile X syndrome exhibit significant visuospatial working memory deficits that extend beyond the effects of differences in IQ. These deficits are correlated with abnormalities in activation in brain areas that are known to be involved in working memory. In addition, FMRP expression is correlated with brain activation in subjects with fragile X syndrome, a finding that may reflect the involvement of this protein in the dynamic response to working memory load. These results bear possible clinical significance in light of behavioral problems exhibited by subjects with fragile X syndrome in the realm of social functioning. As the gene defect in this disorder can be readily quantified, we believe that fragile X syndrome may serve as a model for bridging the gap between the molecular biology of neurogenetic disorders and their neuronal and behavioral manifestations.

ACKNOWLEDGMENTS

Supported by NIMH grants MH-50047 and MH-01142, grant HD-31715 and grant HD-40761 (to Dr. Menon) from the National Institute of Child Health and Human Development, a grant from the M.I.N.D. Institute of the University of California at Davis, and the Lynda and Scott Canel Fund for Fragile X Research. The authors thank Christine Blasey, Ph.D., for assistance with statistical analysis, Karen Patterson for FMR1 gene product analysis, and Pam Dyer for fragile X DNA analysis.

REFERENCES

1. Turner G, Webb T, Wake S, Robinson H: Prevalence of fragile X syndrome. *Am J Med Genet* 1996;64:196–197.
2. Rudelli RD, Brown WT, Wisniewski K, Jenkins EC, Laure-Kamionowska M, Connell F, Wisniewski HM: Adult fragile X syndrome: clinico-neuropathologic findings. *Acta Neuropathol* (Berl) 1985;67:289–295.
3. Hinton VJ, Brown WT, Wisniewski K, Rudelli RD: Analysis of neocortex in three males with the fragile X syndrome. *Am J Med Genet* 1991;41:289–294.
4. Freund LS, Reiss AL: Cognitive profiles associated with the fra(X) syndrome in males and females. *Am J Med Genet* 1991;38:542–547.
5. Grigsby JP, Kemper MB, Hagerman RJ, Myers CS: Neuropsychological dysfunction among affected heterozygous fragile X females. *Am J Med Genet* 1990;35:28–35.
6. Mazzocco MM, Pennington BF, Hagerman RJ: The neurocognitive phenotype of female carriers of fragile X: additional evidence for specificity. *J Dev Behav Pediatr* 1993;14:328–335.
7. Reiss AL, Freund L: Behavioral phenotype of fragile X syndrome: DSM-III-R autistic behavior in male children. *Am J Med Genet.* 1992;43:35–46.
8. Bregman JD, Leckman JF, Ort SI: Fragile X syndrome: genetic predisposition to psychopathology. *J Autism Dev Disord* 1988;18:343–354.
9. Mazzocco MM, Baumgardner T, Freund LS, Reiss AL: Social functioning among girls with fragile X or Turner syndrome and their sisters. *J Autism Dev Disord* 1998;28:509–517.
10. Baddeley AD, Hitch G: Working memory, in *The Psychology of Learning and Motivation.* Edited by Bower GH. New York, Academic Press, 1974, pp. 47–89.
11. Smith EE, Jonides J: Storage and executive processes in the frontal lobes. *Science* 1999;283:1657–1661.
12. Goldman-Rakic PS: Working memory dysfunction in schizophrenia. *J Neuropsychiatry Clin Neurosci* 1994;6:348–357.
13. Smith ML, Milner B: Differential effects of frontal-lobe lesions on cognitive estimation and spatial memory. *Neuropsychologia* 1984;22:697–705.
14. Fuster JM, Alexander GE: Neuron activity related to short-term memory. *Science* 1971;173:652–654.
15. Friedman HR, Goldman-Rakic PS: Coactivation of prefrontal cortex and inferior parietal cortex in working memory tasks revealed by 2DG functional mapping in the rhesus monkey. *J Neurosci* 1994;14(5, part 1):2775–2788.
16. Goldman-Rakic PS: The physiological approach: functional architecture of working memory and disordered cognition in schizophrenia. *Biol Psychiatry* 1999;46:650–661.

17. Goldman-Rakic PS: Cellular basis of working memory. *Neuron* 1995;14:477–485.
18. Fuster JM: *Memory in the Cerebral Cortex: An Empirical Approach to Neural Networks in the Human and Nonhuman Primate*. Cambridge, Mass, MIT Press, 1995.
19. Smith EE, Jonides J, Koeppe RA: Dissociating verbal and spatial working memory using PET. *Cereb Cortex* 1996;6:11–20.
20. McCarthy G, Blamire AM, Puce A, Nobre AC, Bloch G, Hyder F, Goldman-Rakic P, Shulman RG: Functional magnetic resonance imaging of human prefrontal cortex activation during a spatial working memory task. *Proc Natl Acad Sci* USA 1994;91:8690–8694.
21. McCarthy G, Puce A, Constable RT, Krystal JH, Gore JC, Goldman-Rakic P: Activation of human prefrontal cortex during spatial and nonspatial working memory tasks measured by functional MRI. *Cereb Cortex* 1996;6:600–611.
22. Courtney SM, Petit L, Maisog JM, Ungerleider LG, Haxby JV: An area specialized for spatial working memory in human frontal cortex. *Science* 1998;279:1347–1351.
23. Thomas KM, King SW, Franzen PL, Welsh TF, Berkowitz AL, Noll DC, Birmaher V, Casey BJ: A developmental functional MRI study of spatial working memory. *Neuroimage* 1999;10(3, part 1):327–338.
24. Schapiro MB, Murphy DG, Hagerman RJ, Azari NP, Alexander GE, Miezejeski CM, Hinton VJ, Horwitz B, Haxby JV, Kumar A: Adult fragile X syndrome: neuropsychology, brain anatomy, and metabolism. *Am J Med Genet* 1995;60:480–493.
25. Guerreiro MM, Camargo EE, Kato M, Marques-de-Faria AP, Ciasca SM, Guerreiro CA, Netto JR, Moura-Ribeiro MV: Fragile X syndrome: clinical, electroencephalographic and neuroimaging characteristics. *Arq Neuropsiquiatr* 1998;56:18–23.
26. Hjalgrim H, Jacobsen TB, Norgaard K, Lou HC, Brondum-Nielsen K, Jonassen O: Frontal-subcortical hypofunction in the fragile X syndrome (letter). *Am J Med Genet* 1999;83:140–141.
27. Oberle I, Rousseau F, Heitz D, Kretz C, Devys D, Hanauer A, Boue J, Bertheas MF, Mandel JL: Instability of a 550-base pair DNA segment and abnormal methylation in fragile X syndrome. *Science* 1991;252:1097–1102.
28. Taylor AK, Safanda JF, Fall MZ, Quince C, Lang KA, Hull CE, Carpenter I, Staley LW, Hagerman RJ: Molecular predictors of cognitive involvement in female carriers of fragile X syndrome. *JAMA* 1994;271:507–514.
29. Willemsen R, Mohkamsing S, de Vries B, Devys D, van den Ouweland A, Mandel JL, Galjaard H, Oostra B: Rapid antibody test for fragile X syndrome. *Lancet* 1995;345:1147–1148.
30. Wechsler D: Wechsler Intelligence Scale for Children, 3rd ed. San Antonio, TX, Psychological Corp (Harcourt), 1991.
31. Wechsler D: Wechsler Adult Intelligence Scale, 3rd ed. San Antonio, TX, Psychological Corp (Harcourt), 1997.
32. Woodcock RW, Mather N: Woodcock-Johnson Tests of Cognitive Ability: Standard and Supplemental Batteries. Allen, TX, DLM Teaching Resources, 1989.
33. Benton AL, Sivan AB, Hamsher Kd, Varney NR, Spreen O: Judgment of Line Orientation, in *Contributions to Neuropsychological Assessment: A Clinical Manual*. New York, Oxford University Press, 1994, pp. 44–54.

34. Hayes C, Mathias C: Improved brain coil for fMRI and high resolution imaging (abstract), in *Proceedings of the Fourth Annual Meeting of the International Society for Magnetic Resonance in Medicine.* Berkeley, Calif, ISMRM, 1996, pp. 1414.
35. Glover GH, Lai S: Self-navigated spiral fMRI: interleaved versus single-shot. *Magn Reson Med* 1998;39:361–368.
36. Cohen JD, MacWhinney B, Flatt M, Provost J: PsyScope: a new graphic interactive environment for designing psychology experiments. *Behav Res Methods Instrum Comput* 1993;25:257–271.
37. Talairach J, Tournoux P: *Co-Planar Stereotaxic Atlas of the Human Brain: Three-Dimensional Proportional System.* Stuttgart, Germany, Georg Thieme, 1988.
38. Friston KJ, Holmes AP, Poline JB, Grasby PJ, Williams SC, Frackowiak RS, Turner R: Analysis of fMRI time-series revisited. *Neuroimage* 1995;2:45–53.
39. Poline JB, Worsley KJ, Evans AC, Friston KJ: Combining spatial extent and peak intensity to test for activations in functional imaging. *Neuroimage* 1997;5:83–96.
40. Holmes AP, Friston KJ: Generalizability, random effects and population inference (abstract). *Neuroimage* 1998;7:S754.
41. Keppel G, Zedeck S: *Data Analysis for Research Designs: Analysis of Variance and Multiple Regression Correlation Approaches.* New York, WH Freeman, 1989.
42. Duvernoy H: *The Human Brain: Surface, Three-Dimensional Sectional Anatomy.* New York, Springer-Verlag, 1991.
43. Ono M, Kubik S, Abernathey CD: *Atlas of the Cerebral Sulci.* Stuttgart, Germany, Georg Thieme, 1990.
44. Dykens EM, Hodapp RM, Leckman JF: Adaptive and maladaptive functioning of institutionalized and noninstitutionalized fragile X males. *J Am Acad Child Adolesc Psychiatry* 1989;28:427–430.
45. Milner B, Petrides M, Smith ML: Frontal lobes and the temporal organization of memory. *Hum Neurobiol* 1985;4:137–142.
46. Petrides M, Milner B: Deficits on subject-ordered tasks after frontal- and temporal-lobe lesions in man. *Neuropsychologia* 1982;20:249–262.
47. Belger A, Puce A, Krystal JH, Gore JC, Goldman-Rakic P, McCarthy G: Dissociation of mnemonic and perceptual processes during spatial and nonspatial working memory using fMRI. *Hum Brain Mapp* 1998;6:14–32.
48. Carlson S, Martinkauppi S, Rama P, Salli E, Korvenoja A, Aronen HJ: Distribution of cortical activation during visuospatial n-back tasks as revealed by functional magnetic resonance imaging. *Cereb Cortex* 1998;8:743–752.
49. Courtney SM, Ungerleider LG, Keil K, Haxby JV: Object and spatial visual working memory activate separate neural systems in human cortex. *Cereb Cortex* 1996;6:39–49.
50. Klingberg T, O'Sullivan BT, Roland PE: Bilateral activation of fronto-parietal networks by incrementing demand in a working memory task. *Cereb Cortex* 1997;7:465–471.
51. D'Esposito M, Aguirre GK, Zarahn E, Ballard D, Shin RK, Lease J: Functional MRI studies of spatial and nonspatial working memory. *Brain Res Cogn Brain Res* 1998;7:1–13.

52. Callicott JH, Mattay VS, Bertolino A, Finn K, Coppola R, Frank JA, Goldberg TE, Weinberger DR: Physiological characteristics of capacity constraints in working memory as revealed by functional MRI. *Cereb Cortex* 1999;9:20–26.
53. Feng Y, Gutekunst CA, Eberhart DE, Yi H, Warren ST, Hersch SM: Fragile X mental retardation protein: nuclcocytoplasmic shuttling and association with somatodendritic ribosomes. *J Neurosci* 1997;17:1539–1547.
54. Weiler IJ, Irwin SA, Klintsova AY, Spencer CM, Brazelton AD, Miyashiro K, Comery TA, Patel B, Eberwine J, Greenough WT: Fragile X mental retardation protein is translated near synapses in response to neurotransmitter activation. *Proc Natl Acad Sci* USA 1997;94:5395–5400.

9

Memory: An Overview, with Emphasis on Developmental, Interpersonal, and Neurobiological Aspects

Daniel J. Siegel

Objective: *To review recent findings from memory research and related scientific studies and to provide an overview of their implications for clinical practice.* ***Method:*** *Published research data from a range of scientific disciplines are summarized and integrated into a conceptual framework regarding the interpersonal, neurobiological, and subjective nature of the development of memory.* ***Results:*** *Memory is a fundamental property of the human mind that has been the focus of research of a wide range of academic disciplines. Convergent findings from these various studies suggest that the fundamental elements of memory can be best understood by focusing on its origins in the brain and the impact of social communication on its development.* ***Conclusions:*** *An interdisciplinary approach is important for the clinician who seeks to understand the various layers of memory that develop during the early years of life. J. Am. Acad. Child Adolesc. Psychiatry, 2001, 40(9):997-1011.* ***Key Words:*** *memory, implicit memory, explicit memory, autobiographical memory, interpersonal neurobiology, narrative.*

This review will provide clinicians and researchers in child mental health a basic knowledge and conceptual understanding relevant to research on memory or interpretations of clinical assessments of memory functioning. The study of memory is carried out by a wide array of academic disciplines, including those of cognitive psychology, developmental psychology, neuropsychology, cognitive neuroscience, psychiatry, neurology, anthropology, and psycholinguistics. For this reason, a basic review of memory must attempt to "translate" across the different disciplines. This article integrates a number of usually independent disciplines, such as attachment research, cognitive neuroscience, and clinical psychiatry, and demonstrates the usefulness of such a synthetic approach. This review examines the nature of memory, with an emphasis on the neurobiological, developmental, interpersonal, and subjective aspects of this fundamental process of the human mind. More extensive application of this multidisciplinary, "interpersonal neurobiology" view of development, relationships, and mental health can be found in *The Developing Mind: Toward a Neurobiology of Interpersonal Experience* (Siegel, 1999). This perspective enables us to view how the mind develops at the interface of neurophysiological process and interpersonal experience. This article will highlight how memory can be seen as the fundamental way in which the mind develops throughout the life span.

This review focuses on clinically relevant concepts. More comprehensive coverage of research methodologies is listed in the references to this article. The clinical assessment of memory requires developmentally appropriate tasks that can be offered in the form of a mental status examination, memory test batteries, neuropsychological test batteries, or other measures of memory. The details of the administration and interpretation of these clinical assessments can be found in psychiatric textbooks and other basic references. Often, such tasks examine the various dimensions of memory, such as timing (immediate, recent, or remote), aspects of processing (encoding, storage, or retrieval), strategies used (such as rehearsal and retrieval strategies), perceptual modalities required (visual, auditory), context-dependency (in which settings does memory impairment occur?), and ways in which memory performance affects the life of the child or adolescent. This article will offer a bridge between the various empirical research approaches to memory and the clinical implications of these findings for the practitioner.

A GENERAL DEFINITION OF MEMORY

Only recently have we been able to apply the scientific method to understanding the basic elements of memory (Milner et al., 1998; Tulving and Craik, 2000). Common misconceptions about memory include the following: that we are always aware of what we have experienced, that when we remember something we have the feeling of recollection, and that the mind is able to make a sort of photograph of experiences that is stored without further modification. However, the structure of memory is complex and sensitive to both external and internal factors as it constructs the past, the present, and the anticipated future (Ingvar, 1985; Johnson-Laird, 1983).

Memory may be broadly defined as the way past events affect future function. Memory represents the way the brain is affected by experience and subsequently alters its responses. In other words, the brain experiences the world and encodes this interaction in a manner that alters future ways of responding. This process affects both the information and the very nature of the processes that encode such information.

One way of understanding the overlap of developmental and memory processes is that the brain responds to experience by alteration in synaptic strengths or the creation of new synaptic connections. Brain development can also be described by these same synaptic changes. Indeed, experience is often required in order to activate specific genes to be transcribed and produce the proteins that allow structural changes to take place at the neural level. This activity-dependent aspect of development means that the unfolding of brain structure depends on the activation of the neurons themselves. Experience creates neural activity that, in turn, activates the genetic machinery that allows for the alteration of synaptic connections.

INFORMATION PROCESSING AND NEUROBIOLOGY

The brain is composed of spider web-like neural networks capable of firing in a myriad of patterns, called a neural net profile (Tucker, 1992). The structure of the neural net allows it to "learn" by an encoding process that initially activates a specific set of associated neuronal firing patterns that are distributed throughout the brain (McClelland et al., 1995). The connection of neurons in an intricate network, the structure of the brain, allows for learning to occur (Morris, 1989). It is the firing of the components of the network, the circuits of neurons, that alters the probabilities of certain patterns firing in the future. If a certain pattern has been stimulated in the past, the probability of activating a similar profile in the future is enhanced. If the pattern is fired repeatedly, the probability of future activation is further increased. The increased probability is created by changes in the synaptic connections within the network of neurons. Changes at the level of the cell membrane alter the firing probability of specific combinations of neurons (Kandel and Abel, 1995; Martin and Kandel, 1996). The process of "long term potentiation" is one way in which such alteration of connection strengths among neurons occurs (Milner et al., 1998). This process appears to require the coordinated activity of both pre- and postsynaptic neurons and the release of nitric oxide. Duration of changes in the strengths of synaptic connections can vary, from quite brief levels of chemical alterations to extended intervals mediated by structural changes in neural connections.

The specific pattern of firing, the "energy" contained within a certain neural net profile of activated neurons, contains within it "information." This information is often called a "representation." The visual system is able to represent visual images whereas the auditory system is able to create representations of sounds. Furthermore, specific regions may carry out different forms of information processing. Thus, language processing may be mediated by circuits primarily within the left hemisphere, whereas nonverbal representations, such as others' facial expressions, may be carried out primarily within the right hemisphere. More complex representations, such as those of concepts and categories, may be mediated in associational regions of the neocortex while more basic representational processes encoding information about the body, such as respirations and heart rate, may be located in deeper, brainstem regions of the brain.

The activation of neural patterns of firing is thought to create informational processing in the brain. The complex neural network alters the strengths of its interconnections based on patterns of activity. In this manner, the network learns from its past experiences. The increased probability of firing a similar pattern is how the network "remembers." Information is encoded and retrieved through the synaptic changes that direct the flow of energy through the brain.

Experience shapes the structure of the brain through "experience-dependent" brain development. At birth, the infant brain has an overabundance of neurons with relatively few synaptic connections compared with the highly differentiated and interconnected set of connections that will be established in the first few years of life. Developmental neuroscientists describe an interaction between the genetically determined timing and specificity of synapse formation and synaptogenesis driven primarily by experiential stimulation. Some researchers have suggested the term experience-expectant development as the process in which connections among neurons are created primarily by genetic information, with their subsequent maintenance requiring minimal amounts of stimulation, such as exposure to sound or light (Greenough and Black, 1992). Synapse formation involves the activation of genes to produce the proteins that enable connections to be made and maintained. Genes themselves as well as experience can activate the genetic machinery to produce synaptogenesis. The shaping of brain structure is also determined by the pruning or parcellation (reduction) of neurons and synapses that are not stimulated by experience or are destroyed by toxic influences such as excessive stress hormone production.

Memory, as with brain development, involves alterations in the connectivity among neurons (Barnes et al., 1995; Merzenich and Sameshima, 1993; Merzenich et al., 1991; Rakic et al., 1994). Chemical alterations strengthen associations among neurons for short-term encoding; long-term memory involves the activation of the genetic machinery required for the establishment of new synaptic connections. Experience involves the activation of neuronal firing patterns. This neural firing can, in turn, activate genes within the neurons' nuclei that lead to synaptogenesis and the creation and strengthening of the connections among the functionally linked neurons (Kandel, 1998). The term experience-dependent refers to the general processes by which neuronal connections are maintained, strengthened, or created as a result of experience.

"Recent work on plasticity in the sensory cortices has introduced the idea that the structure of the brain, even in sensory cortex, is unique to each individual and dependent on each individual's experiential history" (Milner et al., 1998, p. 463). What we usually think of as "memory" refers to the way in which events can influence the brain and its future activity.

THE PROCESSES OF MEMORY

The initial impact of experience leads to an activation of neuronal firing that is a part of the encoding of a memory. The next stage is the storage of memory, which is the increased probability that a similar profile will be activated again. There is no "storage closet" in the brain in which something is placed and then taken out when needed. Memory storage is the change in probability of activating a particular neural network pattern in the future. Retrieval is the actual activation of that potential neural net profile that resembles, but is not identical with, the profile activated in the past.

The neural net of the brain can activate a set of anatomically and chronologically associated firings in response to the environment. This profile is encoded, stored, and able to be retrieved based on the simple axiom defined by Donald Hebb (1949) that "neurons which fire together at one time will rend to fire together in the future." Another way of phrasing this is that "neurons which fire together, wire together." This is the essence of how the neural net remembers.

Recent studies suggest that given the task of visualizing an object, the parts of the brain responsible for visual processing will become active (Kosslyn, 1994). Thus the mind is able to generate a pattern of neural firing at the time of seeing with the eyes or imagining with the mind. Representations come in many forms, including perceptual ones (like visualizing the Eiffel Tower), semantic ones (like seeing the words "Eiffel Tower" and knowing their meaning), as well as sensory ones (such as feeling hungry) (Perner, 1991).

Our memories are based on the binding together of various aspects of these neuronal activation patterns. These associational linkages make it more likely for items to be activated simultaneously during the retrieval process. This then links together representations with a wide range of internal mental processes unique to each individual. Brain imaging studies suggest that the representation of an experience may be stored in particular regions of the brain, such as the perceptual areas in the posterior part of the neocortex, which were initially activated in response to the experience. Encoding and retrieval processes may be mediated via distinct regions (such as in the left and right orbitofrontal cortex, respectively) (Wheeler et al., 1997). Thus specific regions may mediate a process whereby neural patterns (representations) are activated and then bound together in the act of encoding or recollection (Buckner, 1996; Kapur et al., 1994; Shimamura, 1995). What are stored are the probabilities of neurons firing in a specific pattern—not an actual "thing."

In memory research, the initial impact of an experience on the brain has been called an engram (Schacter, 1996). Scientists have named at least two types of memory. A verbally accessible memory has been called explicit or declarative memory. Another distinct form of memory is called implicit or nondeclarative memory. Researchers have used various names such as Early vs. Late, Non declarative vs. Declarative, Procedural vs. Semantic/Episodic, and Implicit versus Explicit (Buckner et al., 1995; Schacter, 1992; Squire, 1992). For the purposes of this article, we will use the terms implicit and explicit to identify these functionally distinct systems (Table 9.1).

Trace theory describes a similar encoding process. In this view, an engram or memory trace has both a gist (a general notion) and specific details (Schacter, 1996). With time, the details of an experience may begin to fade away and become less "tightly bound" together. The gist, however, may remain quite accurate and easily accessible for retrieval. When trying to retrieve "an original memory," one may be calling up the gist at first and then later trying to reconstruct the details. This reconstruction process may be

TABLE 9.1
Types and Characteristics of Memory

Forms of memory
Early, nondeclarative, procedural, implicit vs.
Late, declarative, episodic/semantic, explicit
Developmental biology of memory
Implicit processing systems (early memory): Present at birth.
Explicit processing systems (late memory):
Semantic: Develops initially by 1 to 2 years of age.
Autobiographical: Progressive development with onset after second year of life.
Implicit memory
A form of memory devoid of the subjective internal experience of "recalling," of self, or of time. Involves mental models and "priming."
Includes behavioral, emotional, perceptual, and perhaps somatosensory memory.
Focal attention not required for encoding.
Is mediated via brain circuits involved in the initial encoding and independent of the medial temporal lobe/hippocampus.
Explicit memory
A form of memory requiring conscious awareness for encoding and having the subjective sense of recollection (and, if autobiographical, of self and time).
Includes semantic (factual) and episodic (autobiographical) memory.
Focal attention needed for encoding.
Hippocampal processing required for storage.
Cortical consolidation makes selected events a part of permanent memory.

Note: Reprinted from chapter 2, Siegel (1999).

profoundly influenced by the present environment, the questioning context itself, and other factors, such as current emotions and our perception of the expectations of those listening to the response (Christianson, 1991). Memory is an active process in which even the most "concrete" experiences, such as recalling an architectural structure, are actually dynamic representational processes. Remembering is not merely the reactivation of an old engram; it is the construction of a new neural net profile with features of the old engram and elements of memory from other experiences as well as influences from the present state of mind.

For the clinician, these issues should be kept in mind when interviewing children about past events, including trauma. The gist of a situation may be recalled with great accuracy, but the details may be more subject to bias from ongoing experience. Recollection can be extremely accurate; it can also be susceptible to the ongoing experiences of social influence and the unfolding of a larger narrative process.

IMPLICIT MEMORY: MENTAL MODELS, BEHAVIORS, IMAGES, AND EMOTIONS

From the first days of life, infants actively perceive the environment around them. Research has shown that they are able to demonstrate recall for experiences in the form of behavioral, perceptual, emotional, and possibly somatosensory learning (Bauer, 1996; Schacter, 1996). Researchers can demonstrate, for example, that babies can turn their heads to a learned stimulus. They can perceive visual patterns and even relate these to other perceptual modalities such as touch or sound (Stern, 1985). If they become frightened by a loud noise associated with a particular toy, they will get upset when shown that toy in the future. These forms of memory are called implicit. They are available early in life and when retrieved are not thought to carry with them the internal sensation that something is being recalled.

Implicit memory involves parts of the brain that do not require conscious processing during encoding or retrieval (Squire et al., 1993). When implicit memory is retrieved, the neural net profiles that are reactivated involve circuits in the brain that are a fundamental part of our everyday experience of life, such as behaviors, emotions, and images. These implicit elements form part of the foundation for our subjective sense of ourselves: we act, feel, and imagine without recognition of the influence of past experience on our present reality.

Implicit memory relies on brain structures that are present at birth and remain available to us throughout life. These structures include the amygdala and other limbic regions for emotional memory, the basal ganglia and motor cortex for behavioral memory, and the perceptual cortices for perceptual memory.

With repeated experiences, the infant's brain—functioning with its rapidly developing neural net, parallel processor—is able to detect similarities and differences across experiences and across modalities of perception. From these comparative processes, the infant's mind is able to make "summations" or generalized representations from repeated experiences as encoded in these areas of the brain. This is a fundamental aspect of learning. These generalizations form the basis of mental models or schemata that help the mind to interpret present experiences as well as to anticipate future ones. Mental models are a basic component of implicit memory.

Mental models help the mind to seek out familiar objects or experiences and to know what to expect from the environment. Deviations from the usual can be ascertained so that the world becomes a familiar and negotiable place to live. Studies of children and adults suggest that perceptual biases are based on these nonconscious mental models (Johnson-Laird, 1983). The brain can be called an "anticipation machine," constantly scanning the environment and trying to determine what will come next (Freyd, 1987). Prior experiences shape our anticipatory models, and thus the term prospective memory has been used to describe how the mind attempts to "remember the future" based on what has occurred in the past (Ingvar, 1985). Readiness for response is enhanced by anticipating the next moment in time, what the world may offer next, and what behavior to initiate in response.

Mental models, the generalizations from past experiences, are the essence of learning. Anticipating the future may be a fundamental component of implicit memory distinct from the more complex and deliberate aspect of planning for the future.

DEVELOPMENTAL IMPLICATIONS OF IMPLICIT MEMORY: ATTACHMENT AND THE EARLY YEARS OF LIFE

By a child's first birthday, repeated patterns of implicit learning are deeply encoded in the brain. Indeed, attachment studies yield striking differences in infants' behavior when they are with each parent. The infant's states of mind when she is with her mother can affect her differently from those that are activated when she is with her father. This may be the origin of the differences that can be seen between an infant's attachment to each parent. By 18 months, the maturation of the child's brain has allowed for the blossoming of comprehension and expression of language.

The patterns of particular states of mind in the infant are encoded as an implicit form of memory. Repeated experiences of terror and fear can be ingrained within the circuits of the brain as states of mind. With chronic occurrence, these states can become more readily activated (retrieved) in the future such that they become characteristic traits of the individual (Perry et al.,

1995). In this way, our lives can be shaped by reactivations of implicit memory that lack a sense that something is being recalled. We simply enter these ingrained states and experience them as the reality of our present experience.

Insights into the ways in which early experiences have shaped the implicit memory system can aid in the understanding of a variety of aspects of human relationships. Being with a particular person can activate distinct mental models that affect the individual's perceptions, emotions, behaviors, and beliefs in response to another person. Each of us filters our interactions with others through the lens of mental models created from patterns of experiences in the past. These models can shift rapidly outside of awareness, sometimes creating abrupt transitions in states of mind and interactions with others. In this way, "transference"—the activation of old mental models and states of mind from our relationships with important figures in the past—happens all of the time in settings both in and outside of the psychotherapy suite.

EXPLICIT MEMORY: FACTS, EVENTS, AND AUTOBIOGRAPHICAL CONSCIOUSNESS

By the second birthday, toddlers have developed a new capacity: to talk about their recollections of the day's events and to remember more distant experiences from the past. This ability to have explicit memory parallels the maturation of the medial temporal lobe (including the hippocampus) and the orbitofrontal cortex (Kelley et al., 1998; Perner and Ruffman, 1995; Schacter et al., 1996; Squire and Zola-Morgan, 1991; Tulving, 1993). When explicit recollections are retrieved, people have the internal sensation of "I am remembering." Two forms of explicit memory are semantic (factual) and episodic (autobiographical or oneself in an episode in time).

The development of the unique aspects of explicit memory involves a number of domains in the child's experiencing. A sense of sequencing, thought to be a function of the hippocampus as a "cognitive mapper," develops during the child's second year of life (Bauer, 1996; Edelman, 1992). Recalling the order in which events occur in the world allows the child to develop a sense of time and of sequence. Children come to expect, with at times intense and passionate reactions to deviations, what is the norm for what comes first and what comes next. Associated with this hippocampal ability is the establishment of an internal map. Loss of hippocampal functioning in animals, for example, leads to loss of memory for running a maze (Squire, 1987). In contrast, enriched environments have been shown to increase the number of neurons in the hippocampus (Kempermann et al., 1997). This cognitive mapper is able to create a sense of the world across time. Explicit memory allows the mind to have a sense of space and time and to remember where things are and when they were there.

As children grow into their second year, they begin to develop a more complex image of themselves in the world. This sense of self has been identified by studies that examine, for example, how children respond to seeing themselves in the mirror with a red mark placed on their face. They notice something different in their reflection, suggesting that they have a mental image of what they usually look like. By 18 months they are able to touch themselves rather than the mirror in exploring the red mark. In the second year, the child is developing a sense of the physical world, time and sequence, and of the self, all of which form the foundation of explicit autobiographical memory (Wheeler et al., 1997). Before this time, events in the child's life may have been remembered ("event memory"), but it is thought that these recollections are of experiences without an enriched sense of self across time, which is the hallmark of autobiographical (episodic) recollection (Bauer and Dow, 1994; Nelson, 1993b).

Recent neuroimaging studies suggest that memory for facts (semantic memory)—including events—is functionally quite distinct from memory of the self across time (episodic) (Wheeler et al., 1997). Semantic memory allows for propositional representations—symbols of external or internal facts that can be declared linguistically or graphically and can be assessed as "true" or "false." Such semantic knowledge has been called noesis and allows us to know about facts in the world. In contrast, autobiographical or episodic memory requires a capacity termed autonoesis (self-knowing) and appears to be dependent on the development of frontal cortical regions of the brain. These regions undergo rapid experience-dependent development during the first few years of life (Schore, 1994) and possibly continuing into adulthood. The ability of the human mind to carry out "mental time travel," to have a sense of recollection of the self at a particular time in the past, awareness of the self in the present, and projections of the self into the imagined future, are the unique contributions of autonoetic consciousness (Wheeler et al., 1997).

By the middle of the third year of life, a child has already begun to join her parents in the mutually constructed tales woven from their real-life events and imaginations (Myers et al., 1987; Nelson, 1993b). The richness of self-knowledge and autobiographical narratives appears to be mediated by the interpersonal dialogues in which caregivers co-construct narratives about external events and the internal, subjective experiences of the characters (Miller et al., 1990; Ochs and Capps, 1996; Oppenheim et al., 1997). In this way, we can hypothesize that attachment experiences—that is, communication with parents and other caregivers—may directly enhance the capacity for autonoetic consciousness in the child. In certain attachment classifications, both parent and child may reveal a paucity in the degree of complexity and coherence of their autobiographical narratives. This finding has been noted in the pairs of "dismissing" adults and their children who have "avoidant" attachments to them (Hesse, 1999; Siegel, 1999).

THE PHASES AND TIMING OF MEMORY

The encoding process for both forms of explicit memory—semantic and episodic—appears to require focal, conscious, directed attention to activate the hippocampus (Moscovitch, 1995). As encoding occurs, stimuli are placed initially in sensory memory, which lasts for about a quarter to half a second. This "sensory buffer" contains the initial neural activations of the perceptual system. Only a selected portion of the items from this huge immediate sensory process are then placed in working memory, lasting up to half a minute (if there is no further rehearsal). If the mind rehearses or refreshes the activity of these activated circuits of working memory, then the items can be either maintained for longer periods in this site (such as practicing a phone number long enough to dial it repeatedly if the line is busy) or placed into longer-term storage. Working memory, similar to the notion of "short-term" memory, corresponds to what clinicians call "immediate" memory.

Working memory has been called the "chalkboard of the mind." Working memory is the mental process involved when we say we are "thinking about something" and allows us to reflect on the present and the past (Baddeley, 1992; Goldman-Rakic, 1993). When we consciously think of a problem or an event, working memory allows us to mentally link together various representations and manipulate them. Imaging studies have implicated the dorsolateral prefrontal cortex as the region thought to be a primary mediator of working memory (Andreasen et al., 1995; Arnsten, 2000; Hendren et al., 2000).

Working memory does not require the transcription and translation processes that enable genes to promote protein production (Milner et al., 1998). Working memory is thought to be mediated by transient chemical alterations in synaptic "connectivity" or the functional strengths of connections among associated neurons. In contrast, encoding into longer-term memory appears to be dependent on gene activation with the resultant production in proteins and alteration in synaptic structure and hence structural neuronal connectivity. The product of such encoding and neural processing leads to the more lasting and stable component, long-term memory.

Long-term explicit memory is thought to be the process by which items are stored for extended periods beyond working memory (Bailey and Kandel, 1995). For example, recalling a close friend's phone number requires that it be placed in long-term storage. Remembering the phone number of a shop you need to call only once requires working memory to hold onto those digits just long enough to dial the number. After the call, the shop's number vanishes from any lasting form of explicit storage. If working memory persisted, we would be bombarded by irrelevant information. Placing a needed item into long-term memory allows us to recall important data. When we ask others to recall their experiences from the past month, we are in effect requesting that they activate a representational process that has been "stored" as an increased probability of firing within a neural net. This is mediated by alterations in synaptic strengths within the network. Recollection can be viewed as the actual activation of this potential or latent representation.

The hippocampus is essential for both encoding into and retrieval from long-term explicit memory. The linkage to the circuits of the dorsolateral prefrontal cortex may be the mechanism for access to working memory whereby representations can be consciously examined, manipulated, and reported to others (Incisa della Rocchetta and Milner, 1993; Gershberg and Shimamura, 1995). Clinicians' assessment of "recent" or "remote" memory often corresponds to researchers' notion of "long-term" memory.

For an element of long-term memory to become a part of permanent explicit memory, a process called cortical consolidation must occur (Abel et al., 1998). Though the specific mechanism has not yet been elucidated, cortical consolidation may require a nonconscious activation or rehearsal process that allows representations to be stored in the "associational cortex" (Kandel, 1989). This region of the cerebral cortex appears to integrate representations from a variety of parts of the brain. In cortical consolidation, information is finally free of the need for the hippocampus for retrieval. This consolidation process appears to depend on the rapid eye movement sleep stage, which is thought to be attempting to make sense of the day's activities (Karni et al., 1992; Winson, 1993). Though filled with a combination of seemingly random activations, aspects of the day's experiences, and elements from the more distant past, dreams may be a fundamental way in which the mind consolidates the myriad of explicit recollections into a coherent set of representations for permanent memory.

Research regarding the details of the consolidation process is still in its infancy (Milner et al., 1998). Cortical consolidation may take weeks, months, or perhaps years to occur. For example, if a teenager has a head injury from a motorcycle accident on the first of December, he may lose recollection of events from November and October but be able to recall those from September and earlier. This is called retrograde amnesia and involves impairment in the ability of his hippocampus to retrieve not-yet-consolidated memories. He may also experience severe difficulty recalling events after the accident, called anterograde amnesia. This is due to the inability of his damaged hippocampus to encode new items into long-term, explicit memory. The teenager's ability to encode or retrieve items from implicit memory may be intact. Implicit memory can be assessed via "indirect" measures of memory, such as those that evaluate "priming." For example, he can learn new skills and have emotional associations to recent events, but he may be unable to recall when he acquired the new knowledge or have any sense of time or self connected with the recollections.

Usually the implicit encoding of an event is associated with its explicit counterpart. Explicit encoding requires focal, conscious attention; it is processed through the initial phases of encoding in working memory and then processed through long-term memory on its way toward cortical consolidation. There are certain situations, however, in which there is a disassociation between implicit and explicit memory. In infantile or childhood amnesia (discussed below), implicit memory is intact but explicit recall, especially episodic memory, is impaired. Other examples include hypnotic amnesia, the effects of certain medications (such as the benzodiazepines), surgical anesthesia, neurological conditions such as Korsakoff syndrome, and divided attention phenomena (e.g., the dichotic listening experiment). Indirect recall is an indirect measure of memory that assesses implicit memory (Schacter, 1996). The subject's brain encodes information implicitly such that the brain is primed, that is, made more likely, to bring up that information when given a cue with no conscious sense of recall of the experience. Without focal attention, items are not encoded explicitly. Implicit memory may be intact, but explicit memory is impaired for that stimulus or event (Schacter, 1992).

THE SUBJECTIVE EXPERIENCE OF MEMORY

The autobiographical narrative process is directly influenced by both implicit and explicit memory. Through autonoetic consciousness we are able to perform "mental time travel," creating representations of the self in the past, present, and future (Wheeler et al., 1997). As the child develops into the third year of life, the orbitofrontal cortex becomes capable of mediating episodic memory and autonoesis. Events are encoded as they are personally experienced as the child moves from having only semantic (factual) knowledge of events to also being able to have episodic (autobiographical) memory (with a sense of self and time). Both implicit mental models and explicit autonoesis enable the mind to prepare for the future.

When either semantic or episodic explicit memory is retrieved, there is an internal sensation of "I am recalling something." This distinguishes explicit from implicit recollection in which there is no such subjective sense of remembrance. Explicit memories take a number of forms. Semantic memory recalls factual information (such as the capitals of the countries of Europe). If we recall that we were once there but cannot summon the sensation of the self in time on the trip, then this reflects only a semantic memory for a personally experienced event. Recent neuroscience studies support the notion that semantic recall of events lacking a sense of self is quite different from episodic recall (Wheeler et al., 1997). Noetic consciousness (knowing the fact that one was once in Europe) is thought to be distinct from autonoetic consciousness (recalling the self-experience of the trip). Episodic recall activates autobiographical memory representations and evokes the sense of the self in time that differentiates it from semantic recollections. These distinctions may be important in understanding the nature of recollections in children and adolescents who have experienced traumatic events.

Within explicit, autobiographical memory we can find a number of variations. For example, a teenager may recall a general sense of herself, say, from her senior year in high school. This generic episodic recollection can be thought of as a summary of a year of specific episodes. In a sense this is a self-concept, or self-schema made conscious, about herself during that year. She may also be able to recall a specific event during that time, such as her last day of high school. In retrieving this memory, she may recall it as an event she can observe from a distance. This is an observer recollection which some might consider a distanced form of episodic retrieval but others would label as an event memory within semantic recall (Schacter, 1996; Wheeler et al., 1997). In contrast, she may recall the event as if she were actually there, a participant or field recollection. In this case, she would be able to see things from her actual perspective. Observer memory appears to involve less emotional intensity than do field recollections. Autonoesis thus evokes elements of the self's lived experience rather than merely the propositional (factual) representations of noetic consciousness.

The distinct experiential aspects of memory are thought to involve different centers of brain activation (Fink et al., 1996). For example, semantic recall appears to involve a dominance of left over right hippocampal activation. Autobiographical recall, in contrast, involves more of the right hippocampus and right orbitofrontal cortex (Wheeler et al., 1997). This distinction may reveal itself when we sense that a fact is known without any feeling that it is a part of our experienced life. This may also help us to understand the finding of increased activation of the right hemisphere in the visual cortical activity during the recollection of unresolved traumatic memories (Rauch et al., 1996).

Recent studies reveal the significant distinctions between semantic and episodic memory (Moscovitch, 1995). For semantic memory, noetic consciousness allows for facts about the world. Noetic awareness is the focusing of attention on a particular aspect of semantic representations. Though semantic and episodic memory have much in common—they are flexibly accessible, have virtually unlimited capacities for representing "data," are encoded with contextual features, and can be retrieved in a declarative manner utilizing language or drawing—they in fact appear to be mediated by somewhat distinct mechanisms (Wheeler et al., 1997).

Autonoetic consciousness is created within the various layers of frontal lobe function (Buckner, 1996). These include an integrating capacity in which more posteriorly stored information can be organized and sequenced into a meaningful set of representations, executive functions that provide a more global control of widely distributed brain processes, and the mediation of self-reflection and social cognition (Tucker et al., 1995). Episodic memory is mediated in circuits with close proximity to those with the integrating executive functions that create social and self-awareness. "Mental time travel" is an actively constructing mental process that creates the self within a social world. Several independent lines of research point to the prefrontal regions—especially the orbitofrontal cortex in the right hemisphere—as a crucial area for integrating memory (Wheeler et al., 1997), attachment (Schore, 1994), emotion (Tucker et al., 1995), bodily representation and regulation (Damasio, 1994), and social cognition (Baron-Cohen, 1995). Children reveal distinct differences in their capacity for autonoetic reflection, which may be due in part to the differential development of their integrating prefrontal regions. Attachment research and developmental psychology studies of memory suggest that interactions between parents and children may have a direct effect on the child's capacity for autobiographical recall. One plausible explanation for this finding is that the prefrontal regions are exquisitely responsive to social experience and are also the regions responsible for autonoesis.

The process of reactivating representations from explicit memory is often dependent on the features of the internal and external environment. When there is a match between retrieval cue and memory representation, the process is called ecphory (Tulving, 1993). Ecphory depends on the features of the eliciting stimulus and the form in which the representation has been "stored" in memory. This effect of the context on the retrieval of explicit memory reveals how retrieval is enhanced when conditions have similarities in the physical world (sights, sounds, smells) or in one's state of mind (emotions, mental models, states of general arousal) to those that were present at the time of the initial encoding. In this way, explicit memory is said to be context-dependent. The hippocampus is able to encode its cognitive mapping onto experiences, giving them a context in which they are both registered and stored. The actual representations of such experiences are thought to be stored in more posterior portions of the brain. The prefrontal regions are thought to perform the process of creating an episodic "retrieval state" in which a match (ecphory) between retrieval cue and stored representation can occur (Wheeler et al., 1997). As children mature, their capacities for developing "retrieval strategies" that enable them to have more elaborate spontaneous or cued recollections may depend on the development of the prefrontal regions. Such development is first seen during the preschool years (Nelson and Carver, 1998).

Individuals may have recollections in which they lack an understanding of how the contextual cues have led to specific events being recalled. The exploration of these memories may be carried out by searching for a match between the features present at the time of retrieval and at the time of the original event. Such a search can sometimes reveal the underlying emotional meaning or gist of a particular recollection. However, the sense of mental time travel by itself does not mean that the recollection is accurate: it merely implies that the prefrontally mediated autonoetic awareness circuits are involved in the activation of stored or internally generated representations—nor that ecphory has occurred. In this manner, the prefrontal regions may attempt to create accurate assemblies of representations. Whether accurate or not, they may carry a sense of the self recalling the past. This can be viewed as an "ecphoric sensation" which has a sense of conviction that the recalled memory is indeed accurate. We can have a clear sense that something happened when in fact it did not. Such subjective sensations may be a part of imagination, dreaming, and accurate or inaccurate recollection.

The richness of recollection we may feel in reflecting on past experiences is shaped in part by the internal or external context cues that can then initiate a cascade of further related recollections. Initial ecphory (retrieval cue matching stored memory representation) is followed by a series of sometimes unpredictable associative linkages influenced by both memory and present experience. These associated recollections and retrieval cues can be woven into the process of remembering and can become a part of the "reconstructed" memory. Representations resembling those of the past are reassembled during the process of recollection. Retrieval is thus a "memory modifier": the act of reactivating a representation can allow it to be stored again in a modified form (Bjork, 1989). The frontal lobes carrying out the integrating, executive, and socially constructive memories of the self can directly shape the nature of autobiographical recollections and life stories. These processes explain one way in which our memories, things we may regard as facts, can actually change over time. This may also explain how repeated questioning regarding a possible experience of abuse can lead a child to confuse recollections of the stories told from retrieval of elements of the initial experience.

Explicit memory is often communicated to us and to others in the form of descriptive words or pictures communicating a story or sequence of events. If involving the sense of self at some time in the past, then this is a part of autobiographical explicit memory. We listen to the words and receive a linguistic message or visualize the pictures and have a conscious sense of the story being told. Recollections usually involve the association of these explicit elements with their implicit counterparts. To sense these it is important to recall (explicitly) that the activation of implicit memory does not have a sense of "something is being remembered." We sense, perceive, or filter our explicit memory through the mental models of implicit memory. We can watch for the shadows that such implicit recollections cast on the stories we tell as well as on nonverbal aspects of behavior and communication. A clinician is thus wise to listen to both the details and the "between-the-line" messages and themes of an individual's unfolding story.

"CHILDHOOD AMNESIA"

For more than a century clinicians have been aware of an impairment in the ability of adults or older children to recall the first years of their lives. Initial impressions placed this "memory barrier" at around 5 years of age. Early psychoanalytic writings, though not supported by modern analytic thinking, suggested that infantile amnesia was due to overwhelming traumatic experiences that were being blocked and that one focus of treatment would be to uncover this "repression barrier" (Freud, 1895).

Developmental psychologists view childhood amnesia differently; they suggest that the immaturity in several domains, including the sense of self and of time, verbal ability, and narrative capacity, might be the limiting factors impairing recall for the period before the age of about 2 to 3 years (Fivush and Hudson, 1990; Newcombe and Fox, 1994; Rovee-Collier, 1993). Neurobiologists have looked at the development of the hippocampus/medial temporal lobe and prefrontal regions during the first years of life as a possible mediator of childhood amnesia (Bacheveller, 1992; Perner and Ruffman, 1995). This view supports the developmental psychologists' observations in providing the likely neurobiological underpinnings to this normal developmental form of amnesia. In this way, explicit memory may require the neural maturation of the hippocampus to allow for the full expression of first semantic and then later, with the development of the prefrontal regions, episodic memory.

Implicit memory is intact at birth; explicit, semantic memory begins before the child's second birthday (Bauer et al., 1994, 1995). A 1-year-old will be able to have implicit recollection of all sorts of experiences (e.g., becoming excited when she hears the car pull into the garage because she knows emotionally that her mother is coming home). She has already developed the capacity for generalized recollections, called general event knowledge (Bauer and Dow, 1994; Nelson, 1993a). Before 18 months she has begun to develop the ability to recall the sequence of events (Bauer, 1996). She thus can encode and retrieve facts from specific experiences. This can be considered a form of semantic memory in which knowledge of specific events can be recalled after a long delay (Bauer et al., 1994).

Studies thus suggest that semantic explicit memory is intact from quite early on. Support for this view comes from recent findings that children, even in their second year of life, have a remarkable ability to retain facts about novel experiences with considerable accuracy (Bauer, 1996).

After about 18 months, a child develops self-referential behaviors that reveal a sense of continuity of the self through time. By the second birthday, she can begin to talk about events that happened to her. As she continues to mature, her sense of self develops more fully and allows for the emergence of episodic memory and the capacity for mental time travel—of remembering herself in specific experiences in the past. As her prefrontal regions develop, this capacity continues to become more complex and sophisticated. These regions continue to develop into adulthood and may explain the deepening capacity for self-awareness and autonoetic consciousness across the life span. Before the preschool years, she can say that she saw a dog that morning or that she went to visit her grandfather at the park. She can narrate her ongoing experience and verbalize and plan for her anticipations of future events. Though now she can talk about her recent recollections, she cannot episodically remember when she was an infant. Some facts that she learned during her second year of life, however, such as the names of objects, may be quite available to her within semantic memory. Also, her complex and rich implicit learning is and will remain intact.

Some authors argue that childhood amnesia should be used to describe not an impairment in general explicit recall, but rather as very specifically due to the developmental lag in the onset of episodic memory (Perner and Ruffman, 1995; Wheeler et al., 1997). In this view, the neurobiological substrate necessary for autonoesis—the hippocampus and orbitofrontal regions—may determine the timing of the onset of autobiographical memory as well as its possibly experience-dependent development within attachment relationships.

Researchers have not yet been able to explain the finding that children beyond 5 years of age may have limited access to elements that were available to them earlier. Thus children at 3 or 4 years of age may have an ease of explicit recall of aspects of their daily lives, yet a few years later they may lack a continuous set of memories for that earlier period. One possibility is that before 5 years of age the consolidation process that transforms long-term memory into permanent memory is not yet mature. Further research is needed to explore the validity of this proposed mechanism.

The development of explicit memory appears to be directly influenced by interpersonal experiences. This view is supported by the finding that children who have more experiences of talking about their memories with their parents are able to recall more details about their lives later on (Bauer and Wewerka, 1995; Fivush, 1996). Memory talk is a common process in which parents focus their attention on the contents of the child's memories. A similar observation is that parents who participate in an elaborative form of communication have children with a richer sense of autobiographical recall. "Elaborative" parents talk with their children about what they, the children, think about the stories which they read together. In contrast "factual" parents, subjects who were found to talk only about the facts of stories, not the child's imagination or response, had a less developed ability for recall (Dunn and Brown, 1991; McCabe and Peterson, 1991; Reese and Fivush, 1993). There is likely a range of communication styles between the extremes of these research categories. Nevertheless, these findings support the general principle that interpersonal experiences appear to have a direct effect on the development of explicit memory. Could these effects be mediated by the experience-dependent growth of the orbitofrontal regions responsible for encoding and retrieval of episodic memory? No studies exploring this possibility have been published.

Are these merely genetic findings revealing that parents give rise to offspring who will share their traits? One must await further studies, such as those that might examine the narratives of identical twins raised apart, to confirm the origin of these differences in narrative style. There is clearly a difference in narrative experience, whatever the origin: some families participate in frequent co-construction of narrative and elaborative memory talk. In reinforcing this kind of experience, parents may facilitate their children's ability to describe their memories and their imagination. In a similar fashion, children raised in families who discussed people's emotional reactions tended to be more interested in and able to understand others' emotions (Bretherton, 1993; Nelson, 1993a). These children are also taught that what they have to say about the contents of their minds is important.

TRAUMA AND MEMORY

Traumatic experiences may involve internal and interpersonal processes that may lead to profound effects on memory (Cicchetti and Toth, 1998). Early and severe traumatic experiences may lead to elevated levels of stress hormones that are toxic to the developing brain and have been found to be associated with impaired brain growth (De Bellis et al., 1999a,b) as well as impaired memory processing (Diamond and Rose, 1994). Some studies of older individuals with posttraumatic stress disorder have revealed a decreased size of the hippocampus that may impair the processing of explicit memory (Bremner et al., 1995). In these ways, trauma may produce direct effects on the brain structures that subsume memory encoding, storage, and retrieval.

The processing of memory, even in the face of intact neural structures, may be functionally impaired in posttraumatic conditions (Bower and Sivers, 1998). For example, unresolved traumatic memory may involve impairment in the cortical consolidation process that leaves the memories of these events out of permanent, explicit memory. Such a blockage in the pathway toward consolidating memory may lead to impediments in the creation of a coherent narrative of the self (Siegel, 1999). This individual may be vulnerable to experiencing intrusive implicit images of past horrors in the form of internal sensations, flashbacks, and nightmares. Nightmares, occurring during the dream stage of sleep (involving active rapid eye movement), may reveal futile attempts of the brain to resolve and consolidate such blocked memory configurations. Dream stages of sleep are thought to play a central role in reorganizing memory and reinforcing the connections between memory and emotion (Hobson, 1992).

Autonoetic consciousness of traumatic events may be disturbed in individuals who have experienced trauma that remains "unresolved" (Siegel, 1999, 2001). This unresolved state of mind has important implications for how the mind functions within the interpersonal relationship of attachment. Some individuals may become flooded by excessive implicit recollections in which they lose the self-monitoring features of episodic recall and feel not as if they are intensely recalling a past event but rather that they are in the event itself (Siegel, 1995, 1996). Under such conditions, a parent may lose the capacity for flexible, attuned responses to a child. This mechanism may be one explanation for the finding that adults with an attachment classification of "unresolved trauma or grief" tend to have children who have a disorganized attachment. Main and Hesse (1990) have proposed that the parent's frightened, frightening, or disorienting behaviors with the child lead to a paradoxical injunction in which the child is terrified by the very figure who is supposed to be the source of comfort and soothing (Main, 1999). Children with disorganized attachment have been shown to be vulnerable to the later development of dissociative symptoms (Carlson, 1998).

In its essence, unresolved trauma or grief can be conceptualized as a lack of cortical consolidation regarding that aspect of an individual's life history and may clinically be seen as the absence of a coherent narrative version of a traumatic experience. Unresolved states remain isolated from the normal integrative functioning of the individual and can impair flexible responsivity and the development of a coherent sense of self. Unresolved trauma leaves the individual prone to an unstable state of potential implicit activations that tend to intrude on the survivor's internal experience and interpersonal relationships. For a parent, such unresolved states of mind can have a devastating effect on the individual's children. Parental disorganization due to unresolved trauma or grief is associated with the child's development of disorganized attachment and risk for dissociative adaptations. Preventive measures involving assessment and intervention at the level of unresolved parental grief and trauma might provide an effective strategy for promoting child mental health (D. J. Siegel and M. Hartzel, unpublished).

MEMORY AND THE ACCURACY OF RECOUNTING

Recounting the elements of autobiographical explicit memory is a social experience that is profoundly influenced by the social interaction. Thus what is recounted is not the same as what is initially remembered and is not necessarily completely accurate in detail. Children may be especially capable of remembering the gist of an experience with great accuracy, but they may be less able to spontaneously recall the details of past events. Therapists, attorneys, judges, and others involved in litigation and investigation around issues of childhood abuse would be wise to be aware of the studies documenting the accuracy of children's memory even in the face of incomplete and, at times, inconsistent reporting (Goodman and Fivush, 1993).

Some individuals, especially young children, may be more susceptible to suggestive influences than others (Schumacher, 1991). The relatively immature retrieval strategies of early childhood may make preschoolers and younger children especially vulnerable to interview pressures (Ceci and Bruck, 1993; Ceci and Huffman, 1997). These factors may also make their accurate testimonies appear to be distorted or inconsistent.

Furthermore, studies suggest that it is possible for an individual to have a firm conviction of the veridicality of a "recollection" of an event that has never occurred. Thus the degree of conviction we have in the accuracy of a memory may not correspond to its accuracy (Ceci and Bruck, 1993). The use of internal corroborations, such as the structure of memory systems and the relationship between implicit and explicit components of memory of an event, may be useful in understanding how past experiences have influenced a patient's life. External corroboration, such as the experience of other family members, police reports, photo albums, and journals, may be useful in creating a fuller picture.

MEMORY AND NARRATIVE

The telling of stories plays a crucial role in the interaction between adult and child (Ochs and Capps, 1996). From early in development, children begin to narrate their lives, telling the sequence of events and internal experiences of their daily existence (Nelson, 1989; Britton and Pellegrini, 1990).

The developmental psychologist Vygotsky (1986) said that the child's internalization of her experiences with parents creates thought. This view reveals the possibility that some of our most cherished personal processes, such as thought or even self-reflection, may have their origins as interpersonal communication.

Many forms of human communication within psychotherapy—from play and drawing with young children to autobiographical reflections with older children and adolescents—involve the co-construction of narrative around the memory talk between individuals.

The narrative process may reflect a core capacity of the individual to integrate a sense of coherence across the many states of mind that exist at a given developmental stage and across time. This central capacity for integration may be one possible explanation for the attachment research finding that the most robust predictor of a child's security of attachment is the coherence of the parent's life narrative as assessed in the research instrument, the Adult Attachment Interview (Hesse, 1999; Siegel, 1999). This finding suggests that adults' narratives reveal a central process that impacts on the nature of their interpersonal communication. As a function of both implicit and explicit memory, narratives reveal how the mind integrates a massive amount of experience across the individual's lifetime. As we explore with our patients the "stories of their lives," we are assessing far more than a mere recounting of events. We are, in reality, reaching to the core of their selves and joining with them in the co-construction of a powerful form of integration that links the past with the present as they anticipate and create their future life experiences.

AFFILIATION

Dr. Siegel is Director, Center for Human Development, Los Angeles, and Associate Clinical Professor of Psychiatry, UCLA School of Medicine.

ACKNOWLEDGMENTS

This article is adapted in part from *The Developing Mind* (Siegel, 1999) with permission from The Guilford Press.

REFERENCES

Abel T., Martin K. C., Bartsch D., Kandel E. R. (1998). Memory suppressor genes: inhibitory constraints on the storage of long-term memory. *Science* 279:338–341.

Andreasen N. C., O'Leary D. S., Cizadlo T. et al. (1995). Remembering the past: two faces of episodic memory explored with positron emission tomography. *Am J Psychiatry* 152:1576–1585.

Arnsten A. F. T. (2000). Genetics of childhood disorders, XVIII: ADHD, part 2: norepinephrine has a critical modulatory influence on prefrontal cortical function. *J Am Acad Child Adolesc Psychiatry* 39:1201–1203.

Bachevelier J. (1992). Cortical versus limbic immaturity: relationship to infantile amnesia. In: *Developmental Behavioral Neuroscience: Minnesota Symposium on Child Psychology*, Vol 24, Gunnar MR, Nelson CA, eds. Hillsdale, NJ: Erlbaum, pp. 129–154.

Baddeley A. (1992), Working memory. *Science* 255:556–559.

Bailey C. H., Kandel E. R. (1995). Molecular and structural mechanisms underlying long-term memory. In: *The Cognitive Neurosciences*, Gazzaniga MS, ed. Cambridge, MA: MIT Press, pp. 19–36.

Barnes C. A., Erickson C. A., Davis S., McNaughton B. L. (1995). Hippocampal synaptic enhancement as a basis for learning and memory: a selected review of current evidence from behaving animals. In: *Brain and Memory: Modulation and Mediation of Neuroplasticity*, McGaugh JL, Weinberger NM, Lynch G, eds. New York: Oxford University Press, pp. 259–276.

Baron-Cohen S. (1995). *Mindblindness: An Essay on Autism and Theory of Mind.* Cambridge, MA: MIT Press.
*Bauer P. J. (1996). What do infants recall of their lives? Memory for specific events by one to two-year-olds. *Am Psychol* 51:29–41.
Bauer P. J., Dow G. A (1994). Episodic memory in sixteen- and twenty-month-old children: specifies are generalized but not forgotten. *Dev Psychol* 30:403–417.
Bauer P. J., Hertsgaard L. A., Dow G.A. (1994). After eight months have passed: long-term recall of events by one and two year-old children. *Memory* 2:353–382.
Bauer P. J., Hertsgaard L. A., Wewerka S. S. (1995). Effects of experience and reminding on long-term recall in infancy: remembering not to forget. *J Exp Child Psychol* 59:260–298.
Bauer P. J., Wewerka S. S. (1995). One to two-year-olds' recall of events: the more expressed, the more impressed. *J Exp Child Psychol* 59:475–496.
Bjork R. (1989). Retrieval inhibition as an adaptive mechanism in human memory. In: *Varieties of Memory and Consciousness: Essays in Honor of Endel Tulving*, Roediger H. L, Craik F. I. M., eds. London: Wiley, pp. 283–288.
Bremner J. D., Randall P., Scott T. M., et al. (1995). MRI-based measures of hippocampal volume in patients with combat-related posttraumatic stress disorder. *Am J Psychiatry* 152:973–981.
Bretherton I. (1993). From dialogue to internal working models: the co-construction of self in relationships. In: *Memory and Affect in Development: The Minnesota Symposia on Child Psychology*, Vol 26, Nelson C. A., ed. Hillsdale, NJ: Erlbaum, pp. 237–264.
Britton B. K., Pellegrini A. D. (1990). *Narrative Thought and Narrative Language.* Hillsdale, NJ: Erlbaum.
Bower G. H., Sivers H. (1998). Cognitive impact of traumatic events. *Dev Psychopathol* 10:625–654.
Buckner R. L., (1996). Beyond HERA: contributions of specific prefrontal brain areas to long-term memory retrieval. *Psychon Bull Rev* 3:149–158.
Buckner R. L., Petersen S. E., Ojemann J. G., Miezin F. M., Squire L. R., Raichle M. E. (1995). Functional anatomical studies of explicit and implicit memory retrieval tasks. *J Neurosci* 15:12–29.
Carlson E. A. (1998). A prospective longitudinal study of attachment disorganization/ disorientation. *Child Dev* 69:1107–1128.
Ceci S., Bruck M. (1993). Suggestibility of the child witness: a historical review and synthesis. *Psychol Bull* 113:403–439.
Ceci S., Huffman M. L., (1997), How suggestible are preschool children? Cognitive and social factors. *J Am Acad Child Adolesc Psychiatry* 36:948–958.
Christianson S. A., ed. (1991). *Handbook of Emotion and Memory.* Hillsdale, NJ: Erlbaum.
*Ciccheti D., Toth S., eds. (1998). Risk, trauma, and memory (special issue). *Dev Psychopathol* 10(4).
Damasio A. (1994). *Descarte's Error: Emotion, Reason, and the Human Brain.* New York: Grosset/Putnam.
De Bellis M. D., Baum A. S., Birmaher B et al. (1999a). AE Bennett Research Award: developmental traumatology. part I: biological stress systems. *Biol Psychiatry* 45:1259–1270.

De Bellis M. D., Keshavan M. S., Clark D. B., et al. (1999b). AE Bennett Research Award: developmental traumatology, part II: brain development. *Biol Psychiatry* 45:1271–1284.

Diamond D. M., Rose G. (1994). Stress impairs LTP and hippocampal dependent memory. *Ann NY Acad Sci* 746:411–414.

Dunn J., Brown J. (1991). Relationships, talk about feelings, and the development of affect regulation in early childhood. In: *The Development of Emotion Regulation and Dysregulation*, Garber J., Dodge K. A., eds. Cambridge, England: Cambridge University Press, pp. 89–110.

Edelman G. (1992). *Bright Air, Brilliant Fire*. New York: Basic Books.

Fink G. R., Markowowitsch H. J., Reinkemeier M., Bruckbauer T., Kessler J., Wolf Dieter H. (1996), Cerebral representation of one's own past: neural networks involved in autobiographical memory. *J Neurosci* 16:4275–4282.

Fivush R. (1996). Constructing narrative, emotion, and self in parent—child conversations about the past. In: *The Remembering Self Construction and Accuracy in the Self-Narrative*, Neisser U., Fivush R., eds. Cambridge, England: Cambridge University Press, pp. 136–157.

Fivush R., Hudson J. A., eds. (1990). *Knowing and Remembering in Young Children*. New York: Cambridge University Press.

Freud S. (1895). Project for a Scientific Psychology. In: *The Standard Edition of the Complete Psychological Works of Sigmund Freud*, Vol. 1, Strachey J., ed. & trans. London: Hogarth Press, pp. 281–397.

Freyd J. J., (1987). Dynamic mental representations. *Psychol Rev* 94:427–438.

Gershberg F. B., Shimamura A. P. (1995). The role of the frontal lobes in the use of organizational strategies in free recall. *Neuropsychologia* 13:1305–1333.

Goldman-Rakic P. S., (1993). Working memory and the mind. In: *Mind and Brain: Readings from Scientific American Magazine*, September, Freeman W. H., ed. New York: Freeman, pp. 66–77.

Goodman L., Fivush R. (1993), *Child Victims, Child Witnesses*. New York: Guilford.

Greenough W. T., Black J. E., (1992). Induction of brain structure by experience: substrates for cognitive development. In: *Developmental Behavioral Neuroscience: The Minnesota Symposia on Child Psychology*, Vol. 24, Gunnar M. R., Nelson C. A., eds. Hillsdale, NJ: Erlbaum, pp. 155–200.

Hebb D. O., (1949). *The Organization of Behavior: A Neuropsychological Theory*. New York: Wiley.

Hendren R. L., De Backer I., Pandina G. J. (2000). Review of neuroimaging studies of child and adolescent psychiatric disorders from the past 10 years. *J Am Acad Child Adolesc Psychiatry* 39:815–828.

*Hesse E. (1999). The Adult Attachment Interview: historical and current perspectives. In: *Handbook of Attachment: Theory, Research, and Clinical Applications*, Cassidy J., Shaver P. R., eds. New York: Guilford, pp. 395–433.

Hobson J. (1992). The brain as a dream machine: an activation-synthesis hypothesis of dreaming. In: *Essential Papers on Dreams*, Lansky M., ed. New York: New York University Press, pp. 452–473.

Incisa della Rocchetta A., Milner B. (1993). Strategic search and retrieval inhibition: the role of the frontal lobes. *Neuropsychologia* 31:503–524.

Ingvar D. H., (1985). "Memory of the future": an essay on the temporal organization of conscious awareness. *Hum Neurobiol* 4:127–136.

Johnson-Laird P. N., (1983). *Mental Models: Towards a Cognitive Science of Language, Inference, and Consciousness*. Cambridge, MA: Harvard University Press.

Kandel E. R., (1989). Genes, nerve cells, and the remembrance of things past. *J Neuropsychiatry Clin Neurosci* 1:103–125.

Kandel E. R. (1998). A new intellectual framework for psychiatry. *Am J Psychiatry* 155:457–469.

Kandel E. R., Abel T. (1995). Neuropeptides, adenylyl cyclase, and memory storage. *Science* 268:825–826.

Kapur S., Craik F. I. M., Tulving E., Wilson A. A., Houle S., Brown G. M., (1994). Neuroanatomical correlates of encoding in episodic memory: levels of processing effect. *Proc Natl Acad Sci* USA 91:2012–2015.

Karni A., Tanne D., Rubenstein B. S., Askenasi J. J., Sagi D. (1992). No dreams, no memory: the effect of REM sleep deprivation on learning a new perceptual skill. *Soc Neurosci Abstr* 18:387.

Kelley W. M., Miezin F. M., McDermott K. B., et al. (1998). Hemispheric specialization in human dorsal frontal cortex and medial temporal lobe for verbal and nonverbal memory encoding. *Neuron* 20:927–936.

Kempermann G., Kuhn H. G., Gage F. H. (1997). More hippocampal neurons in adult mice living in an enriched environment. *Nature* 386:493–495.

Kosslyn S. M., (1994). *Image and Brain: The Resolution of the Imagery Debate*. Cambridge, MA: MIT Press.

Main M. (1999). Epilogue: attachment theory: eighteen points with suggestions for future studies. In: *Handbook of Attachment: Theory, Research, and Clinical Applications*, Cassidy J., Shaver P. R., eds. New York: Guilford, pp. 845–884.

Main M., Hesse E. (1990). Parents' unresolved traumatic experiences are related to infant disorganized status: is frightened and/or frightening parental behavior the linking mechanism? In: *Attachment in the Preschool Years*, Greenberg M., Cicchetti D., Cummings M., eds. Chicago: University of Chicago Press, pp. 161–182.

Martin K. C., Kandel E. R. (1996). Cell adhesion molecules, CREB, and the formation of new synaptic connections (comment). *Neuron* 4:567–570.

McCabe A., Peterson C. (1991). Getting the story: a longitudinal study of parental styles in eliciting narratives and developing narrative skill. In: *Developing Narrative Structure*, McCabe A., Peterson C., eds. Hillsdale, NJ: Erlbaum, pp. 217–253.

McClelland J. L., McNaughton B. L., O'Reilly R. C., (1995). Why there are complementary learning systems in the hippocampus and neocortex: insights from the successes and failures of connectionist models of learning and memory. *Psychol Rev* 102:419–457.

Merzenich M. M., Grajski K. A., Jenkins W. M., Recanzone G. H., Peterson B. (1991). Functional cortical plasticity: cortical network origins of representations changes. *Cold Spring Harb Symp Quant Biol* 55:873–887.

Merzenich M. M., Sameshima K. (1993). Cortical plasticity and memory. *Curr Opin Neurobiol* 3:187–196.

Miller P. J., Potts R., Fung H., Hoogstra L., Mintz J. (1990). Narrative practices and the social construction of self in childhood. *Am Ethnol* 17:292–311.

*Milner B., Squire L. R., Kandel E. R. (1998). Cognitive neuroscience and the study of memory. *Neuron* 20:445–468.

Morris R. G. M., ed. (1989). *Parallel Distributed Processing: Implications for Psychology and Neurobiology.* Oxford, England: Clarendon.

Moscovitch M. (1995). Recovered consciousness: a hypothesis concerning modularity and episodic memory. *J Clin Exp Neuropsychol* 17:276–290.

Myers N. A., Clifton R. K., Clarkson M. G. (1987). When they were very young: almost threes remember two years ago. *Infant Behav Dev* 10:123–132.

Nelson C. A., ed. (1993a). *Memory and Affect in Development: The Minnesota Symposia on Child Psychology,* Vol. 26. Hillsdale, NJ: Erlbaum.

Nelson C. A., Carver L. J. (1998). The effects of stress and trauma on brain and memory: a view from developmental cognitive neuroscience. *Dev Psychopathol* 10:793–810.

Nelson K., ed. (1989). *Narratives From the Crib.* Cambridge, MA: Harvard University Press.

Nelson K. (1993b). Events, narratives, memory: what develops? In: *Memory and Affect in Development: The Minnesota Symposia on Child Psychology,* Vol. 26, Nelson C. A., ed. Hillsdale, NJ: Erlbaum, pp. 124.

Newcombe N., Fox N. A. (1994). Infantile amnesia: through a glass darkly. *Child Dev* 65:31–40.

Ochs E., Capps L. (1996). Narrating the self. In: *Annual Review of Anthropology,* Durham W., Valentine Daniels E., Schieffelin B., eds. Palo Alto, CA: Annual Reviews Inc. 25:19–43.

Oppenheim D., Nir A., Warren S., Emde R. N. (1997). Emotion regulation in mother-child narrative co-construction: associations with children's narratives and adaptation. *Dev Psychol* 33:284–294.

Perner J. (1991). *Understanding the Representational Mind.* Cambridge, MA: MIT Press.

Perner J., Ruffman T. (1995). Episodic memory and autonoetic consciousness: developmental evidence and a theory of childhood amnesia. *J Exp Child Psychol* 59:516–548.

Perry B. D., Pollard R. A., Blakely T. L., Baker W. L., Viglinate D. (1995). Childhood trauma, the neurobiology of adaptation, and "use-dependent" development of the brain: how states become traits. *Infant Ment Health J* 16:217–291.

Rakic P., Bourgeois J. P., Goldman-Rakic P. S. (1994). Synaptic development of the cerebral cortex: implications for learning, memory, and mental illness. *Prog Brain Res* 102:227–243.

Rauch S. L., van der Kolk B. A., Fisler R. E., et al. (1996). A symptom provocation study of posttraumatic stress disorder using positron emission tomography and script-driven imagery. *Arch Gen Psychiatry* 53:380–387.

Reese E., Fivush R. (1993). Parental styles of talking about the past. *Dev Psychol* 29:596–606.

Rovee-Collier C. (1993). The capacity for long-term memory in infancy. *Curr Dir Psychol Sci* 2:130–135.

Schacter D. L., (1992). Understanding implicit memory: a cognitive neuroscience approach. *Am Psychol* 47:559–569.
Schacter D. L., (1996). *Searching for Memory: The Brain, the Mind, and the Past.* New York: Basic Books.
Schacter D. L., Alpert N. M., Savage C. R., Rauch S. L., Albert M. S. (1996). Conscious recollection and the human hippocampal formation: evidence from positron emission tomography. *Proc Natl Acad Sci* USA 93:321–325.
Schore A. N. (1994). *Affect Regulation and the Origin of the Self: The Neurobiology of Emotional Development.* Hillsdale, NJ: Erlbaum.
Schumacher J. F. (1991). *Human Suggestibility: Advances in Theory, Research and Applications.* New York: Routledge.
Shimamura A. P. (1995). Memory and frontal lobe function. In: *The Cognitive Neurosciences*, Gazzaniga M. S., ed. Cambridge, MA: MIT Press, pp. 803–814.
Siegel D. J. (1995). Memory, trauma, and psychotherapy: a cognitive science view. *J Psychother Pract Res* 4:93–122.
Siegel D. J. (1996). Cognition, memory, and dissociation. *Child Adolesc Psychiatr Clin N Am* 5:509–536.
*Siegel D. J. (1999). *The Developing Mind: Toward a Neurobiology of Interpersonal Experience.* New York: Guilford.
Siegel D. J. (2001). Toward an interpersonal neurobiology of the developing mind: attachment relationships, "mindsight," and neural integration. *Infant Ment Health J* 22:67–94.
Squire L. R. (1987). *Memory and Brain.* New York: Oxford University Press.
Squire L. R. (1992). Declarative and nondeclarative memory: multiple brain systems supporting learning and memory. *J Cogn Neurosci* 4:232–243.
Squire L. R., Knowlton B., Musen G. (1993). The structure and organization of memory. *Annu Rev Psychol* 44:453–495.
Squire L. R., Zola-Morgan S. (1991).The medial temporal lobe memory system. *Science* 153:2380–2386.
Stern D. N. (1985). *The Interpersonal World of the Infant.* New York: Basic Books.
Tucker D. M. (1992). Developing emotions and cortical networks. In: *Developmental Behavioral Neuroscience: Minnesota Sympossium on Child Psychology*, Vol. 24, Gunnar M. R., Nelson C. A., eds. Hillsdale, NJ: Erlbaum, pp. 75–128.
Tucker D. M., Luu P., Pribram K. H. (1995). Social and emotional self-regulation. *Ann N Y Acad Sci* 769:213–239.
Tulving E. (1993). Varieties of consciousness and levels of awareness in memory. In: *Attention, Selection, Awareness, and Control: A Tribute to Donald Broadbent*, Baddeley A., Weiskrantz L., eds. London: Oxford University Press, pp. 283–299.
Tulving E., Craik F. I. M. (2000). *The Oxford Handbook of Memory.* New York: Oxford University Press.
Vygotsky L. (1986). *Thought and Language.* Cambridge, MA: MIT Press.
*Wheeler M. A., Stuss D. T., Tulving E. (1997). Toward a theory of episodic memory: the frontal lobes and autonoetic consciousness. *Psychol Bull* 121:331–354.
Winson J. (1993). The biology and function of rapid eye movement sleep. *Curr Opin Neurobiol* 3:243–248.

10

Infant Temperament and the Brainstem Auditory Evoked Response in Later Childhood

Sue A. Woodward, Mark H. McManis, Jerome Kagan, Patricia Deldin, Nancy Snidman, Melissa Lewis, and Vali Kahn

Brainstem auditory evoked responses (BAERs) were evaluated on 10- to 12-year-old children (N = 56) who had been classified as high or low reactive to unfamiliar stimuli at 4 months of age. BAER measurement was selected because high reactive infants tend to become inhibited or fearful young children, and adult introverts have a faster latency to wave V of the BAER than do extroverts. Children previously classified as high reactive at 4 months had larger wave V components than did low reactive children, a finding that possibly suggests greater excitability in projections to the inferior colliculus. The fact that a fundamental feature of brainstem activity differentiated preadolescent children belonging to two early temperamental groups supports the value of gathering physiological data in temperament research.

The theoretical definition of human temperament lies at the interface of behavior and biology. Despite the dual nature of this construct, most research on temperament relies solely on behavioral variables derived from parental reports or direct observations. Although these measures provide critical information, technical advances make it feasible to add biological measures to assessments of behavior. This empirical strategy can be of importance because as children grow, the expected association between the behavioral and biological correlates of infant temperament is more difficult to detect in the laboratory setting, in part because the defining behaviors seen in very young children become masked by the influences of socialization. Consequently, physiological measures might be of help in discriminating among older children who possess different temperaments early in life but have become more behaviorally homogeneous. In this study of 10- to 12-year-old children categorized in infancy as high or low reactive to unfamiliar stimuli, we examined the importance of combining measures of physiology and behavior.

The categories of high and low reactive refer to two temperamental profiles that are observed at 4 months of age. The two groups are defined by behavioral differences in motor activity and distress in response to unfamiliar visual, auditory, and olfactory stimuli (Kagan, 1994). High reactive infants display vigorous motor activity combined with crying in response to unfamiliar stimuli, whereas low reactive infants show minimal motor activity and minimal distress in response to the same events. Recent statistical analyses support the categorical (vs. dimensional) nature of these two temperamental types (Stern et al., 1994; Woodward et al., 2000).

The two 4-month temperamental classifications predict level of fearful behavior during later childhood. Specifically, high reactive 4-month-old infants are more likely when confronted with unfamiliar objects, events, places, or people in their 2nd year to show a profile—called *behaviorally inhibited*—characterized by withdrawal, hesitation, or crying. Low reactive infants are biased to show the complementary profile—called *behaviorally uninhibited*—of relatively rapid approach to unfamiliar events combined with affective spontaneity when interacting with strangers (Kagan & Snidman, 1991). Peripheral physiological measures also differentiate these two groups and are in accord with the hypothesis that these two behavioral profiles are characterized by different levels of excitability of motor and autonomic targets. Fearful and/or shy children, compared with fearless and/or sociable children, show higher reactivity in sympathetic targets of the cardiovascular system, especially larger increases in blood pressure and heart rate in response to orthostatic stress and greater constriction of the arteriovenous anastomoses of the fingertips following cognitive challenge (Kagan, Reznick, & Snidman, 1987; Kagan, Snidman, & Peterson, 2000; Snidman, Kagan, Riordan, & Shannon, 1995).

However, the overt behavioral differences in timidity and sociability between the two groups of toddlers become less dramatic with development. By 4½ years of age, most children from both infant groups have developed less extreme behavioral profiles, presumably a result of social experiences with parents, peers, and teachers. In one sample, only 15% of high reactive infants remained consistently shy or fearful over three laboratory visits from 14 months to 4½ years of age. It is important to note that not one high reactive infant became a consistently fearless child, and only one low reactive infant became consistently subdued or fearful at all ages (Kagan, Snidman, & Arcus, 1998).

It is not known, however, whether high or low reactive infants will continue to differ physiologically as they approach adolescence. This knowledge is critical for a deeper understanding of the physiological systems associated with these temperamental types. In addition, discovering sensitive physiological markers might help identify purer phenotypes (e.g., children who are shy or fearful as a result of a temperamental predisposition rather than environmental circumstances). Finally, research has demonstrated that 7-year-old children who were high reactive infants are at risk for developing anxious symptoms (e.g., fear of being kidnapped or reluctance to sleep over at a friend's house) (Kagan & Snidman, 1999). Similarly, children who were very fearful at 2 years are at higher risk for adolescent social anxiety (Kagan, Snidman, Zentner, & Peterson 1999; Schwartz, Snidman, & Kagan, 1999). Consequently, a more complete understanding of the physiology linked to infant temperamental types may prove useful in the identification of children at risk for anxious psychopathology.

The brainstem auditory evoked response (BAER), typically elicited by presenting a series of clicks through earphones, is a potentially relevant physiological variable because research on humans demonstrates that variation in the magnitude and latency of wave V differentiates among related personality and clinical categories. The BAER is reflected in a series of seven waves believed to correspond to the successive reactions of discrete structures of the auditory nerve and brainstem. These evoked reactions reflect the first stages of auditory processing and are considered by most to be independent of attention or related cognitive processes (Chiappa, 1997; Hall, 1992).

Of relevance to this report are findings that introverts have a shorter wave V latency than do extroverts (Bullock & Gilliland, 1993; Stelmack & Wilson, 1982; Swickert & Gilliland, 1998) and that adults with panic disorder show a larger amplitude wave V than do controls (Iwanami, Isono, Okajima, & Kamaijima, 1997). Children who are very shy and/or fearful are more likely to become introverted adults, whereas fearless children are more likely to become extroverted (Kagan, 1994). Further, children born to parents with panic disorder are more likely than controls to become shy and avoidant (Rosenbaum et al., 1993). The fact that high reactive infants tend to become subdued or fearful children suggests the hypothesis that children who were high reactive infants should have an enhanced wave V (faster latency or greater amplitude) compared with children who were low reactive infants.

METHOD

Participants

Participants were 56 10- to 12-year-old children who were part of a longitudinal study and were categorized previously as high or low reactive at 4 months of age: 32 high reactives (15 boys and 17 girls) and 24 low reactives (16 boys and 8 girls). In addition, most (91%) were also seen in the laboratory at 14 months and 21 months to have their fear behaviors to unfamiliar stimuli assessed. All participants were healthy Caucasian infants born at term to middle-class mothers, most of whom were college educated and who had limited their intake of tobacco, alcohol, and caffeine during pregnancy.

Previous Assessments (4, 14, and 21 Months)

At 4 months of age, the infants were assessed for behavioral reactivity to unfamiliar stimuli with a standard protocol. Each infant, seated in an infant chair, was exposed first to the mother looking at the infant and then, with the mother outside the perceptual field of the infant, to a series of visual, auditory, and olfactory stimuli (e.g., colorful mobiles, a tape recording of a voice speaking nonsense syllables over trials of increasing loudness, and dilute butyl alcohol on a cotton swab held near the infant's nose). The battery lasted approximately 30 minutes if no breaks were needed for feeding or soothing. Frequency of motor movements (individual limb movements, bilateral limb extensions, and back arches) and of crying and fretting (total seconds crying combined with number of trials with fussing) in response to the episodes was quantified reliably from videotape (for motor movements, $r = .84$; for crying, $r = .77$; and for fretting, $r = .83$) (Arcus & Kagan, 1995; for more details on procedure, variable coding, or results, see Kagan, 1994). Infants who displayed both high motor activity and high levels of distress were classified as high reactive, whereas infants displaying both minimal motor activity and minimal distress were categorized as low reactive. Infants in two other groups (high motor activity with low distress and low motor activity with high distress) were not included in the current study of 10- to 12-year-olds because there were no firm hypotheses regarding them.

The children were assessed in the laboratory for fearful behavior in response to unfamiliar people, events, and objects at 14 months and 21 months. Assessments were similar at both ages and included events such as (a) an unfamiliar woman wearing a gas mask and approaching the child, (b) placement of electrocardiogram electrodes on the child's body, and (c) the examiner inviting the child to imitate novel actions. The frequency of fear responses (operationalized as fretting or crying in response to a novel event, failing to approach a novel object or person despite encouragement by the examiner, or refusing to imitate an examiner's action) were coded reliably from videotape (at 14 months, $r = .89$; at 21 months, $r = .93$) (Arcus & Kagan, 1995). For the 14-month visit, the range of possible fear responses was 0 to 13; for the 21-month visit, the range was 0 to 12 (see Kagan, 1994, for details).

10-12-Year Assessment

The children completed a 3-hour battery of physiological and behavioral tasks that included the brainstem procedure. For this procedure, the child was seated in a small reclining chair with his or her neck supported by a pillow. The examiner asked the child to close his or her eyes and relax as if trying to fall asleep and explained that the child would hear a clicking sound in the right ear through earphones (Telephonics TDH-49). Two blocks of 2,200 alternating-polarity 0.1-ms clicks (70 dB SPL for Block 1; 80 dB SPL for Block 2) were presented at a rate of 27/s. Each block lasted approximately 1.5 minutes, and there was a 1-minute break between blocks.

Prior to the brainstem procedure, participants were screened for ear health and function. The screening included obtaining an ear-health history from the parent, visual inspection of the ear, tympanometry, and a hearing test (a two-interval, two-alternative, forced-choice staircase procedure at 500 Hz and then at 2,000 Hz adapted from Buus, Florentine, & Poulsen, 1997). The 56 participants, out of a possible 63, were within the normal range on all measures,[1] and none was on medication that could have affected the central nervous system.[2] In addition, face measurements (vertex-gnathion height and bizygomatic width taken with sliding calipers) were gathered to control for possible facial skeletal differences between temperamental groups that could potentially affect the BAER.

The brainstem data were collected with silver surface electrodes at Cz, A1, and A2 (according to the international 10/20 system) (Jasper, 1958). The recording epoch was 37 ms; 10 ms were utilized for analysis. Wave-forms were amplified with an Isolated Bioelectric Amplifier (SA Instrumentation Co., San Diego, CA) and analog band-pass filtered at .08 to 3,000 Hz. The data were digitized at 10,000 Hz and digitally refiltered at 30 to 3,000 Hz. The peaks and troughs of waves I, III, and V from the reference electrode ispilateral to the stimulated ear and waves III and V from the reference electrode contralateral to the stimulated ear were identified with a computer algorithm and checked manually by a coder who was unaware of participant category (see Figure 10.1).

---

[1]Of the 7 children excluded from the study, 2 were for technical problems (1 high reactive); 3 exceeded 3 SDs above the mean on the hearing test (2 high reactives); 1 had off-scale tympanometry readings for the right ear (peak pressure < -120 daPa; low reactive); and 1 had a history of hearing problems (low reactive).

[2]In addition to monitoring medication on all of our participants, we assessed caffeine consumption on the last 36 of the 56 children. Of the 36, only 6 (2 low reactives) had consumed caffeine on the day of testing, ranging from 4 sips of Coke to 8 oz (237 ml) of Coke or iced tea. T tests revealed that there were no significant differences between those who had consumed caffeine and those who had not on any of the latency or amplitude measures. In addition, removal of those individuals who had consumed caffeine from the analyses did not alter the findings of this study.

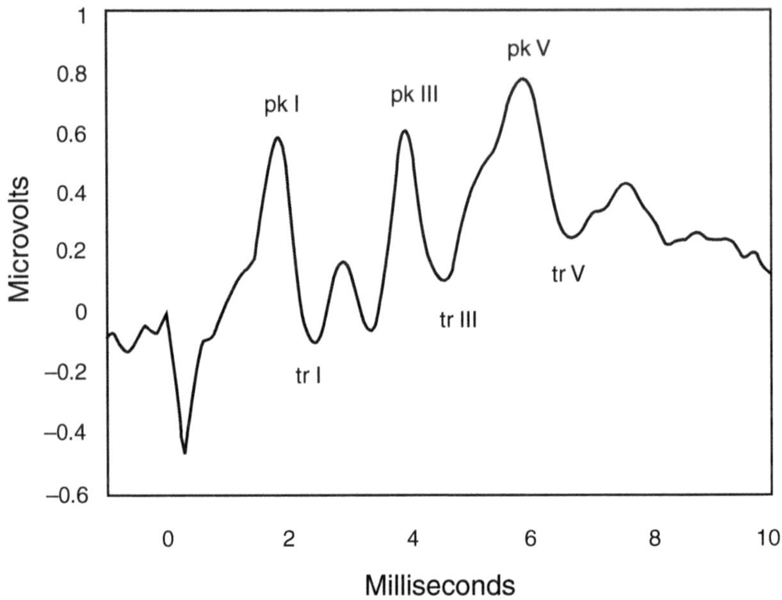

Figure 10.1. Example of an averaged brainstem auditory evoked response for a single 10-year-old child in response to 2.200 70-dB clicks recorded from the ipsilateral lead. Amplitude of wave V was measured as the amplitude change from the trough (tr) of wave III to the peak (pk) of wave V.

Two behavioral variables were assessed: number of smiles and number of spontaneous comments (unprovoked remarks or elaborations) made to the female examiner. These variables have proven to be reliable indicators of social uncertainly at 4 and 7 years and differentiated children who were previously categorized as high and low reactive in infancy (Kagan, 1994). Videotapes of the session were coded for the number of spontaneous comments and smiles made by each child to the examiner during the initial tasks of the battery, which lasted about 18 minutes. These tasks included an ear examination, recording of blood pressure, application of heart rate electrodes, and instructions and practice trials for a test of auditory acuity. We limited the coding of spontaneous comments and smiles to the initial tasks for two reasons. First, the initial contact with the unfamiliar examiner should have generated maximal social uncertainty. Second, the majority of the procedures administered after the first 18 minutes required that the child be quiet, and therefore there were few opportunities to talk to or smile at the examiner. The intercoder reliability (r) based on the independent coding of 20 children was .88 for comments and .91 for smiles.

Results

As predicted, children who had been categorized as high reactive at 4 months had significantly larger wave V amplitudes (measured as the change in amplitude from the trough of wave III to the peak of wave V)[3] than children previously classified as low reactive. We conducted a repeated measures multivariate analysis of covariance: both decibel levels and the reference electrodes ipsilateral and contralateral to the stimulated ear were within-subject factors; infant temperamental category and gender were between-subjects factors; and facial skeletal profile (bizygomatic width over vertex-gnathion height) and auditory threshold (for both 500 and 2,000 Hz) were covariates. The analysis revealed a significant main effect for infant temperamental category, $F(1, 43) = 8.01$, $p = .007$. Figure 10.2 displays the mean wave V amplitude differences for each lead at each decibel level: these values were consistently higher for high reactives. No other main effects were significant. In addition, no significant differences were found for latency or other amplitude measures of waves I, III, and V (see Tables 10.1 and 10.2). The expected shorter latency to peak of wave V for 80 dB than for 70 dB was found across all children: ipsilateral, $t(54) = 6.64$, $p < .001$; contralateral, $t(52) = 5.03$, $p < .001$. Finally, there was only one significant gender difference found for any of the latency or amplitude measures: faster latency to wave I peak for girls at the ipsilateral lead at 70 dB, $t(53) = 2.02$, $p = .05$.

We also computed the proportion of children in each group whose mean wave V amplitudes (average of the four wave V variables: the two stimulus decibel levels at both the ipsilateral and contralateral leads) were above the median value. The median wave V amplitude for all children was 0.66 microvolts ($M = 0.68$). Significantly more high reactive (66%) than low reactives (27%) had an average wave V amplitude that exceeded the median: $\chi^2(1, N = 51) = 7.32$, $p = .007$.

We conducted an analysis of earlier behavior for 51 of the 56 children who had been assessed at 14 and 21 months to determine whether frequency of fear reactions to unfamiliar events in the 2nd year predicted wave V amplitude. The average wave V amplitude was positively correlated with mean number of fears in the 2nd year, $r(51) = .41$, $p = .003$. This relation was significant for high reactives, $r(29) = .32$, $p = .048$ (one-tailed), but not for low reactives, who had a restricted range of fear scores (0 to 3, $M = 1.35$).

Finally, although there were no significant differences between high and low reactives for the mean number of smiles and spontaneous comments made to the examiner at the 10- to 12-year visit, the groups differed when

[3]The reader should note that this is not the traditional method for wave V amplitude calculation (typically measured as the amplitude of the peak minus the following trough). See the Discussion section of this chapter for details.

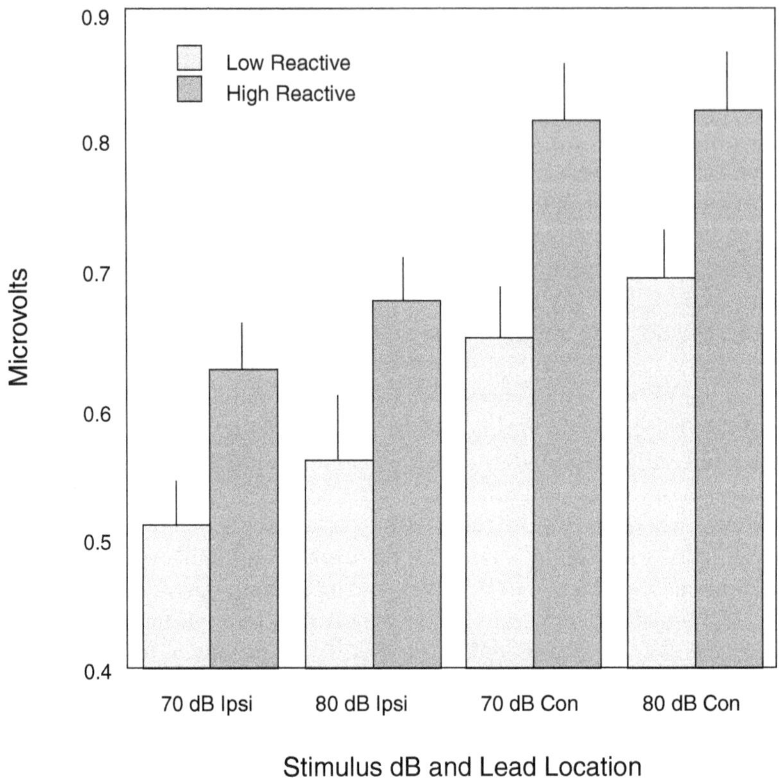

Figure 10.2. Mean amplitude of wave V (as measured from trough of wave III) for contralateral (Con) and ipsilateral (Ipsi) leads at 70 dB and 80 dB. A repeated measures multivariate analysis of covariance using both decibel levels and both ipsilateral and contralateral leads was significant for infant temperament (see text) and demonstrated that children who were previously high reactive infants (black bars) had greater wave V amplitude than children who were low reactive infants (gray bars).

we divided the distributions of smiles and comments into terciles. More high than low reactives were in the lowest terciles (as compared to the middle and upper terciles combined) for spontaneous comments (44% vs. 17%), χ^2 (1, N = 56) = 4.61, p = .03. A similar trend existed for smiles: 41% of high reactives were in the lowest tercile compared with 21% of low reactives, χ^2 (1, N = 56) = 2.46, p = .12. There was no correlation between the average wave V and the number of smiles, r (51) = .07, or spontaneous comments, r (51) = .04.

TABLE 10.1
Latencies to the Peaks of Waves I, III, and V and the Interpeak Latencies by Temperamental Category at Each Lead and Decibel Level

Lead, decibel level, and temperamental category		Peak I		Peak III		Peak V		I–III		III–V		I–V	
	n	*M*	*SD*	*M*	*SD*	*M*	*SD*	*M*	*SD*	*M*	*SD*	*M*	*SD*
Ipsi, 70 dB													
HR	32	1.90	0.14	4.09	0.24	5.97	0.16	2.19	0.24	1.89	0.22	4.08	0.21
LR	23	1.93	0.11	4.12	0.25	6.00	0.20	2.19	0.23	1.88	0.15	4.07	0.18
Ipsi, 80 dB													
HR	32	1.82	0.12	3.96[a]	0.17	5.88	0.15	2.15[a]	0.17	1.92[a]	0.16	4.06	0.20
LR	24	1.80	0.08	4.02[a]	0.17	5.89	0.14	2.23[a]	0.17	1.86[a]	0.12	4.09	0.14
Con, 70 dB													
HR	30	—	—	3.89	0.18	6.08	0.18	—	—	2.19[a]	0.21	—	—
LR	23	—	—	3.93[a]	0.29	6.16	0.17	—	—	2.22[a]	0.27	—	—
Con, 80 dB													
HR	32	—	—	3.86[b]	0.17	6.02	0.19	—	—	2.17[b]	0.20	—	—
LR	24	—	—	3.80[a]	0.17	6.05	0.15	—	—	2.26[a]	0.14	—	—

Note: Ipsi = the reference electrode ipsilateral to the stimulated ear; Con = the reference electrode contralateral to the stimulated ear (for the contralateral lead, the peak of wave I was not measured); HR = children classified as high reactive at 4 months; LR = children classified as low reactive at 4 months.
[a] Sample size for this mean is $n - 1$.
[b] Sample size for this mean is $n - 3$.

DISCUSSION

The data revealed differences in the BAERs of preadolescent children that were in accord with their infant temperamental categories. Specifically, children who were high reactive infants had larger wave V amplitudes than children who were low reactive infants. This result implies that these two temperamental groups differ in a significant property of brainstem function. However, this study does not reveal the nature of that difference.

There are a number of possible explanations for this result. The first, which we favor, is that the amygdala and its projections to the inferior colliculus are consistently more excitable in children who were high reactive infants than in children who were low reactive infants. As a result, children who were high reactive infants had larger wave V magnitudes. This hypothesis is in accord with our theory of infant reactivity, derived from the animal literature, which links the defining behaviors of infant reactivity (motor movements and

TABLE 10.2
Amplitudes of Waves I, III, and V by Temperamental Category at Each Lead and Decibel Level

Lead, decibel level, and temperamental category		Amplitude I (t)		Amplitude III (t)		Amplitude V (t)		Amplitude V	
	n	*M*	*SD*	*M*	*SD*	*M*	*SD*	*M*	*SD*
Ipsi, 70 dB									
HR	32	0.37	0.18	0.24	0.15	0.58	0.20	0.63	0.20
LR	23	0.31	0.11	0.25	0.16	0.55	0.14	0.51	0.15
Ipsi, 80 dB									
HR	32	0.42	0.17	0.31[a]	0.13	0.66[a]	0.20	0.68[a]	0.19
LR	24	0.46	0.14	0.28[a]	0.15	0.65	0.16	0.56[a]	0.24
Con, 70 dB									
HR	30	—	—	0.27	0.12	0.39	0.18	0.82	0.23
LR	23	—	—	0.24[a]	0.20	0.32[a]	0.12	0.65	0.19
Con, 80 dB									
HR	32	—	—	0.25[b]	0.15	0.42	0.19	0.82	0.25
LR	24	—	—	0.30[a]	0.15	0.34	0.13	0.70	0.18

Note: Amplitude V is measured from the trough of wave III to the peak of wave V and is the wave V variable discussed in the Results and Discussion of this article. Amplitudes I (t), III (t), and V (t) are measured according to the more traditional system: for example, Amplitude I (t) is the peak of wave I minus the trough of wave I. Ipsi = the reference electrode ipsilateral to the stimulated ear; Con = the reference electrode contralateral to the stimulated ear (for the contralateral lead, the peak of Wave I was not measured); HR = children classified as high reactive at 4 months; LR = children classified as low reactive at 4 months.

[a] Sample size for this mean is n – 1.

[b] Sample size for this mean is n – 3.

distress) to distinct regions of the amygdala. Specifically, projections from the basolateral area of the amygdala to the central pallidum regulate motor activity, and projections from the central nucleus of the amygdala to the central gray mediate distress cries in animals (Rolls, 1992; Rolls & Williams, 1987; Vogt & Barbas, 1988). Thus, it is reasonable to hypothesize that infants who show a combination of high motor activity and frequent distress to unfamiliar stimuli—high reactives—might have lower thresholds of activation in the basolateral and central areas of the amygdala than do low reactive infants, who show minimal levels of both motor activity and distress.

The current BAER results are potentially consistent with this explanation of infant reactivity because the limbic structures hypothesized to be the foundation of the temperamental differences project indirectly to brainstem sites that are thought to be the origin of the BAER (Brandao et al., 1999; Klepper & Herbert, 1991; Meller & Dennis, 1991; Price & Amaral, 1981; Rizvi,

Ennis, Behbehani, & Shipley, 1991). The fifth component in the BAER is presumed to reflect the activity of the inferior colliculus (Durrant, Martin, Hirsch, & Schwegler, 1994; Hashimoto, Ishiyama, Yoshimoto, & Nemoto, 1981; Moller, Jannetta, & Jho, 1994). Specifically, the peak of wave V is believed to represent the termination of the lateral lemniscus on the inferior colliculus (Moller et al., 1994). In addition, there is a slow wave that peaks simultaneously with wave V (Levine et al., 1993), also captured by our wave V measurement, that is thought to reflect activity of the inferior colliculus (Hashimoto, 1982).

Studies utilizing tracing techniques have shown that the amygdala of many species projects indirectly (via the periaqueductal gray or locus ceruleus) to the inferior colliculus (Brandao et al., 1999; Klepper & Herbert, 1991; Meller & Dennis, 1991; Price & Amaral, 1981; Rizvi et al., 1991). Further, lesions of the central nucleus of the amygdala raise the elicitation threshold in the inferior colliculus for responses, like freezing, that are often used to index a fear state in animals (Maisonnette, Kawasaki, Coimbra, & Brandao, 1996). These data imply that variation in amygdala excitability can influence the responsiveness of the inferior colliculus and, therefore, the magnitude and/or latency of wave V.

We recognize, however, that the empirical affirmation of our prediction that children who were high reactive infants would have an enhanced wave V does not constitute proof of the speculated mechanisms described above. We include this interpretation because it was an *a priori* reason for the current research. However, a number of equally viable alternative mechanisms could also explain our results.

First, the inferior colliculus, which is part of a primitive fear circuit and the origin of wave V, might be inherently more excitable in children who were high reactive as infants than in children who were low reactive as infants. Second, structures other than the amygdala could prime the inferior colliculus more consistently in high reactives. One such structure is the locus ceruleus, a brainstem region that responds to novelty and affects the inferior colliculus (Klepper & Herbert, 1991). Alternatively, Stelmack and Wilson, who found a faster latency to the peak of wave V for introverts than for extroverts, hypothesized that a difference in peripheral nervous system mechanisms accounted for their BAER findings (Stelmack 1997; Stelmack & Wilson, 1982). Finally, Gilliland and colleagues, who also demonstrated faster latency to wave V among introverts, speculated that their BAER findings were associated with group differences in the arousability of the ascending reticular activating system, a brainstem region with connections to the inferior colliculus (Bullock & Gilliland, 1993; Matthews & Gilliland, 1999; Swickert & Gilliland, 1998).

Regardless of which brainstem region is responsible for the current findings, an important question for future research is raised: Would high reactive infants have shown a larger wave V than low reactive infants if we had measured the BAER at 4 months of age? Although we believe that is likely, it is also possible that the experiences associated with being a high reactive infant and a fearful toddler caused brainstem sites to become more excitable. Future longitudinal assessments of BAERs should address this question.

Even though more high reactive than low reactive children had very low values for spontaneous comments and smiles, most high reactives were not excessively shy or timid when they came to the laboratory at 10 to 12 years of age. Although more sensitive behavioral measures on a larger sample size might have differentiated these two groups more clearly, the data support the notion that behavioral distinctions between temperamental groups become increasingly subtle with development, and physiological variables therefore become a critical addition to traditional behavioral batteries. This suggestion may be especially relevant for the identification of children at risk. Children who were high reactive infants, and/or fearful and shy toddlers, are at greater risk for anxious behaviors and social anxiety in later childhood or adulthood (Kagan & Snidman, 1999; Kagan et al., 1999; Schwartz et al., 1999). Because wave V magnitude appears to be a sensitive marker of a temperamental bias for infant reactivity, regardless of contemporary sociability, measurement of wave V as part of a larger test battery might help identify children and adolescents who are vulnerable to the development of anxious psychopathology.

REFERENCES

Arcus, D., & Kagan, J. (1995). Temperamental and craniofacial variation in the first two years. *Child Development, 66,* 1529–1540.

Brandao, M. L., Anseloni, V. Z., Pandossio, J. E., De Araujo, J. E., & Castilho, V. M. (1999). Neurochemical mechanisms of the defensive behavior in the dorsal midbrain. *Neuroscience and Biobehavioral Reviews, 23,* 863–875.

Bullock, W. A., & Gilliland, K. (1993). Eysenck's arousal theory of introversion-extroversion: A converging measures investigation. *Journal of Personality and Social Psychology, 64,* 113–123.

Buus, S., Florentine, M., & Poulsen, T. (1997). Temporal integration of loudness, loudness discrimination, and the form of the loudness function. *Journal of the Acoustical Society of America, 101,* 669–680.

Chiappa, K. H. (1997). *Evoked potentials in clinical medicine.* Philadelphia: Lippincott-Raven.

Durrant, J. D., Martin, W. H., Hirsch, B., & Schwegler, J. (1994). 3CLT ABR analyses in a human subject with unilateral extirpation of the inferior colliculus. *Hearing Research, 72,* 99–107.

Hall, J. W. (1992). *Handbook of auditory evoked responses.* Boston: Allyn & Bacon.

Hashimoto, I. (1982). Auditory evoked potentials recorded directly from the human VIIIth nerve and brain stem: origins of their fast and slow components. In P. A. Buser, W. A. Cobb, & T. Okuma (Eds.), *Kyoto symposia* (EEG Suppl. No. 36, pp. 305–313). Amsterdam: Elsevier Biomedical Press.

Hashimoto, I., Ishiyama, Y., Yoshimoto, T., & Nemoto, S. (1981). Brainstem auditory-evoked potentials recorded directly from human brainstem and thalamus. *Brain, 104,* 841–859.

Iwanami, A., Isono, H., Okajima. Y., & Kamaijima, K. (1997). Auditory event-related potentials in panic disorder. *European Archives of Psychiatry and Clinical Neuroscience, 247,* 107–111.

Jasper, H. H. (1958). The ten-twenty electrode system of the International Federation. *Electoencephalography and Clinical Neurophysiology, 10,* 371–375.

Kagan, J. (1994). *Galen's prophecy.* New York: Basic Books.

Kagan, J., Reznick, J. S., & Snidman, N. (1987). The physiology and psychology of behavioral inhibition in children. *Child Development, 58,* 1459–1473.

Kagan, J., & Snidman, N. (1991). Infant predictors of inhibited and uninhibited profiles. *Psychological Science, 2,* 40–44.

Kagan, J., & Snidman, N. (1999). Early childhood predictors of adult anxiety disorders. *Biological Psychiatry, 46,* 1536–1541.

Kagan, J., Snidman, N., & Arcus, D. (1998). Childhood derivatives of high and low reactivity in infancy. *Child Development, 69,* 1483–1493.

Kagan, J., Snidman, N., & Peterson, E. (2000). Temperature asymmetry and behavior. *Developmental Psychobiology, 37,* 186–193.

Kagan, J., Snidman, N., Zentner, M., & Peterson, E. (1999). Infant temperament and anxious symptoms in school age children. *Development and Psychopathology, 11,* 209–224.

Klepper, A., & Herbert, H. (1991). Distribution and origin of noradrenergic and serotonergic fibers in the cochlear nucleus and inferior colliculus of the rat. *Brain Research, 557,* 190–201.

Levine, R. A., Gardner, J. C., Fullerton, B. C., Stufflebeam, S. M., Carlisle, E. W., Furst, M., Rosen, B. R., & Kiang, N. Y. S. (1993). Effects of multiple sclerosis brainstem lesions on sound lateralization and brainstem auditory evoked potentials. *Hearing Research, 68,* 73–88.

Maisonnette, S. S., Kawasaki, M. C., Coimbra, N. C., & Brandao, M. L. (1996). Effects of lesions of amygdaloid nuclei and substantia nigra on aversive responses induced by electrical stimulation of the inferior colliculus. *Brain Research Bulletin, 40,* 93–98.

Matthews, G., & Gilliland, K. (1999). The personality theories of H. J. Eysenck & J. A. Gray: a comparative review. *Personality and Individual Differences, 26,* 583–626.

Meller, S. T., & Dennis, B. J. (1991). Efferent projections of the periaqueductal gray in the rabbit. *Neuroscience, 40,* 191–216.

Moller, A. R., Jannetta, P. J., & Jho, H. D. (1994). Click-evoked responses from the cochlear nucleus: a study in humans. *Electroencephalography and Clinical Neurophysiology, 92,* 215–224.

Price, J. L., & Amaral, D. G. (1981). An autoradiographic study of the projections of the central nucleus of the monkey amygdala. *Journal of Neuroscience, 1,* 1242–1259.

Rizvi, T. A., Ennis, M., Behbehani, M. M., & Shipley, M. T. (1991). Connection between the central nucleus of the amygdala and the midbrain periaqueductal gray: topography and reciprocity. *Journal of Comparative Neurology, 303,* 121–131.

Rolls, E. J. (1992). Neurophysiology and functions of the primate amygdala. In J. P. Aggelton (Ed.), *The amygdala: neurobiological aspects of emotion, memory, and mental dysfunction* (pp. 143–166). New York: Wiley-Liss.

Rolls, E. J., & Williams, G. V. (1987). Neuronal activity in the ventral striatum of the primate. In M. B. Carpenter & A. Jayarama (Eds.), *The basal ganglia* (pp. 349–356). New York: Plenum Press.

Rosenbaum, J. F., Biederman, J., Bolduc-Murphy, E. A., Faraone, S. A., Chaloff, J., Hirshfeld, D. R., & Kagan, J. (1993). Behavioral inhibition in childhood: a risk factor for anxiety disorders. *Harvard Review of Psychiatry, 1,* 2–16.

Schwartz, C. E., Snidman, N., & Kagan, J. (1999). Adolescent social anxiety as an outcome of inhibited temperament in childhood. *Journal of the American Academy of Child and Adolescent Psychiatry, 38,* 1008–1015.

Snidman, N., Kagan, J., Riordan, L., & Shannon, D. (1995). Cardiac function and behavioral reactivity during infancy. *Psychophysiology, 32,* 199–207.

Stelmack, R. M. (1997). The psychophysics and psychophysiology of extraversion and arousal. In H. Nyborg (Ed.), *The scientific study of human nature: tribute to Hans J. Eysenck at eighty* (pp. 388–403). New York: Elsevier Science.

Stelmack, R. M., & Wilson, K. G. (1982). Extraversion and the effects of frequency and intensity of the auditory brainstem evoked response. *Personality and Individual Differences, 3,* 373–380.

Stern, H., Arcus, D., Kagan, J., Rubin, D. B., & Snidman, N. (1994). Statistical choices in infant temperament research. *Behaviormetrika, 21,* 1–17.

Swickert, R. J., & Gilliland, K. (1998). Relationship between the brainstem auditory evoked response and extraversion, impulsivity, and sociability. *Journal of Research in Personality, 32,* 314–330.

Vogt, B. A., & Barbas, H. (1988). Structure and connections of the cingulate vocalization region in the rhesus monkey. In J. D. Newman (Ed.), *The physiological control of mammalian vocalization* (pp. 203–228). New York: Plenum Press.

Woodward, S. A., Lenzenweger, M. F., Kagan, J., Snidman, N., & Arcus, D. (2000). Taxonic structure of infant reactivity: evidence from a taxometric perspective. *Psychological Science, 11,* 300–305.

11

Temperamental Contributions to Social Behavior: The Moderating Roles of Frontal EEG Asymmetry and Gender

Heather A. Henderson, Nathan A. Fox, and Kenneth H. Rubin

Objectives: *Infant temperament is thought to provide one of the fundamental bases for social and emotional development. Few studies have examined the direct and indirect influences of early temperament and physiological disposition on later development.* ***Method:*** *This article presents results of a longitudinal study that took place between the years 1989 and 1996 in which the relations between maternal reports of negative reactivity at 9 months of age and maternal ratings and laboratory observations of social wariness and sociability at 4 years of age (n = 97) were examined. Also examined were the moderating roles of (1) frontal electroencephalogram (EEG) asymmetry as assessed at 9 months of age and (2) the child's gender.* ***Results:*** *Negative reactivity predicted social wariness for infants with right frontal EEG asymmetry, but not for those with left frontal EEG asymmetry and for boys but not girls. The only significant predictor of sociability was gender. Specifically, at 4 years of age girls were rated higher on the measure of sociability than were boys.* ***Conclusion:*** *The findings are discussed in terms of the roles of frontal EEG asymmetry and gender in moderating the impact of temperamental negative reactivity on later social behavior.*

Temperament is used to describe individual differences in styles of responding, both emotionally and motorically, that are present from birth, constitutionally based, and relatively stable over time (Rothbart and Derryberry, 1981; Thomas et al., 1968). These individual differences are thought to provide the basis for the emergence of trajectories of social and emotional development (Rothbart and Bates, 1998). However, the specific nature of these trajectories depends not only on the temperamental characteristics of an infant, but on intervening social and developmental processes. One of the primary goals in the study of infant temperament is to identify such processes that link early temperament to later behavior.

Despite variation among researchers in their emphasis on specific dimensions of temperament, most current models of temperament include some aspect of negative reactivity (e.g., Buss and Plomin, 1984; Goldsmith and Campos, 1982; Rothbart and Derryberry, 1981; Thomas et al., 1968). Negative reactivity is used to describe signs of distress including crying, fussing, and motoric agitation. Using standardized assessment procedures, individual differences in infant irritability have been identified in the neonatal period and these early differences are predictive of later differences in global negative reactivity (Crockenberg, 1981; Riese, 1987). Negative reactivity has been implicated as the temperamental precursor for the later display of behavioral inhibition in response to novel objects, people, and events (Buss and Plomin, 1984; Calkins et al., 1996; Engfer, 1993; Kagan and Snidman, 1991).

In considering the relations between early temperament and later social and emotional development, the majority of longitudinal studies follow a direct linkage model, in which early temperament is thought to be directly and linearly related to later adjustment (e.g., Caspi and Silva, 1995; Kagan et al., 1984). The degree of discontinuity in temperament-adjustment linkages is, however, quite high. The variable outcomes of infants who are similar in temperament, even those in the extremes, suggest that other factors such as parent–child interactions and out-of-home care experiences may moderate the link between early temperament and adjustment. As such, temperament may be linearly related to social outcomes, albeit through indirect processes, such that the relations are moderated by other variables (Rothbart and Bates, 1998). Certain types of temperament, and even extreme temperament, may not reflect a risk for maladjustment per se, but rather a catalyst, which in combination with other factors, define trajectories of social and emotional development. In this report we consider the influence of endogenous (frontal EEG asymmetry) and exogenous (gender) variables on the predictability of social behaviors during the preschool years from maternal temperament reports of negative reactivity gathered during the first year of life.

Frontal EEG asymmetry reflects the difference in the degree of activation between the left and right frontal regions. Patterns of frontal EEG asymmetry are thought to relate to the tendency to approach or withdraw from novel or stressful events (Fox, 1991, 1994). A variety of data from adult clinical and normal populations, as well as from infant and child studies, suggest that the two sides of the frontal cortex may be differentially specialized for approach or withdrawal tendencies. These behavioral tendencies have often been associated with the experience or expression of emotion (e.g., Davidson, 1992; Davidson and Fox, 1982). A number of these studies indicate that the left frontal area is associated with behaviors facilitating approach such as fine motor behavior, language, and the expression of certain positive emotions (Fox and Davidson, 1984; Kinsbourne, 1978). In contrast, the right frontal area is associated with behaviors facilitating withdrawal from novel or stressful stimuli such as gross motor movement, autonomic reactivity, and the expression of certain negative affects (Fox and Davidson, 1984). These approach-withdrawal tendencies may bias the individual's interactions with the environment such that they may initiate or withdraw from stressful situations or unfamiliar social exchanges.

For example, preschool children who displayed elevated amounts of reticent and anxious behavior during interactions with unfamiliar peers exhibited increased electrical activity in the right frontal region (right frontal EEG asymmetry) compared with their more sociable peers (Fox et al., 1995). And in a sample of school-age children, increases in anxiety when placed in a situation designed to elicit social stress were paralleled by increases in right frontal EEG asymmetry (Schmidt et al., 1999). Based on these data and on the role that frontal asymmetry seems to play as an endogenous influence on social behavior, we hypothesized that for infants who displayed patterns of right frontal EEG asymmetry, negative reactivity would be positively related to social wariness and negatively related to sociability at 4 years of age.

There are parallel data linking activity in left frontal cortex to approach behaviors and the expression of associated affect and sociability. For example, Fox et al. (in press) reported that young children who displayed consistently high levels of sociability across the toddler years were more likely to exhibit left frontal EEG asymmetry. Based on these patterns of data, we hypothesized that for infants who displayed patterns of left frontal EEG asymmetry, negative reactivity would not be predictive of social wariness or sociability.

Another potential influence on the relation between negative reactivity and social behavior may be gender. Some reports suggest that the link between temperament and social development may be particularly strong for boys (e.g., Crockenberg and Smith, 1982; Fagan, 1990). One reason for this may be that parents respond differently to boys' and girls' expressions of the same behaviors and emotions (Mills and Rubin, 1990). This may be especially true for temperamental characteristics that describe behaviors with strong culturally prescribed gender stereotypes (Hinde et al. 1985; Stevenson-Hinde and Glover, 1996). In Western cultures there appears to be a perception that distress and fearfulness are more acceptable for girls than for boys. For example, Hinde et al. (1985) found that shy preschool-age boys had significantly poorer relationships both at home and at school compared with equally shy girls. Furthermore, Rubin et al. (1993) reported that socially wary, fearful, and withdrawn boys, not girls, were more likely to express loneliness and perceive themselves as being socially incompetent and as having poor social relationships. These differences have been attributed, in part, to parents' gender stereotypes. Fearfulness in boys may not be congruent with parental expectations and may lead to greater concern and overly intrusive interactions with caregivers (Park et al., 1997). Parental concern and attention may serve to amplify temperamental patterns of behavior by preventing the child from developing effective strategies for coping with negative emotion (e.g., Arcus et al., 1992; Park et al., 1997; Rubin et al., 1997). We thus hypothesized that the relation between negative reactivity and social wariness would be stronger for boys than for girls.

In summary, in this study we examined the influence of maternal reports of negative reactivity in the first year of life on measures of sociability and social wariness taken at 4 years of age. Social wariness is used to describe one form of social withdrawal that is characterized by social reticence, which involves the combination of low levels of social interaction and the frequent production of anxious, onlooking, and unoccupied behaviors (Coplan et al., 1994). In contrast to other forms of solitary play, social reticence has been associated with overt indications of anxiety, poor performance on cooperative group tasks, and an inability to regulate negative emotions (Coplan et al., 1994; Rubin et al., 1995). In addition to examining the direct relations between early reactivity and later social behavior, we examined whether this relation was modified by (1) patterns of frontal EEG asymmetry as assessed during infancy and (2) the child's gender. We hypothesized that the relations between negative reactivity and social wariness would be stronger for infants displaying patterns of right frontal EEG asymmetry compared with the relations for infants displaying patterns of left frontal EEG asymmetry. We further hypothesized that negative reactivity would be more predictive of social wariness for boys than for girls.

METHOD

Participants

The participants in the current study were 139 infants and their mothers, from two independent cohorts, who were taking part in a longitudinal study of the relations between temperament, psychophysiology, and social and emotional development. Participants were recruited via mailing lists. Families were sent a general letter asking them whether they were interested in a study on child development. Families that mailed back a brief demographic questionnaire were contacted by telephone for a laboratory appointment. In this article we report on the 97 infants (46 males and 51 females) who had complete data at both 9 months and 48 months of age. The families were white and of middle-class background, living in the greater Washington, D.C., area. Approximately 68% of the mothers and 72% of the fathers were college-educated. Approximately one third of the children were first-born.

Of the 42 children excluded from analysis, 23 were excluded because they did not return to the laboratory for the 48-month visit and 19 because they were missing data at 9 months of age (12 were missing EEG data and 7 were missing maternal reports of temperament). Comparisons between the children who were included versus excluded from the analysis due to missing data did not suggest that attrition was selective based on any of our predictor or outcome variables. Specifically, the 23 children who did not return to the laboratory at 48 months did not differ from the others in terms of 9-month maternal reports of negative reactivity, 9-month EEG, or sex distribution. Similarly, the 12 infants who did not have EEG data at 9 months were no different from the infants who did in terms of maternal reports of 9-month negative reactivity or any of the 48-month outcome measures.

PROCEDURES

Nine-Month Assessment. At 9 months of age infants and their families visited the laboratory, at which time brain electrical activity (EEG) was recorded from the infants; mothers completed the Infant Behavior Questionnaire (Rothbart, 1981, 1986), an 87-item parent rating form in which parents are asked to rate the frequency of specific infant behaviors as they occurred in the previous week. Following Rothbart (1986), the Fear and Distress to Limitations subscales were summed and used as an index of Negative Reactivity (see also Park et al., 1997).

EEG Data Collection. To minimize fussing and movement during EEG data collection, the infants sat on their mothers' laps directly in front of a table on which a metal bingo wheel was placed. An experimenter placed different numbers of brightly colored balls (1, 3, or 7) in the wheel and spun the wheel for a series of six trials, each lasting 20 seconds. These trials were separated by 10-second intervals in which the experimenter tapped the balls on the outside of the bingo wheel in order to keep the infant's attention between trials. EEG was recorded for the entire 3-minute period. Previous work has found that recording epochs of this duration provide estimates of EEG power with good internal consistency (Lund et al., 1995) and a reliable estimate of the subject's frontal asymmetry index related to a bias toward approach or withdrawal behaviors (Fox et al., 1992; Tomarken et al., 1990).

Prior to the recording of EEG from each subject, a 0.477 V_{RMS} 10-Hz signal was input into each of the channels and this amplified signal was recorded for calibration purposes. EEG was recorded from the following sites (F3, F4, P3, P4, C3, C4, O1, O2) by placing a Lycra stretch cap of an appropriate circumference on the infant's head. The EEG data were digitized at a rate of 512 Hz and then rereferenced using software to an average reference configuration. The digitized EEG data were artifact-scored on the basis of visual inspection of the signal in order to remove portions of the EEG record marked by eye movement or motor movement. All instances of artifact were removed from all channels of the EEG record prior to subsequent analysis.

The rereferenced, artifact-scored EEG data were submitted to a discrete Fourier transform analysis that used a Hanning window with 50% overlap. The result of this analysis was to produce power in picowatt ohms (or microvolts squared) for each channel. Spectral power data in single-hertz frequency bins from 1 to 12 Hz were computed for each of the stimulus conditions at each of the collection sites. Power in the 4- to 6-Hz frequency band was computed for each site by summing the single-hertz bins in these three frequencies. The 4- to 6-Hz band is where the majority of power was localized. The measure of power was log-transformed to normalize the distribution, and the asymmetry index was computed as the difference between right and left sites (e.g., LN [F4] – LN [F3]). In this report we present data from the frontal and parietal sites.

Forty-eight-Month Assessment. Children and their families returned to the laboratory when the children were 4 years old. The children were scheduled to visit the laboratory in groups of four children who were of the same gender and similar in age (within 3 months), but who were unfamiliar to one another. The procedures and methods used to observe the children's social behaviors with one another were identical with those used with earlier cohorts of children (e.g., Fox et al., 1996; Rubin et al., 1995). Of particular interest in this study were the children's behaviors during two unstructured free-play sessions: the first occurred soon after the children arrived at the laboratory and the second took place approximately 25 minutes after the first. The experimenter began each play session by explaining to the children that they were free to play with any of the toys they wished. She then left the room, and the children were left undisturbed for the full 15-minute period, unless they needed assistance.

Behavioral Coding. Behaviors in both the free-play sessions were coded with the Play Observation Scale (Rubin, 1985, 2000; Rubin and Coplan, 1998). Ten-second intervals were coded for social participation (unoccupied, onlooking, solitary play, parallel play, conversation, group play) and the cognitive quality of play (functional, dramatic, and constructive play; exploration; games with rules). This resulted in approximately 90 coding intervals per child in each of the two free-play sessions. For both cohorts, three independent observers coded the Play Observation Scale. Intercoder reliability on a randomly selected group of children totaling 30% of the entire sample was calculated between pairs of observers using the Cohen κ. For the full variable matrix, including social and cognitive play categories, κ values ranged from 0.81 to 0.94 for the first cohort, and 0.87 to 0.94 for the second cohort.

During this visit, mothers completed the Colorado Child Temperament Inventory (CCTI) (Buss and Plomin, 1984; Rowe and Plomin, 1977). The CCTI is a 30-item parent report that assesses maternal perceptions of dispositional characteristics along six dimensions. Of interest were the Shyness and Sociability dimensions. As a measure of behavior problems, mothers completed the Child Behavior Checklist (CBCL) (Achenbach and Edelbrock, 1983). The CBCL is a 113-item checklist in which parents use a 3-point scale to rate how descriptive a series of behavior problems are of their own child. The scale is reduced into two broad-band factors assessing Internalizing and Externalizing behavior problems.

RESULTS

Formation of Aggregate Measures of Social Wariness and Sociability at 48 Months

At 48 months of age, aggregate measures of social wariness and sociability were formed on the basis of a combination of maternal reports and observed behaviors during play with unfamiliar peers in the laboratory. Reticent behavior during free play was calculated by summing the standardized proportions of onlooking and unoccupied behaviors during both free-play sessions (Coplan et al., 1994). Prior to being used in correlational analyses, the observed reticence variable was transformed using a natural logarithm function to reduce the positive skew of the data and better approximate a normal distribution. Observed reticence was highly correlated with maternal reports of shyness ($r_{97} = 0.54$, $p < .001$), and the two variables were standardized and summed to create a composite measure of social wariness. As in previous reports examining the relations between social wariness and other indices of social and emotional adjustment (e.g., Coplan et al., 1994; Fox et al., 1996), the aggregate measure of social wariness was positively correlated with Internalizing behavior problems on the CBCL ($r_{93} = 0.41$, $p < .001$). Despite the positive correlation between Internalizing and Externalizing behavior problem scores on the CBCL ($r_{93} = 0.47$, $p < .001$), the aggregate measure of social wariness was not correlated with Externalizing behavior problems ($r_{93} = -0.01$, not significant).

Social behavior during free play was calculated by summing the standardized proportions of all group-play activities as well as conversations. Observed social play was correlated with maternal reports of CCTI sociability ($r_{97} = 0.31$, $p < .01$), and a composite measure of sociability was computed by standardizing and summing the measures of observed and maternal report of sociability.

The resulting composite measure of sociability was negatively correlated with the social wariness composite ($r_{97} = -0.62$, $p < .001$).

HIERARCHICAL REGRESSION ANALYSES

We conducted separate hierarchical multiple regression analyses to examine the predictive relations between negative reactivity in infancy and social wariness and sociability in the preschool years. Hierarchical analyses allowed for an examination of possible moderating effects linking negative reactivity to later social behaviors, once controlling for the main effects of negative reactivity. For each analysis, the predictors were entered into the regression equation in the following order: (1) 9-month negative reactivity, (2) 9-month frontal EEG asymmetry, (3) gender, (4) negative reactivity × frontal EEG asymmetry, (5) negative reactivity × gender, and (6) negative reactivity × frontal EEG asymmetry × gender. No main or interaction effects were found when the identical analyses were run with the parietal EEG asymmetry data, confirming the specificity of the EEG asymmetry effects to the frontal sites.

PREDICTING 48-MONTH SOCIAL WARINESS

The results of the hierarchical regression analysis predicting social wariness are presented in Table 11.1. The full model accounted for 18% of the variance in social wariness ($F_{6,90} = 3.35$, $p < .01$). The main effect of negative reactivity approached significance, reflecting the zero-order correlation between maternal reports of negative reactivity at 9 months and the composite measure of social wariness at 48 months ($r_{97} = 0.18$, $p = .08$). The interactions between negative reactivity and frontal asymmetry, and negative reactivity and gender, both accounted for unique proportions of variance in the prediction of social wariness over and above that accounted for by the main effects of the predictors. The three-way interaction (negative reactivity × frontal EEG asymmetry × gender) did not contribute further to the prediction of social wariness.

The interaction between negative reactivity and frontal asymmetry accounted for an additional 7% of the variance in social wariness. To interpret the interaction, infants were divided into two groups based on their 9-month asymmetry scores. Infants with frontal asymmetry scores less than 0 (indicative of right EEG asymmetry) formed the right frontal group, and infants with frontal asymmetry scores greater than 0 (indicative of left frontal EEG asymmetry) formed the left frontal group. The correlations between 9-month negative reactivity and 4-year social wariness were computed separately for these two groups. For the right frontal group, there was a significant and positive

TABLE 11.1
Summary of Hierarchical Regression Analysis for Variables Predicting Social Wariness at 48 Months ($N = 97$)

Predictors	β	ΔR^2	F for ΔR^2
1. 9-Month negative reactivity	.18	0.03	3.11†
2. 9-Month frontal asymmetry	–.12	0.01	1.40
3. Gender	–.08	0.01	0.56
4. Negative reactivity × asymmetry	–1.30	0.07	7.12**
5. Negative reactivity × gender	–1.10	0.04	4.73*
6. Neg react × asym × gender	.69	0.02	2.15
Multiple $R = 0.43$			
Total $R^2 = 0.18$			
$F_{6.90} = 3.35$**			

†$p < .10$; *$p < .05$; **$p < .01$

correlation ($r_{39} = 0.40$, $p = .01$). In contrast, for the left frontal group the correlation was nonsignificant ($r_{58} = –0.01$, $p > .10$). The magnitude of the two correlations was compared using Fisher z scores; because the hypotheses were directional, one-tailed tests were used to test the significance. This analysis revealed that the two correlations differed significantly ($z = 2.03$, $p = .02$).

To interpret the interaction between negative reactivity and gender, the correlation between negative temperament and social wariness was examined separately for boys and girls. For boys, there was a significant and positive correlation ($r_{46} = 0.34$, $p = .02$), but for girls the correlation was nonsignificant ($r_{51} = 0.01$, $p > .10$). The one-tailed z test of the difference between the magnitude of correlations was significant ($z = 1.65$, $p = .05$).

PREDICTING 4-YEAR SOCIABILITY

The results of the hierarchical regression analysis predicting sociability are presented in Table 11.2. Following an identical order of entry for the predictor variables and their interaction terms, the full model for sociability was significant ($F_{6,90} = 2.44$, $p < .05$). The main effect of negative reactivity approached significance ($\Delta R^2 = 0.03$, $p = .07$); however, the main effect of gender accounted for the greatest proportion of unique variance ($\Delta R^2 = 0.05$, $p = .03$). Unlike the analysis for social wariness, neither frontal EEG asymmetry nor gender significantly moderated the effects of negative reactivity on later sociability. Thus, despite the strong negative correlation between the composite measures of sociability and social wariness, the moderated linkage model including negative reactivity, frontal EEG asymmetry, and gender was specifically predictive of later social wariness.

TABLE 11.2
Summary of Hierarchical Regression Analysis for Variables Predicting Sociability at 48 Months ($N = 97$)

Predictors	β	ΔR^2	F for ΔR^2
1. 9-Month negative reactivity	–.18	0.03	3.29†
2. 9-Month frontal asymmetry	.09	0.01	0.72
3. Gender	.22	0.05	4.85*
4. Negative reactivity × asymmetry	.63	0.02	1.64
5. Negative reactivity × gender	.52	0.01	1.00
6. Neg react × asym × gender	–.79	0.03	2.71
Multiple $R = 0.37$			
Total $R^2 = 0.14$			
$F_{6,90} = 2.24$*			

†$p < .10$; *$p < .05$

DISCUSSION

A primary goal in the study of infant temperament is to understand better the processes through which early individual differences in temperament impact upon later social and emotional development and adaptation. Although there are several reports in the literature that show direct relations between early negative reactivity and the display of social wariness at later ages, these relations are modest at best. Clearly, the complexities associated with the measurement of both infant temperament and early social behavior may contribute to the modest levels of prediction over time. However, this aside, the more challenging task is to identify theoretically relevant variables that help determine the varied developmental pathways leading from early temperament to later social behavior (e.g., Park et al., 1997; Rothbart and Bates, 1998).

The data from the current study indicate that maternal report of negative reactivity during the first year of life, by itself, did not significantly predict either sociability or social wariness. Although the zero-order correlations did not reach conventional levels of significance, they were in the expected directions, with a positive relation between negative reactivity and later social wariness and a negative relation between negative reactivity and later sociability. Furthermore, both frontal EEG asymmetry and gender moderated the relation between negative reactivity and social wariness. The same interaction effects did not contribute to the prediction of sociability. The measure of social wariness reflects a specific form of low sociability, one that is associated with a combination of low levels of social interaction and negative affect and behavior problems of an internalizing nature (Coplan et al., 1994; Fox et al., 1996).

Negative emotionality was predictive of social wariness for infants who also displayed a pattern of right frontal EEG asymmetry at 9 months of age, but not for infants with a pattern of left frontal EEG asymmetry. These data follow a stress-diathesis model that involves both inborn temperament and frontal EEG asymmetry (Schmidt & Fox, 1998). High levels of negative reactivity in early infancy reflect a stressor for infants and their caregivers, and right frontal EEG asymmetry, insofar as it reflects a bias to withdraw from novel or stressful stimuli, provides the diathesis that sets an infant on a pathway toward social wariness. Alternately, left frontal EEG asymmetry may serve as a protective factor that sets a highly reactive infant on a different pathway in which the child develops strategies involving approach and positive emotions. It is important to note that highly reactive infants with left frontal EEG asymmetry did not become highly social compared with their peers, as evidenced by the fact that the negative reactivity-by-frontal EEG asymmetry interaction did not contribute to the prediction of sociability. Rather, left frontal EEG asymmetry served to attenuate the relation between negative reactivity and later social wariness to practically zero.

The influence of negative reactivity on social wariness was also moderated by gender. Specifically, negative reactivity during infancy was positively related to social wariness for boys, but not for girls. Several independent reports indicate that caregivers interact in qualitatively different ways with highly reactive sons vs. daughters (MacDonald & Parke, 1984; Stevenson-Hinde & Glover, 1996). Together such studies suggest that socially withdrawn and highly reactive boys may have more negative and less engaging interactions with their caregivers compared with socially withdrawn and highly reactive girls.

STUDY LIMITATIONS

There are a number of limitations to the current study that should be noted. First, negative reactivity and EEG asymmetry were assessed once when the infant was 9 months of age. Although both measures have demonstrated reliability and validity, it would have been preferable to measure each repeatedly during the early infancy period. Second, negative reactivity was measured via maternal report that may provide data that are different from direct behavioral observations of temperament. Third, EEG is only an indirect measure of brain functioning. While it is impractical at this point to use more sophisticated neuroimaging techniques with normally developing infants, the conclusions regarding localization and function should be regarded with caution. Finally, in this study we did not assess mother–infant interaction. Lack of these data tempers our interpretation about the mechanisms accounting for the effects of gender and asymmetry as they moderate infant negative reactivity over time.

CLINICAL IMPLICATIONS

Perhaps the most important immediate clinical implication of our work is that it highlights the importance of temperamental differences in understanding the etiology of internalizing behaviors in young children. Clinicians should attend to young infants' dispositions toward irritability and negative emotionality and consider factors in the infant's environment that may serve to moderate the expression of this disposition over time. Given the finding that negative reactivity was predictive of social reticence for boys, but not girls, and that previous reports have described a pattern of parental oversolicitousness in the parents of shy boys, clinicians may wish to help parents establish patterns of interaction that will encourage independence and effective self-regulation among highly negative boys. In addition, although our sample consisted of children from middle-class families who fell within the normal ranges of temperament and behavior problems, we believe our study has implications for infants and young children in at-risk samples. For example, it has been reported that infants of depressed women exhibit a pattern of right frontal EEG asymmetry (Field et al., 1995). Given our findings, clinicians should pay particular attention to patterns of temperamental negative reactivity in infants who may be predisposed to a pattern of right frontal EEG asymmetry or a bias toward withdrawing from novelty. Finally, it is important to note that social wariness was best predicted by the combination of early temperament with either frontal EEG asymmetry or gender, rather than by early temperament alone. Simple fussiness or irritability does not predict risk for maladaptive social behavior. It is the interaction of this temperamental bias with other biological and social factors that best accounts for variability in social outcome.

ACKNOWLEDGMENTS

This research was supported by grants from the John D. and Catherine T. MacArthur Foundation and the NIH (HD 32666 and HD 17899) to Dr. Fox.

REFERENCES

Achenbach TM, Edelbrock CS (1983). Manual for the Child Behavior Checklist and Revised Child Behavior Profile. Burlington: University of Vermont Department of Psychiatry.

Arcus D, Gardner S, Anderson C (1992). Infant reactivity, maternal style, and the development of inhibited and uninhibited behavioral profiles. In: Temperament and Environment. Symposium conducted at the Biennial Meeting of the International Society for Infant Studies, Miami, FL, April.

Buss AH, Plomin R (1984). Temperament: Early Developing Personality Traits. Hillsdale, NJ: Erlbaum.

Calkins SD, Fox NA, Marshall TR (1996). Behavioral and physiological antecedents of inhibition in infancy. *Child Dev* 67:523–540.

Caspi A, Silva PA (1995). Temperamental qualities at age three predict personality traits in young adulthood: longitudinal evidence from a birth cohort. *Child Dev* 66: 486–498.

Coplan RJ, Rubin KH, Fox NA, Calkins SD, Stewart SL (1994). Being alone, playing alone, and acting alone: distinguishing among reticence and passive and active solitude in young children. *Child Dev* 65:129–137.

Crockenberg S, Smith P (1982). Antecedents of mother–infant interaction and infant irritability in the first three months of life. *Infant Behav Dev* 5:105–119.

Crockenberg SB (1981). Infant irritability, mother responsiveness, and social support influences on the security of infant–mother attachment. *Child Dev* 52:857–865.

Davidson RJ (1992). Anterior cerebral asymmetry and the nature of emotion. *Brain Cogn* 20:125–151.

Davidson RJ, Fox NA (1982). Asymmetrical brain activity discriminates between positive and negative affective stimuli in human infants. *Science* 218:1235–1237.

Engfer A (1993). Antecedents and consequences of shyness in boys and girls: a 6-year longitudinal study. In: Social Withdrawal, Inhibition, and Shyness in Childhood, Rubin KH, Asendorf JB, eds. Hillsdale, NJ: Erlbaum, pp. 49–79.

Fagan J (1990). The interaction between child sex and temperament in predicting behavior problems of preschool-age children in day care. *Early Child Dev Care* 59:1–9.

Field T, Fox NA, Pickens J, Nawrocki T (1995). Relative right frontal EEG activation in 3- to 6-month-old infants of depressed mothers. *Dev Psychol* 31:358–363.

Fox NA (1991). If it's not left, it's right: electroencephalogram asymmetry and the development of emotion. *Am Psychol* 46:863–872.

Fox NA (1994). Dynamic cerebral processes underlying emotion regulation. *Monogr Soc Res Child Dev* 59:152–166.

Fox NA, Bell MA, Jones NA (1992). Individual differences in response to stress and cerebral asymmetry. *Dev Neuropsychol* 8:161–184.

Fox NA, Davidson RJ (1984). Hemispheric substrates for affect: a developmental model. In: The Psychobiology of Affective Development, Fox NA, Davidson RJ, eds. Hillsdale, NJ: Erlbaum, pp. 353–382.

Fox NA, Henderson HA, Rubin KH, Calkins SD, Schmidt LA (in press). Continuity and discontinuity behavioral inhibition and exuberance: psychophysiological and behavioral influences across the first four years of life. *Child Dev.*

Fox NA, Rubin KH, Calkins SD et al., (1995). Frontal activation asymmetry and social competence at four years of age. *Child Dev* 66:1770–1784.

Fox NA, Schmidt LA, Calkins SD, Rubin KH, Coplan RJ (1996). The role of frontal activation in the regulation and dysregulation of social behavior during the preschool years. *Dev Psychopathol* 8:89–102.

Goldsmith HH, Campos JJ (1982). Toward a theory of infant temperament. In: The Development of Attachment and Affiliative Systems, Emde RN, Harmon RJ, eds. New York: Plenum, pp. 161–193.

Hinde RA, Stevenson-Hinde J, Tamplin A (1985). Characteristics of 3- to 4-year-olds assessed at home and their interactions in preschool. *Dev Psychol* 21:130–140.

Kagan J, Reznick JS, Clarke C, Snidman N, Garcia-Coll C (1984). Behavioral inhibition to the unfamiliar. *Child Dev* 58: 2212–2225.

Kagan J, Snidman N (1991). Infant predictors of inhibited and uninhibited profiles. *Psychol Sci* 2:40–44.

Kinsbourne M (1978). Evolution of language in relation to lateral action. In: Asymmetrical Function of the Brain, Kinsbourne M, ed. London: Cambridge University Press, pp. 553–566.

Lund TR, Sponheim SR, Iacono WG, Clementz BA (1995). Internal consistency reliability of resting EEG power spectra in schizophrenic and normal subjects. *Psychophysiology* 32:66–71.

MacDonald K, Parke RD (1984). Bridging the gap: parent–child play interaction and peer interactive competence. *Child Dev* 55:1265–1277.

Mills RS, Rubin KH (1990). Parental beliefs about problematic social behaviors in early childhood. *Child Dev* 61:138–151.

Park S, Belsky J, Putnam S, Crnic K (1997). Infant emotionality, parenting, and 3-year inhibition: exploring stability and lawful discontinuity in a male sample. *Dev Psychol* 33:218–227.

Riese ML (1987). Longitudinal assessment of temperament from birth to 2 years: a comparison of full-term and preterm infants. Infant Behav Dev 10:347–363.

Rothbart MK (1981). Measurement of temperament in infancy. *Child Dev* 52:569–578.

Rothbart MK (1986). Longitudinal observation of infant temperament. *Dev Psychol* 22:356–365.

Rothbart MK, Bates JE (1998). Temperament. In: Handbook of Child Psychology, Vol 3: Social, Emotional, and Personality Development, Eisenberg N, ed; Damon W, series ed, New York: Wiley, pp. 105–176.

Rothbart MK, Derryberry D (1981). Development of individual differences in temperament. In: Advances in Developmental Psychology, Lamb ME, Brown AL, eds. Hillsdale, NJ: Erlbaum, pp. 37–86.

Rowe DC, Plomin R (1977). Temperament in early childhood. *J Pers Assess* 41:150–156.

Rubin KH (1985). Social play and social development. In: Play and Child Development, Caldwell Brown C, Gottfried A, eds. New York: Johnson & Johnson Publications, pp. 88–96.

Rubin KH (2000). The Play Observation Scale (POS) (Revised). University of Maryland (e-mail: krubin@rubinlab.umd.edu).

Rubin KH, Chen X, Hymel S (1993). Socio-emotional characteristics of aggressive and withdrawn children. *Merrill-Palmer* Q 49:518–534.

Rubin KH, Coplan R (1998). Social play in early childhood: an individual differences perspective. In: Play in Early Child Education, Spodek B, Saracho ON, eds. New York: SUNY Press, pp. 144–170.

Rubin KH, Coplan RJ, Fox NA, Calkins SD (1995). Emotionality, emotion regulation, and preschoolers' social adaptation. *Dev Psychopathol* 7:49–62.

Rubin KH, Hastings PD, Stewart S, Henderson HA, Chen X (1997). The consistency and concomitants of inhibition: some of the children, all of the time. *Child Dev* 68:467–483.

Schmidt LA, Fox NA (1998). The development and outcomes of childhood shyness: a multiple psychophysiologic measure approach. *Ann Child Dev* 13:1–20.

Schmidt LA, Fox NA, Shulkin J, Gold PW (1999). Behavioral and physiological correlates of self-presentation in temperamentally shy children. *Dev Psychobiol* 35:119–135.

Stevenson-Hinde J, Glover A (1996). Shy girls and boys: a new look. *J. Child Psychol Psychiatry* 37:181–187.

Thomas A, Chess S, Birch HG (1968). Temperament and Behavior Disorders in Children. New York: New York University Press.

Tomarken AJ, Davidson RJ, Henriques JB (1990). Resting frontal brain asymmetry predicts affective responses to films. *J Pers Soc Psychol* 59:791–801.

Part III

CLINICAL ISSUES

12

Pervasive Developmental Disorders in Preschool Children

Suniti Chakrabarti and Eric Fombonne

Context: *Prevalence rates of autism-spectrum disorders are uncertain, and speculation that their incidence is increasing continues to cause concern.* ***Objective:*** *To estimate the prevalence of pervasive developmental disorders (PDDs) in a geographically defined population of preschool children.* ***Design, Setting, and Participants:*** *Survey conducted July 1998 to June 1999 in Staffordshire, England. The area's 15,500 children aged 2.5 to 6.5 years were screened for developmental problems. Children with symptoms suggestive of a PDD were intensively assessed by a multidisciplinary team, which conducted standardized diagnostic interviews and administered psychometric tests.* ***Main Outcome Measure:*** *Prevalence estimates for subtypes of PDDs.* ***Results:*** *A total of 97 children (79.4% male) were confirmed to have a PDD. The prevalence of PDDs was estimated to be 62.6 (95% confidence interval, 50.8 to 76.3) per 10,000 children. Prevalences were 16.8 per 10,000 for autistic disorder and 45.8 per 10,000 for other PDDs. The mean age at diagnosis was 41 months, and 81% were originally referred by health visitors (nurse specialists). Of the 97 children with a PDD, 25.8% had some degree of mental retardation and 9.3% had an associated medical condition.* ***Conclusions:*** *Our results suggest that rates of PDD are higher than previously reported. Methodological limitations in existing epidemiological investigations preclude interpretation of recent high rates as indicative of increased incidence of these disorders although this hypothesis requires further rigorous testing. Attention is nevertheless drawn to the important needs of a substantial minority of preschool children.*

Autism is a severe developmental disorder involving deviance and often delay in the development of language or communication skills; social interactions and reciprocity; and imagination, play, and interests.[1] Since the first epidemiological survey of autism was conducted in the mid-1960s in England,[2] more than 30 surveys have been performed worldwide.[3,4] Rates of autism typically have been reported in the range of 4 to 6 per 10,000 although these figures increased in surveys conducted in the last 15 years.[4,5] These estimates do not account for a large group of children falling short of strict diagnostic criteria for autism (pervasive developmental disorders [PDDs]) and whose development poses similar assessment and educational challenges.

Although the apparent increased prevalence of autism may reflect improved detection and recognition of autism and its variants, it might also index a secular change in the incidence of the disorder. The role of genetic factors in the origin of autism does not favor such a hypothesis,[6] however. Moreover, no survey has thus far concentrated specifically on preschool children. Obtaining a reliable estimate in this age group is particularly important since early intensive preschool education might improve the outcome in autism.[7,8] Accordingly, the goals of this study were to estimate the prevalence of PDDs in preschool children in a geographically defined population.

METHODS

Site and Target Population

The study was conducted at the child development centers in Stafford, Cannock, and Wightwick in the Midlands, England, and it received approval from the South Staffordshire Health Authority local ethics committee. These child development centers serve the entire preschool and early school population of one National Health Service Trust. The survey was conducted from July 1998 to June 1999 although some initial clinical assessments were performed from 1994 onward. The area is a mixture of urban, rural, and semi-industrial areas. There is a stable population of indigenous British people with a small (1.4%), mostly Asian, immigrant population. The total population living in the area covered by the National Health Service Trust was 320,000 people in June 1998. The target population included all children (N = 15,500) born between January 1, 1992, and December 31, 1995, living within the target area on June 6, 1998.

Case Identification and Definition: 4 Stages

Stage 1. The national framework of Child Health Surveillance recommends the screening by health professionals of all U.K. children at birth; at age 6 weeks; and between ages 6 and 9 months, 18 and 24 months, and 3¼ and 3½ years. In the study population, all the neonatal and 6-week screenings were performed by pediatricians or general practitioners and the 7-month screening by health visitors, who are nurse specialists experienced in working with children and families. Health visitors or physicians performed the 18- to 24- month and 3¼- to 3½-year screening. Screening was conducted in accordance with the guidelines of the "Health for All Children" report,[9] which emphasizes continuity of care, making observations, checking history, eliciting parental concerns, offering health advice and guidance, and moving away from prescriptive tests. The primary care worker may also have had the opportunity to listen to and discuss any concerns about the child's progress during the immunization visits at 2, 3, 4, and 13 months. Besides health visitors, speech and language therapists, pediatricians, general practitioners, and other professionals contributed to the referral process, especially for children older than 3 years. The study was coordinated through the child development centers that processed all the referrals of preschool children.

The participating professionals underwent training sessions on early identification of developmental problems and received written guidelines for referral of children with developmental or behavioral problems. The guidance to those making referrals for the initial screenings was left purposefully general to include children with any likely serious developmental, behavioral, or physical problems. This procedure also ensured maximal sensitivity for PDD case finding. The guidelines for the initial screen were to refer all children with more than mild or transient problems in one or more areas of development, including personal-social, fine or gross motor, speech and language, play skills and attention, concentration, and behavioral difficulties. Referrals were sought as soon as any problem was identified, usually by the age of 2 to 2½ years or earlier.

Stage 2. Children referred at this initial stage underwent a second screening carried out by a developmental pediatrician (S.C.) or by the child development team, consisting of a pediatrician; a specialist health visitor; and speech and language, physical, occupational, and play therapists. Parents or main caretakers were involved in each stage of the screening. Any urgent referrals were fast-tracked to the developmental pediatrician or a multidisciplinary team.

Stage 3. Children who failed the second screening were selected for a 2-week assessment conducted by a multidisciplinary team. During these assessments, a play therapist led a group of four children with their participating parents in 2-hour sessions of structured activities as well as free play. A developmental pediatrician (S.C.) took a detailed developmental history and conducted a comprehensive medical and neurodevelopmental examination. Children were assessed by a speech and language therapist, a pediatric physical therapist, an occupational therapist, a dental nurse, a dietitian, and a nurse specialist trained in behavioral intervention for children with PDDs and other learning problems. Hearing was assessed by an audiological physician, and vision was screened by an orthoptist. At the end of this assessment, a clinical diagnostic formulation was made by the lead pediatrician.

All screening and evaluation steps undertaken at stages 1, 2, and 3 were part of a normal screening procedure implemented by the local service. Permission for extra data collection associated with research was sought either at the end of stage 3 or shortly after entering stage 4. About 75% of parents provided written informed consent. The rest provided oral informed consent.

Stage 4. Children strongly suspected of having a PDD diagnosis were further assessed with standardized diagnostic measures and psychometric assessments. The Autism Diagnostic Interview-Revised (ADI-R)[10–12] is a semistructured diagnostic interview for use with caregivers of children with a possible PDD diagnosis. The ADI-R was administered by the developmental pediatrician (S.C.), who has been trained in its use. The ADI-R algorithm generates scores for the areas of social interaction, communication (verbal and nonverbal), repetitive behaviors, and age of recognition of first abnormalities for which appropriate cutoff points are available. The ADI-R algorithm is compatible with *Diagnostic and Statistical Manual of Mental Disorders, Fourth Edition (DSM-IV)* diagnostic criteria. A total ADI-R score is obtained by summing the scores in the three domains of developmental deviance.

Children diagnosed as having a PDD subsequently underwent a formal psychometric assessment by a senior educational psychologist. All tests were performed in 1999 and early 2000. The tests used were the Wechsler Preschool and Primary Scale of Intelligence[13] and the Merrill-Palmer[14] tests. Intellectual functioning was estimated according to performances on the nonverbal scales of the Wechsler Preschool and Primary Scale of Intelligence or with the quotient derived from the Merrill-Palmer test. Mental retardation was defined according to conventional levels of severity (i.e., mild, 50 to 69; moderate, 35 to 49; severe, 20 to 34, and profound, below 20).

The final diagnostic determination was derived from a review of all existing data by the pediatrician who knew all children well. Diagnosis was made with *DSM-IV* diagnostic criteria[1] for PDD including autistic disorder (AD), Asperger syndrome, Rett syndrome, childhood disintegrative disorder, and pervasive developmental disorder-not otherwise specified (PDD-NOS).

Reliability Study

All ADI-R interviews were videotaped or audiotaped. A subset of 38 ADI-R videotapes was selected at random and blindly rated by three trained raters (including E.F.). Interrater reliability for domain scores as measured by the intraclass correlation coefficient[15] was 0.82 for social interactions, 0.87 for nonverbal communication, 0.85 for verbal communication (based on a subset of 28 children with a sufficient language level), 1.59 for repetitive behaviors, and 0.86 for the total ADI-R score. Agreement on the proportion of subjects scoring higher than each of the predetermined cutoffs was high for all domains (social interactions, 92.1%; nonverbal communication, 90.0%; verbal communication, 85.7%; repetitive behavior, 81.6%; and onset before age 3 years, 97.4%). Blinded raters were also asked to provide an independent global diagnostic judgment about the presence or absence of a PDD on the parental interview. Independent raters confirmed the presence of a PDD in all 38 children, yielding a 100% agreement with the original pediatrician's diagnoses.

Biological Investigations

Following the 2-week assessment, systematic laboratory investigations were performed, which included full blood cell count; plasma chemistry; serum calcium, thyrotropin and thyroxine, and creatine kinase levels; plasma and urine amino acid chromatogram; urine organic acids; chromosomes; fragile X testing; and electroencephalogram. The skin of children with suggestive birthmarks was examined with UV light to detect markers of tuberous sclerosis. In a small number of cases, brain imaging using computed tomographic or magnetic resonance imaging scans was performed on clinical suspicion of a possible neurological problem.

Statistical Analyses

Between-group comparisons for continuous variables were performed with both nonparametric (Kruskal-Wallis) and parametric 1-way analyses of variance followed by post hoc Scheffe pairwise comparisons. Because *p* values were almost identical, the results of parametric analyses are subsequently presented. χ^2 tests were used for categorical variables. Throughout, a conventional *p* value of .05 was retained as the level of statistical significance. Asymptotic 95% confidence intervals (CIs) for prevalence estimates were obtained with STATA software version 6.[16]

RESULTS

Prevalence

The details of case ascertainment in this investigation are summarized in Figure 12.1. Of the 576 children referred to a child development center for a stage 1 assessment, 103 children were clinically diagnosed as having PDD at the stage 3 assessment. Of these 103 children, 99 parents agreed to take part

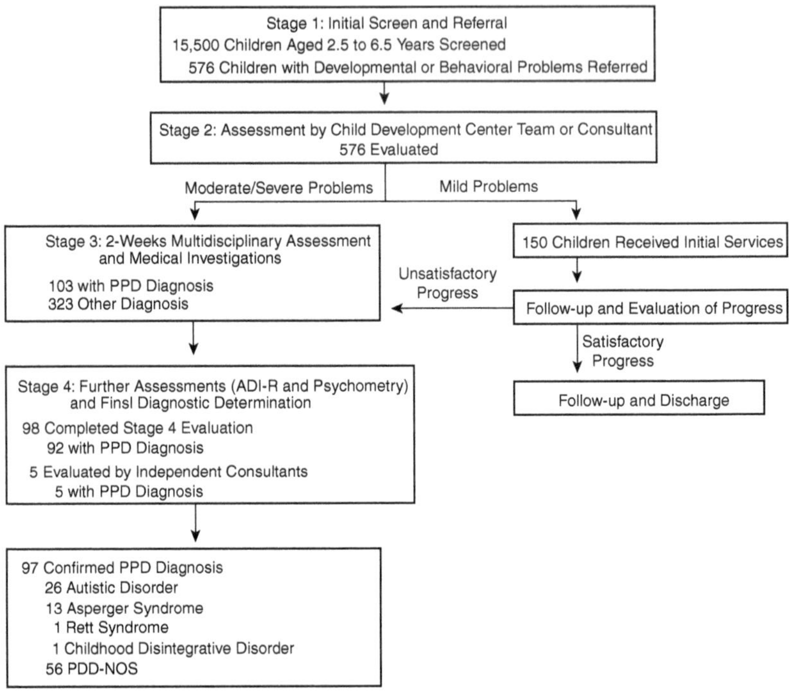

Note: PPD indicates pervasive developmental disorder; ADI-R, Autism Diagnostic Interview-Revised; and PDD-NOS, pervasive developmental disorder-not otherwise specified.

Figure 12.1. Screening Process and Sample Selection.

in the ADI-R interview and 4 parents refused. One interview was deferred indefinitely for external circumstances, and 98 interviews were finally carried out (95 videotaped, 3 audiotaped).

Of the 5 children who did not receive an ADI-R interview, a final PDD diagnosis was subsequently confirmed by an independent educational psychologist or child psychiatrist (2, AD; 3, PDD-NOS). Of the 98 children with ADI-R data, 6 children did not fulfill strict ADI-R diagnostic criteria for a PDD at stage 4. Thus, at the completion of stage 4, 97 children were diagnosed as having PDD, resulting in a prevalence estimate of 62.6 (95% CI, 50.8 to 76.3) per 10,000 children for all PDDs. Further analysis by PDD subtype led to the following estimates: for 26 children with AD, the prevalence was 16.8 (95% CI, 11.0 to 24.6) per 10,000; for 13 with Asperger syndrome, 8.4 (95% CI, 4.5 to 14.3) per 10,000; for 1 girl with Rett syndrome, 0.6 (95% CI, 0.02–3.6) per 10,000; for 1 boy with childhood disintegrative disorder, 0.6 (95% CI, 0.02 to 3.6) per 10,000; and for 56 with PDD-NOS, 36.1 (95% Cl,

27.3 to 46.9) per 10,000. For the 71 children with a PDD diagnosis other than AD, the prevalence was 45.8 (95 % CI, 35.8 to 57.7) per 10,000 children.

ADI-R Mean Scores

The mean (SD) age of 92 children with available ADI data was 58.1 (13.0) months at interview. Excluding the boy with childhood disintegrative disorder and the girl with Rett syndrome, comparison of scores across the three remaining diagnostic subgroups yielded significant differences in all domains except for the repetitive behaviors domain (Table 12.1). Post hoc tests showed that children with AD had consistently higher scores than the two other groups, which in turn did not differ from each other. All children met the requirement of an onset before age 3 years.

Referral Source and Age at Diagnosis

Thirty-four percent of the 97 referrals came from pediatricians, 32.9% from speech and language therapists, 21.6% from health visitors, 5.1% from

TABLE 12.1
Mean Autism Diagnostic Interview-Revised (ADI-R) Scores by Diagnostic Subgroup*

	AD (*N* = 24)	PDD-NOS (*N* = 53)	Asperger Syndrome (*N* = 13)	Fisher Statistic	*p* Value†	AD vs PDD-NOS *p* Value‡	AD vs Asperger Syndrome *p* Value‡	PDD-NOS vs Asperger Syndrome *p* Value‡
Social interaction	22.3 (4.9)	13.6 (5.2)	13.4 (3.3)	28.2	<.001	<.001	<.001	.99
Communication (nonverbal)	11.5 (2.2)	6.4 (3.5)	7.3 (2.8)	23.2	<.001	<.001	.001	.62
Repetitive behavior	5.3 (2.1)	5.3 (2.5)	6.0 (2.3)	0.5	.63	…	…	…
Total ADI-R score	42.1 (5.8)	30.6 (8.9)	31.9 (5.6)	17.9	<.001	<.001	.001	.85

*Data are presented as mean (SD) unless otherwise indicated. AD indicates autistic disorder; PDD-NOS, pervasive developmental disorder–not otherwise specified. Ellipses indicate that Fisher statistic was not significant. The 2 children with a diagnosis of either childhood disintegrative disorder or Rett syndrome and the 5 children without ADI-R interviews were not included in the analysis. The range of ADI-R scores for social interaction was 2 to 30; communication (nonverbal), 0 to 14; repetitive behaviors, 1 to 12; and total ADI-R, 18 to 54.

†Fisher statistic from analysis of variance and *p* value.

‡Results of post hoc Scheffé tests.

general practitioners, and 6.2% from miscellaneous sources. However, a closer look at referral patterns showed that most of the referrals to pediatricians and speech therapists were initiated by health visitors; thus, taking these data in combination, 79 (81%) of the 97 children were originally identified by the health visitor as having a problem requiring further assessment. The average age of children at referral was 35.7 months (range, 11 to 63 months), and the average age at initial clinical diagnosis was 41 months (range, 21 to 78 months). Analyses of variance were performed to test for differences in age at referral and age at diagnosis in the 95 children with AD, Asperger syndrome, or PDD-NOS diagnoses. A significant effect of diagnosis was found for age at referral ($F_{2, 92} = 11.3$; $p < .001$). Pairwise comparisons showed that mean age at referral for children with AD (30.0 months) was significantly lower than for children with PDD-NOS (37.2 months; $p = .03$) or with Asperger syndrome (47.5 months; $p < .001$). Age at referral of children with PDD-NOS was also significantly lower than in those children with Asperger syndrome ($p = .01$). For age at diagnosis, a significant effect of diagnostic subgroup was also found ($F_{2, 92} = 12.0$; $p < .001$). Post hoc Scheffé tests similarly indicated significantly lower mean age at diagnosis for children with AD (34.6 months) vs. children with PDD-NOS (43.1 months; $p = .005$) and lower age at diagnosis for children with Asperger syndrome (51.8 months; $p < .001$), whereas children with PDD-NOS had significantly lower mean age at diagnosis than those with Asperger syndrome ($p = .04$).

Clinical Correlates

The sample included 77 boys (79.4%) with no significant difference ($\chi^2_2 = 0.33$; $p = .85$) in the proportion of boys in the AD (76.9%), Asperger syndrome (84.6%), and PDD-NOS (80.4%) groups. Of the 97 children, 29 (29.9%) had no functional use of language defined as the daily spontaneous use of three-word phrases. The proportion of children without functional language was, however, strongly associated with diagnostic subtype (AD, 69.2%; Asperger syndrome, 0%; PDD-NOS, 16.1%; $\chi^2_2 = 30.6$; $p < .001$).

Of the 97 children, 37 children underwent Merrill-Palmer testing and 56, Wechsler Preschool and Primary Scale of Intelligence testing. Four children could not be tested for practical reasons. Overall, 24 (25.8%) of 93 children had some degree of mental retardation. The two children with childhood disintegrative disorder and Rett syndrome scored in the moderate range of mental retardation. However, patterns of cognitive functioning varied according to diagnosis (Table 12.2) and, combining together all levels of mental retardation, a significant difference was found for the presence or absence of mental retardation between the 3 PDD subtypes ($\chi^2_2 = 40.6$; $p < .001$), the AD group

TABLE 12.2
Intellectual Functioning by Diagnostic Subgroup*

	AD (N = 26)	PDD-NOS (N = 53)	Asperger Syndrome (N =12)
Normal range	8(30.8)	49(92.4)	12 (100)
Mild to moderate retardation	13(50.0)	4(7.6)	0
Severe to profound retardation	5(19.2)	0	0

*Data are presented as number (percentage). AD indicates autistic disorder; PDD-NOS, pervasive developmental disorder–not otherwise specified. The two subjects with either childhood disintegrative disorder or Rett syndrome and the four children who could not be tested are not included in this analysis.

having more frequent and severe cognitive delays than the Asperger syndrome and PDD-NOS groups.

In the sample, five children had a sibling with another PDD (including one twin pair). Four of the sibling pairs were in the age range of this study and were included in the prevalence pool. Of the sibling pairs, three sets were diagnosed with both pairs having PDD-NOS, one set with AD and PDD-NOS, and one set with Asperger syndrome and AD. Based on the total number of siblings across all 93 families (N = 220, including the 97 participating children), the sibling risk is estimated at 3.94% (5/127) in this study.

Associated Medical Conditions

The results of medical investigations in this sample are summarized in Table 12.3. There was no case of deafness, blindness, or fragile X disorder, and only one child had tuberous sclerosis. Six of eight children with an abnormal medical result had mental retardation. Overall, the proportion of children with any abnormal medical result was 9.3%.

COMMENT

Most other surveys [5,17] estimated the prevalence of children with PDD to be nearer to 20 per 10,000 children than the 62.6 per 10,000 prevalence in our study. This rate is, however, consistent with the 57.9 and 67.4 per 10000 estimates reported in two recent investigations.[18,19] These three surveys have all used intensive screening procedures, focused on children younger than 10 years, and used modern standardized diagnostic measures such as the ADI-R[10–12] or the Autism Diagnostic Observation Schedule-Generic.[20] The somewhat lower estimate of 26.1 per 10,000 and 30.1 per 10,000 among children aged 5 to 9 years obtained in another U.K. survey[21] probably reflects

TABLE 12.3
Associated Medical Conditions in Children with Pervasive Developmental Disorder

Sex	Diagnosis	Age at Diagnosis, mo	IQ	Medical Condition
Male	Autism	44	31	Tuberous sclerosis
Female	PDD-NOS	49	83	Hydrocephalus with premature thelarche
Male	PDD-NOS	39	100	Hydrocephalus with aqueduct stenosis and vermian hypoplasia
Male	Autism	42	65	*XYY* Karyotype
Female	PDD-NOS	39	44	*XXX* Karyotype
Female	Autism	57	44	Cerebral palsy, abnormal EEG results, no overt seizures
Female	POD-NOS	50	85	Cerebral palsy
Female	POD-NOS	56	68	Bardet-Biedl syndrome, sleep disturbance with parasomnia-like events
Male	Childhood disintegrative disorder	78	38	Left monoplegia, epilepsy with continuous EEG disturbance from right hemisphere, small infarct in right parietal area

*PDD-NOS indicates pervasive developmental disorder–not otherwise specified; EEG, electroencephalogram.

methodological differences in an investigation that was focusing primarily on common childhood psychiatric disorders. Thus, the latter survey did not rely on screening procedures and diagnostic measures specific to PDDs. It is worth noting that four U.K. surveys of children in the same age groups conducted at the same time and in the same country showed a six-fold variation in prevalence rates, emphasizing how powerfully various methods used in a survey affect prevalence estimates.[4] The findings also point to the probable lack of sensitivity of case finding procedures in earlier surveys resulting in underestimation of rates. Therefore, the prevalence of PDDs seems to be about 60 per 10,000 children, an estimate that draws attention to the needs of a substantial minority of children.

Whether the higher prevalence rates reported recently arose from a secular increase in the incidence of the disorder or merely reflect a broadening of the concept of PDD together with improved detection and recognition cannot be assessed from these data. Comparison of prevalence rates obtained from cross-sectional surveys conducted at different times are confounded by changes in diagnostic concepts and criteria, changes in the efficiency of case finding procedures (as already shown above), and improved awareness in both the lay and professional public about the autism-spectrum conditions.[4] In one survey, comparison of rates between successive birth cohorts was performed holding constant case definition and identification methods, and no evidence could be produced of an increase over time.[22] Reports of increased numbers of children with PDD by providers of educational services have also been quoted as evidence of an epidemic of autism[23,24] although several analyses of these claims refuted their validity.[25–27] One factor accounting for increased rates lies in the decreasing age at diagnosis, which occurred during the last 30 years.[23,25,28] Assuming no change in the underlying incidence and a steady prevalence pool, this trend could explain the increasing numbers of young children seen in clinical settings and identified in surveys, particularly since those surveys usually relied on service providers to detect known cases rather than on systematic population screening.

In our survey, AD accounted for only 27% of the cases with these children showing much greater cognitive and language impairments. By contrast, the majority of cases were found at the mild end of the autistic spectrum, with the PDD-NOS and Asperger syndrome groups accounting for 71.1% of the cases. High proportions of PDDs were also found in recent surveys (46.8%[18] and 40%[19]). Prior surveys focused on a narrow definition, which led to the exclusion of these milder forms although it has been recognized for some time that they represented a group as sizable if not bigger than that of autism.[5] The inclusion of these milder variants certainly may account for a substantial part of the increase in prevalence rates.

Children with a PDD thus present as a whole as less impaired than what has been classically described. Although the average rate of mental retardation was near 75% in previous autism surveys,[5] this rate has fallen to much lower figures of 40%[18] and 55%[19] in large epidemiological series of PDD and was 26% in this survey. Moreover, there appears to be a downward trend for the rate of mental retardation within the group narrowly defined as autism (i.e., 50% in the Brick Township study among 3- to 10-year-olds[19] and 25% among 3- to 5-year-olds in a Finnish survey[29]).

This shift has important implications for intervention since the majority of these children will require education in mainstream schools with provision of individual support. In addition, it is possible that very early intervention in autism and PDD might be associated with a much better cognitive outcome in the short term. Evidence of the beneficial impact of intensive educational programs between the ages of 2 and 4 years has accumulated recently,[7,8] and the notion of a critical period for a maximal effect of intensive educational interventions clearly requires further examination. Parents recognize the first developmental abnormalities before the second birthday in the majority of cases,[30,31] and one encouraging result from this survey was that four fifths of PDD cases were identified at a very early age by trained health visitors, indicating that early population screening programs could detect a high proportion of children with PDDs before the age of 2 years. Instruments with adequate levels of sensitivity and specificity are currently being developed,[18,32,33] which may make that goal attainable. Such screening must be supported with appropriate assessment services combining special expertise in autism and multidisciplinary skills,[32] as was the case in our population.

Consistent with a major role of genetic factors in PDD,[6,34] identified medical abnormalities were found in less than 10% of our sample. Moreover, the abnormalities reported in this sample might not be causally implicated in the development of PDD and might have occurred simply as random findings in a population submitted to intensive medical work-up. Nevertheless, the rate of 10% for medical abnormalities of potential etiological significance is consistent with prior findings deriving from both clinical[35,36] and epidemiological surveys.[3,5] The rate of sibling recurrence obtained in this study is also consistent with figures of 3% to 7% reported by other investigators,[34] and although the absolute magnitude of the risk remains small, a comparison with the population prevalence points toward a large increase in the risk of autism or PDD in families with an already affected child.

Some limitations of this study must be mentioned. First, clinical assessment of children was not performed with standardized diagnostic techniques although such instruments were available for parental interviews and cognitive testing. It is unlikely that this would affect the prevalence estimates obtained in this study since experienced clinicians agreed 100% on the presence of a PDD in the whole sample. Availability of these assessments might nevertheless have provided a different breakdown of the diagnosis into various diagnostic subcategories. Assessing young children with PDDs is a complex task and guidelines to draw the line between high-functioning autism, Asperger syndrome, and PDD-NOS remain to be firmly established. Second, there is a possibility that some children might have been missed despite the intensive screening efforts used in the survey. This might particularly apply to some cases of Asperger syndrome that are sometimes not detected before school age and might have led to some underestimation of the prevalence. Conversely, some children diagnosed as having mild forms of PDD-NOS may turn out on follow-up assessments to have more transient developmental problems. This might have produced an inflation of the prevalence estimate. Whether these two problems might cancel each other remains to be seen, but we are committed to reassess this sample at age 8 to 10 years to address these issues and to obtain a more stable estimate.

AUTHOR CONTRIBUTIONS

Study concept and design; analysis and interpretation of data; drafting of the manuscript; critical revision of the manuscript for important intellectual content; and administrative, technical, or material support: Chakrabarti, Fombonne. Acquisition of data and obtained funding: Chakrabarti. Statistical expertise and supervision: Fombonne.

FUNDING/SUPPORT

Funding for this study was provided by the First Community Health Trust.

ACKNOWLEDGMENTS

We are grateful to the First Community Trust board and its executive directors for supporting this research. We especially thank the parents and children in the research group without whose cooperation and help this research would not have been possible. We also thank all the staff of the child development centers for their support and Sally Williams, BSc, senior educational psychologist of Staffordshire LEA, who conducted all the psychometric assessments of the children. Frank Devine, RGN, RNM, behavior nurse specialist, helped enormously by his meticulous observation and recording of the children's behavior, as well as by providing support to the children's families. We also thank Marianne Murin and Simon Wallace for taking part in the reliability study.

AUTHOR AFFILIATIONS

Child Development Centre, Central Clinic, Stafford, England (Dr. Chakrabarti); and Department of Child & Adolescent Psychiatry, MRC Child Psychiatry Unit, Institute of Psychiatry, King's College, London, England (Dr. Fombonne).

REFERENCES

1. American Psychiatric Association. *Diagnostic and Statistical Manual of Mental Disorders, Fourth Edition.* Washington, D.C.: American Psychiatric Association; 1994.
2. Lotter V. Epidemiology of autistic conditions in young children, I: prevalence. *Soc Pysch.* 1966;1:124–137.
3. Fombonne E. Epidemiological surveys of autism: a review. *Psychol Med.* 1999;29:769–786.
4. Fombonne E. Epidemiological estimates and time trends in rates of autism. *Mol Psychiatry.* In press.
5. Fombonne E. Epidemiological investigations of autism and other pervasive developmental disorders. In Lord C, ed. *Educating Children With Autism.* Washington, D.C.: National Academy of Sciences Press: 2001.
6. Bailey A, Le Couteur A, Gottesman I, et al., Autism as a strongly genetic disorder: evidence from a British twin study. *Psychol Med.* 1995;25:63–77.

7. Rogers S. Brief report: early intervention in autism. *J Autism Dev Disord.* 1996;26:243–246.
8. National Academy of Sciences. *Report of the Committee on Educational Interventions in Children With Autism:* Educating Children With Autism. Washington, D.C.: National Academy of Sciences Press: 2001.
9. Hall D, ed. *Health for All Children: Report of the Third Joint Working Party on Child Health Surveillance*. 3rd ed. Oxford. England: Oxford University Press; 1996.
10. Lord C, Rutter M, Le Couteur A. Autism Diagnostic Interview-Revised: a revised version of a diagnostic interview for caregivers of individuals with possible pervasive developmental disorders. *J Autism Dev Disord.* 1994;24:659–685.
11. Le Couteur A, Rutter M, Lord C, et al., Autism Diagnostic Interview: a standardized investigator-based instrument. *J Autism Dev Disord*. 1989;19:363–387.
12. Fombonne E. Diagnostic assessment in a sample of autistic and developmentally impaired adolescents. *J Autism Dev Disord*. 1992;22:563–581.
13. Wechsler D. *Manual for Wechsler Pre-school and Primary Scale of Intelligence-Revised (British Amendments)*. Kent, England: The Psychological Corp: 1990.
14. Stutsman R. *Merrill-Palmer Scale of Mental Tests Preprints of Part III, Mental Measurement of Pre-school Children*. Chicago, III: Stoelting Co: 1948.
15. Bartko J. On various intraclass correlation reliability coefficients. *Psychol Bull.* 1976;83:762–765.
16. STATA Corp. *Statistic/Data Analysis*. College Station, TX: STATA Press; 1997.
17. Wing L. Gould J. Severe impairments of social interaction and associated abnormalities in children: epidemiology and classification. *J Autism Dev Disord.* 1979;9:11–29.
18. Baird G, Charman T, Baron-Cohen S, et al., A screening instrument for autism at 18 months of age: a 6-year follow-up study. *J Am Acad Child Adolesc Psychiatry.* 2000;39:694–702.
19. Centers for Disease Control and Prevention. *Prevalence of Autism in Brick Township, New Jersey,* 1998. Atlanta, GA: Centers for Disease Control and Prevention 2000. Community Report. Available at http://www.cdc.gov/nceh/cddh/dd/rpttoc.htm. Accessibility verified May 15, 2001.
20. Lord C, Risi S, Lambrecht L, et al., The Autism Diagnostic Observation Schedule-Generic: a standard measure of social and communication deficits associated with the spectrum of autism. *J Autism Dev Disord.* 2000;30:205–223.
21. Fombonne E, Simmons H, Ford T, Meltzer H, Goodman R. Prevalence of pervasive developmental disorders in the British nationwide survey of child mental health. *J Am Acad Child Adolesc Psychiatry,* in press.
22. Fombonne E, du Mazaubrun C, Cans H, Grand H. Autism and associated medical disorders in a French epidemiological sample. *J AM Acad Child Adolesc Psychiatry.* 1997;36:1561–1569.
23. California Department of Developmental Services. *Changes in the Population of Persons With Autism and Pervasive Developmental Disorders in California's Developmental Services System: 1987 Through 1998.* Report to the Legislature; March 1, 1999. Available at: http://www.dds.ca.gov. Accessibility verified May 30, 2001.
24. Wakefield A. MMR Vaccination and autism [letter]. *Lancet.* 1999;354:949–950.

25. Fombonne E. Is there an epidemic of autism? *Pediatrics*. 2001;107:411–413.
26. Dales L, Hammer SJ, Smith NU. Time trends in autism and MMR immunization coverage in California. *JAMA*. 2001;285:1183–1185.
27. Immunization Safety Review Committee. *Measles-Mumps-Rubella Vaccine and Autism*. Washington, D.C.: Institute of Medicine; 2001.
28. Howlin P., Moore A. Diagnosis in autism: a survey of over 1200 patients in the UK. *Autism*. 1997;1:135–162.
29. Kielinen M, Linna SL, Moilanen I. Autism in northern Finland. *Eur Child Adolesc Psychiatry*. 2000;9: 162–167.
30. De Giacomo A, Fombonne E. Parental recognition of developmental abnormalities in autism. *Eur Child Adolesc Psychiatry*. 1998;7:131–136.
31. Rogers JS, Di Lalla D. Age of symptom onset in young children with pervasive developmental disorders. *J Am Acad Child Psychiatry*. 1990;29: 207–216.
32. Filpek PA, Accardo PJ, Baranek GT, et al., The screening and diagnosis of autistic spectrum disorders [published correction appears in *J Autism Dev Disord*. 2000;30:81]. *J Autism Dev Disord*. 1999;29:439–484.
33. Stone W, Coonrod E, Ousley O. Screening tool for autism in two-year-olds (STAT): development and preliminary data. *J Autism Dev Disord*. 2000;30:607–612.
34. Szatmart P, Jones M, Zwaigenbaum L, MacLean J. Genetics of autism: overview and new directions. *J Autism Dev Disord*. 1998;28:351–368.
35. Barton M, Volkmar F. How commonly are known medical conditions associated with autism? *J Autism Dev Disord*. 1998;28:273–278.
36. Rutter M, Bailey A, Bolton P, Le Couteur A. Autism and known medical conditions: myth and substance. *J Child Psychol Psychiatry*. 1994;35:311–322.

13

Open Trial of Risperidone in 24 Young Children with Pervasive Developmental Disorders

Gabriele Masi, Angela Cosenza, Maria Mucci, and Paola Brovedani

Objective: *To describe tolerability and efficacy of risperidone in very young children with pervasive developmental disorders.* ***Method:*** *Twenty-four children aged 3.6 to 6.6 years (mean 4.6 years ± 8 months) enrolled during 1999 and 2000 participated in a 16-week open-label trial with risperidone monotherapy. Outcome measures included the Children's Psychiatric Rating Scale (CPRS), Childhood Autism Rating Scale (CARS), Clinical Global Impression-Improvement (CGI-I), and Children's Global Assessment Scale (C-GAS).* ***Results:*** *Two subjects did not complete the trial because of side effects. The optimal dose was 0.5 mg/day. After the treatment a 21% improvement in CPRS and a 14% improvement in CARS total scores was found. Items related to behavioral control (hyperactivity, fidgetiness, rhythmic motions) and affect regulation (lability of affect, angry affect) improved more than 25%. Based on improvement of at least 25% on the CPRS and a score of 1 or 2 on the CGI-I, eight subjects were considered responders. Functional impairment (C-GAS) improved more than 25%. Thirteen subjects (54%) were free of any side effects; in the other participants risperidone was well tolerated. Only three subjects had a weight gain greater than 10%.* ***Conclusions:*** *Low-dose risperidone may positively affect symptoms in young autistic children, improving disruptive/hyperactive behavior and affective dysregulation. Further controlled studies in this age group are warranted.*

As part of integrated treatment programs, different medications with an effect on the dopaminergic and serotonergic systems were used in patients with pervasive developmental disorders (PDD) (McDougle et al., 2000). The dopamine receptor antagonist haloperidol was extensively studied in children with PDD, and it was associated with improvement in hyperactivity, aggression, and temper tantrums (Anderson and Campbell, 1989; Perry et al., 1989). High sensitivity to side effects, namely extrapyramidal symptoms and tardive dyskinesia, have limited their use in autistic children (Campbell et al., 1997). Furthermore, neuroleptics are less effective on the core symptoms of autism: social withdrawal, lack of emotional reciprocity, and absent or stereotyped language (Locascio et al., 1991).

Newer antipsychotics, called atypical antipsychotics, with dopamine and serotonin receptor antagonism (clozapine, risperidone, olanzapine, and quetiapine) are more effective in reducing both positive and negative symptoms of schizophrenia, with a significantly lower risk of acute extrapyramidal effects and tardive dyskinesia (Armenteros et al., 1997; Kumra et al., 1997a). Risperidone, a potent antagonist of dopamine D2, serotonin 2A, and other serotonin receptors, was found to enhance social interaction in preclinical studies (Corbett et al., 1993) and to reduce negative symptoms in schizophrenic patients (Chouinard et al., 1993). Some core symptoms of autistic syndrome may be considered comparable with the negative symptoms of schizophrenia (Fisman and Steele, 1996), and they may be more sensitive to atypical antipsychotics (McDougle et al., 2000).

Studies have been conducted with risperidone in PDD children older than 10 years of age (Findling et al., 1997; Fisman and Steele, 1996, McDougle et al., 1997; Nicolson et al., 1998; Perry et al., 1997; Zuddas et al., 2000). Even if an early diagnosis and a timely, effective treatment are crucial elements for a good prognosis (Volkmar et al., 1996), only sparse data are available on pharmacological treatments in preschool children.

Casaer et al. (1994) reported a preliminary investigation of pharmacokinetics and safety (but not efficacy) of risperidone in six young autistic children (mean age 4.7) who received a single oral dose of the drug at 0.015 mg/kg daily (three subjects) or 0.030 mg/kg daily (three subjects). The medication was well tolerated, although five children had dose-related somnolence. In McDougle and coworkers' (1997) study of 18 patients, 3 children were aged 6 years or younger. Only a young boy without mental retardation was much improved on the Clinical Global Impression (CGI), while two severely mentally retarded girls did not show any change or were minimally worse. Findling et al. (1997) administered risperidone to six autistic children aged 5 to 9 years, with good efficacy and safety. In a study by Nicolson et al. (1998), 4 of the 10 children were younger than 6 years of age, and they responded positively to treatment. Posey et al. (1999) recently described a significant behavioral improvement in two autistic children aged less than 2 years following treatment with risperidone. In our preliminary study (Masi et al., 2001), risperidone was safe and moderately effective in 10 preschool children with PDD.

Psychopharmacological treatment of very young patients is a major topic of current research. However, several specific questions are largely unanswered, as current knowledge stems from an extrapolation of information from older children, adolescents, or adults (Jensen et al., 1999). First, little is known about the pharmacodynamic effect on the developing brain of drugs administered for extended periods of time during the first years of life, when dramatic developmental changes in neurotransmitters and receptors occur. Some animal data suggest the possibility of permanent up- or down-regulation of receptor systems as a function of exposure to psychotropic drugs in the developing mammalian brain (Vitiello and Jensen, 1995). Second, the greater immaturity of biological systems may modify not only drug response (in terms of pharmacokinetics and/or pharmacodynamics), but also sensitivity to specific therapeutic or untoward effects. These considerations are nonspecific to psychotropic medications, but they are common to pediatric pharmacology as a whole (Vitiello, 1998). Third, a careful medical assessment is crucial to provide a baseline for physiological parameters that may be affected by drug treatment. The specificity of this medical work-up, as well as the minimal frequency of the monitoring, needs further research in this age range. Fourth, when long-term studies are carried out, a possible alternative explanation for observed results in very young children is that psychological or biological changes may occur naturally with time. A developmental approach to interpreting treatment data is needed, considering what we know about normal physical and psychological development. The advisability of incorporating *in vivo* measures of affective, social, and behavioral change during the treatment is crucial in very young and very disturbed children; unfortunately, sensitivity to detect changes in the real world is still unclear for most of these instruments. Finally, all these considerations raise important ethical concerns both in clinical practice and in clinical trials (Jensen, 1998). The off-label medication use in preschool children is a widespread problem that applies not only to psychoactive drugs, but also to 80% of all medications (American Academy of Pediatrics, Committee on Drugs, 1996), which are often administered without a solid knowledge base from clinical trials. These clinical trials in very young children imply other ethical considerations, for example whether or not to use placebo (Jensen, 1998). When safety and efficacy data are lacking, and/or when there is uncertainty regarding whether a medication is a valid alternative, placebo should be preferentially used (Jensen, 1998). Long-term, well-designed, controlled studies on large samples of affected young children should expand the current knowledge on these issues.

The aim of this study was to assess the safety and efficacy of risperidone monotherapy in a sample of preschool children with PDD and persistent uncontrolled behavior. To our knowledge, this is the largest case series of young children with PDD who were treated with an atypical antipsychotic.

METHOD

Subjects

All children aged between 3 and 6.11 years referred to our Division of Child Neurology and Psychiatry as inpatients or outpatients during 1999 and 2000 were screened for psychiatric disorders; historical information, clinical interviews, and symptom ratings according to *DSM-IV* criteria (American Psychiatric Association, 1994) were used. Our clinic is a university research hospital with a national catchment for children and adolescents with a wide range of neuropsychiatric disorders. The children were referred by community-based child and adolescent psychiatrists or pediatricians or by family members. Of all these patients, a consecutive sample of 43 children received a diagnosis of PDD, according to *DSM-IV* diagnostic criteria and Childhood Autism Rating Scale (CARS) score greater than 30 (Schopler et al., 1980). All diagnoses were made by two independent investigators. To improve the reliability and validity of the diagnosis and for the purpose of consensus, clinical data were reviewed by the team of interviewers. When questions arose, patients were reassessed. Twenty-four of these children were considered eligible for the risperidone study, according to severity of symptoms, exclusion criteria (comorbid medical or neurological conditions), and informed consent to treatment from the parents. The other 19 children with PDD did not participate in the study because of refusal of treatment proposal ($N = 9$), families' inability to comply with the follow-up procedures ($N = 6$), and concurrent medical disorders such as epileptic seizures ($N = 4$). Demographic (mean age, gender) and clinical variables (baseline scores on the CARS and Children's Psychiatric Rating Scale [CPRS], intellectual measures) did not differentiate enrolled and nonenrolled children.

The subjects were 21 boys and 3 girls, aged 3.6 to 6.6 years (mean = 4.6 years ± 8 months), 19 with an autistic disorder, 5 with PDD not otherwise specified. All subjects but one had mental retardation (Table 13.1). None of the subjects had a diagnosed genetic, metabolic, or neurological etiology for the PDD. All participants showed severe psychiatric symptoms, unimproved after previous nonpharmacological interventions. Five of these subjects had previously been treated unsuccessfully with vitamin B_6 and/or magnesium; one patient had been treated unsuccessfully with thioridazine. The children were free of other medications for the duration of the study, and they started risperidone treatment after at least a 4-week medication-free interval. All subjects participated in the study after written informed parental consent had been obtained. The study was approved by the human subjects committee of our hospital. We did not request an investigational new drug application from the U.S. Food and Drug Administration.

TABLE 13.1
Clinical Characteristics of Children with Pervasive Developmental Disorders Treated with Risperidone

Patient No.	*DSM-IV* Diagnosis	Age[a]	Gender	Mental Retardation	Drug (mg/day)	Side Effects	C-GAS (Baseline)	C-GAS (4 months)	Clinical Global Improvement
1	Autistic disorder	4y	M	Severe	0.50	None	19	29	Much improved
2	Autistic disorder	4y 2m	M	Severe	0.50	Increased appetite; agitation	18	24	Minimally improved
3	PDD–NOS	4y 8m	M	Moderate	0.50	Dystonia; increased appetite	23	35	Much improved
4	Autistic disorder	5y	M	Severe	0.25	Increased appetite; enuresis	21	27	Minimally improved
5	Autistic disorder	3y 9m	M	Severe	0.25	Tachycardia	18	—[b]	—[b]
6	Autistic disorder	6y 6m	F	Severe	0.50	None	18	30	Much improved
7	Autistic disorder	3y 11m	M	Moderate	0.25	Diarrhea; loss of appetite	25	34	Minimally improved
8	Autistic disorder	4y 8m	M	Severe	0.50	Loss of appetite	21	38	Very much improved
9	Autistic disorder	4y 3m	M	Moderate	0.75	None	18	30	Much improved
10	Autistic disorder	4y 3m	M	Severe	0.50	Enuresis; increased appetite	15	18	Unchanged
11	PDD–NOS	4y 5m	F	Mild	0.25	Sedation; loss of appetite	27	—[b]	—[b]
12	Autistic disorder	4y 9m	M	Moderate	0.50	Enuresis	20	32	Much improved
13	Autistic disorder	4y 11m	M	Moderate	0.50	None	19	20	Unchanged
14	PDD–NOS	5y 10m	F	None	0.75	None	35	40	Minimally improved
15	Autistic disorder	5y 2m	M	Severe	0.50	None	17	25	Minimally improved

(*Continued*)

TABLE 13.1
(Continued)

Patient No.	*DSM-IV* Diagnosis	Age[a]	Gender	Mental Retardation	Drug (mg/day)	Side Effects	C-GAS (Baseline)	C-GAS (4 months)	Clinical Global Improvement
16	Autistic disorder	5y 3m	M	Severe	0.50	None	15	23	Minimally improved
17	PDD–NOS	4y 6m	M	Moderate	0.50	None	19	30	Much improved
18	Autistic disorder	3y 6m	M	Moderate	0.50	None	18	25	Minimally improved
19	Autistic disorder	5y 8m	M	Moderate	0.50	None	19	26	Minimally improved
20	Autistic disorder	3y 8m	M	Moderate	0.50	Increased appetite	18	30	Much improved
21	PDD–NOS	4y	M	Moderate	0.33	Agitation; increased appetite	20	26	Minimally improved
22	Autistic disorder	4y 1m	M	Mild	0.50	None	17	24	Minimally improved
23	Autistic disorder	4y 6m	M	Moderate	0.50	None	18	26	Minimally improved
24	Autistic disorder	3y 8m	M	Severe	0.50	None	18	21	Unchanged

Note: PDD–NOS = pervasive developmental disorder–not otherwise specified; C-GAS = Children's Global Assessment Scale.

[a]y = years; m = months.

[b]Dropout.

Physical and Laboratory Assessment

Baseline assessment consisted of medical history and neurological and physical examinations including weight, heart rate, pulse monitoring, and blood pressure. Screening procedures included a complete blood cell count (CBC); measurement of electrolytes, blood urea nitrogen, fasting glucose, and creatinine; liver function tests; electrocardiogram (ECG); and electroencephalogram (EEG) during sleep. CBC, blood chemistry analyses, and physical examination were repeated every 4 weeks and at the end of the 16-week risperidone trial. An ECG was repeated after 1 and 3 months, and an EEG at the end of the study. The progression of the clinical condition after hospital discharge was monitored through visits or telephone contacts with parents and pediatricians, a few days after the start of risperidone administration, then at least weekly. A side effects checklist was used to assess tolerability.

Behavioral Rating Scales

Behavioral symptoms were assessed in each subject by two independent examiners at baseline and again at the end of the 16-week treatment. Even if the clinical course of the patients was monitored by visits and telephone calls, this monitoring did not follow a fixed-interval schedule, as many patients resided far from the hospital. A more structured psychiatric assessment was conducted at the end of the study, to collect more homogeneous data. In the second assessment, however, information from parents about the whole period of treatment was also considered. The child and adolescent psychiatrists were highly experienced in diagnosis and treatment of young children with PDD and had been properly trained in the use of the diagnostic instruments. The standardized assessment continued after prolonged observations of play interactions with parents and/or examiners, during 5 to 6 days of hospitalization. Children enrolled in the study attended a preschool for 4 hours per day, partly with their parent(s), partly with a teacher. Behavioral and social-emotional skills were directly observed by two trained child and adolescent psychiatrists during these play and interactive activities. Semistructured 60-minute play sessions with a familiar adult were also videotaped, and two different child and adolescent psychiatrists independently rated the target behaviors. We computed coefficients of agreement between the trained raters and two child and adolescent psychiatrists who reviewed the videotapes. Diagnoses of PDD achieved values higher than 0.88; the mean value was 0.95.

Comprehensive rating scales including multiple items relevant for various behavioral aspects for a range of patients were selected to detect changes in specific behavioral-emotional domains (Arnold et al., 2000). The diagnostic work-up included the following:

Children's Psychiatric Rating Scale. The CPRS (Fish, 1985) is a 73-item scale scored from 0 to 6. We have used a smaller subset of the scale, including 14 selected items, which has been proved to be effective for assessment and classification of behavioral symptoms in autistic children, according to construct validity, sensitivity, and specificity of scores (Overall and Campbell, 1988). The CPRS can be considered an effective means for assessing changes during pharmacological trials (Campbell and Palij, 1985). The selected items were underproductive speech; fidgetiness; hyperactivity; hypoactivity; abnormal object relationships; withdrawal; negative, uncooperative behavior; angry affect; nonspontaneous relation to examiner; lability of affect; low voice; loud voice; other speech deviance; and rhythmic motions.

Childhood Autism Rating Scale. The CARS (Schopler et al., 1980) is a 15-item scale with items rated from 1 to 4 measuring autistic behavior. Scores in different items can be computed to achieve a more precise clinical profile. The sum of the scores for the 15 items is used to obtain a broad measure of severity. A score of 37 or higher is considered indicative of severe autistic behavior; a score between 30 and 36.5 is considered indicative of mild to moderate autistic disorder. The CARS is considered an objective, behaviorally based rating system with demonstrated reliability and validity (DiLalla and Rogers, 1994; Garfin et al., 1988). Even though this instrument was developed to aid in the diagnostic process, it has been shown to be sensitive to developmental changes in autistic symptoms (Mesibov et al., 1989) and to treatment effects (Masi et al., 2001; Nicolson et al., 1998; Rogers and Lewis, 1989; Zuddas et al., 2000).

Clinical Global Impression-Improvement. The CGI-I (Guy, 1976), a single item recorded at the end of the study, rates behavior from 7 (very much worse) to 1 (very much improved). This instrument has been extensively used in psychopharmacological studies of children and adolescents with PDD (Findling et al., 1997; Masi et al., 2001; McDougle et al., 1997; Nicolson et al., 1998; Zuddas et al., 2000).

Children's Global Assessment Scale. The Children's Global Assessment Scale (C-GAS) (Shaffer et al., 1983) describes the severity of functional impairment on a scale from 0 (severe impairment) to 100 (superior functioning). It was designed for use with children from 4 to 16 years of age; scores greater than 70 indicate normal functioning. The use of the C-GAS as a measure of change in children and adolescents with PDD has been reported (Fisman and Steele, 1996; Zuddas et al., 2000).

Assessment of Intellectual Functioning. Scales for the assessment of intellectual functioning at baseline were the Griffiths Developmental Scales (Griffiths, 1970) and Leiter International Performance Scale (Leiter, 1979).

Reliability between the research raters was preliminarily controlled for the outcome measures (CPRS, CARS, CGI, and C-GAS), independently scoring the first 15 patients with PDD. The intraclass correlation coefficient was computed at baseline and at the end of the 16-week trial, and it was considered satisfactory for all the measures (> 0.075). Two independent investigators assessed all the children, then the clinical data and videotapes were reviewed by the interviewer team for the purpose of consensus.

Patients were considered responders when they satisfied both of the following two conditions: CGI-I score 1 or 2 (very much improved or much improved) and at least a 25% decrease of CPRS total score.

Design and Dosing Regimen

The design was an open-label, nonblind study of risperidone monotherapy. Children were treated with risperidone for 16 weeks. All subjects were started on a dose of 0.25 mg at bedtime. Subsequent titration was 0.25 mg, with increments no more frequently than at weekly intervals, depending on clinical response and occurrence of side effects. A maximum dose of 0.75 mg or 0.04 mg/kg daily was not exceeded. Mean dosage was 0.49 mg (SD 0.1).

Statistical Analyses

Descriptive analyses were used as appropriate. Baseline and 16-week scores on the CARS, CPRS, and C-GAS were compared by using the paired-samples t test ($p < .05$, two-tailed). To minimize type I errors, we applied Bonferroni correction within measures, but not across measures, setting α at .003. Student t test ($p < .05$, two-tailed) was used to compare responders and nonresponders.

RESULTS

Two subjects did not complete the study, as parents requested discontinuation of the treatment because of side effects. After 2 weeks of treatment one child experienced marked sedation and hyporexia. Before discontinuing treatment, the child's parents had reported an improvement in self-injurious behaviors, which worsened again when the medication was interrupted. The parents of the other child decided to discontinue risperidone after 7 days of treatment (dosage 0.25 mg/day) because of episodes of tachycardia after drug intake. The child did not have similar episodes after discontinuing the drug. The child's ECG and symptoms did not change during treatment.

The following data describe the results of the 16-week treatment in the 22 children who completed the trial. CPRS scores (total score and score in 14 selected items) at baseline and at the end of the trial are reported in Table 13.2. CPRS total score at baseline was 52.73 (SD 4.63) and at the study's end was 41.59 (SD 5.88) ($t = 11.9$, $df = 21$, $p < .001$) (21% improvement). The following areas improved significantly after 16 weeks of treatment ($p < .001$): fidgetiness, hyperactivity, withdrawal, negative and uncooperative behaviors, angry affect, nonspontaneous relation to examiner, lability of affects, and rhythmic motions. The areas that improved more than 25% were hyperactivity (34.4%), fidgetiness (30.7%), angry affect (30.7%), lability of affect (28.6%), withdrawal (26.1%), and rhythmic motions (25.7%).

A smaller improvement was observed in the CARS domains, as reported in other studies (Zuddas et al., 2000). Total score and scores in the 15 items of the CARS at baseline and at the study's end are reported in Table 13.3. The CARS total score at baseline was 45.6 (SD 4.2); CARS total score after treatment was 39.2 (SD 4.2) ($t = 11.04$, $df = 21$, $p < .001$) (14% improvement). The CARS scales that significantly improved after 16 weeks of treatment ($p < .001$) were relating to people; emotional response; body use; taste, smell,

TABLE 13.2
Children's Psychiatric Rating Scale: Baseline and 16-Week Scores

	Baseline Score		16-Week Score				
	Mean	SD	Mean	SD	*t* Score	*df*	*p*
Underproductive speech	5.01	1.02	4.68	1.04			
Fidgetiness	4	0.92	2.77	1.02	9.40	21	< .001
Hyperactivity	4.64	0.79	3.04	0.78	12.64	21	< .001
Hypoactivity	0.63	1.14	0.54	1.06			
Abnormal object relationships	4.86	0.89	4.5	0.86			
Withdrawal	4.86	0.56	3.59	0.59	10.84	21	< .001
Negative, uncooperative	4.68	0.78	3.63	0.84	7.51	21	< .001
Angry affect	3.41	1.22	2.36	0.9	8.52	21	< .001
Unspontaneous relation to examiner	5.09	0.68	4.04	0.9	6.79	21	< .001
Lability of affect	4.64	0.85	3.31	0.89	7.93	21	< .001
Low voice	0.59	1.18	0.5	1.01			
Loud voice	2.18	1.1	1.86	1.03			
Other speech deviance	3.41	1	3.23	0.92			
Rhythmic motions (stereotypic)	4.59	0.85	3.41	0.85	8.34	21	< .001
Total score	52.73	4.63	41.59	5.88	11.9	21	< .001

Note: Bonferroni correction, $\alpha = .003$.

TABLE 13.3
Childhood Autism Rating Scale: Baseline and 16-Week Scores

	Baseline Score		16-Week Score				
	Mean	SD	Mean	SD	*t* Score	*df*	*p*
Relating to people	3.25	0.48	2.66	0.45	6.5	21	< .001
Imitation	3.16	0.7	2.95	0.69			
Emotional response	3.30	0.4	2.66	0.32	7.78	21	< .001
Body use	3.25	0.4	2.61	0.43	7.78	21	< .001
Object use	3.23	0.4	3.09	0.43			
Adaptation to change	3	0.51	2.75	0.55			
Visual response	2.70	0.45	2.57	0.49			
Listening response	2.66	0.56	2.43	0.47			
Taste, smell, touch	2.77	0.84	2.36	0.64	4.5	21	< .001
Fear or nervousness	2.75	0.51	2.39	0.58	3.86	21	< .001
Verbal communication	3.45	0.57	3.39	0.57			
Nonverbal communication	3.09	0.52	2.57	0.52	5.46	21	< .001
Activity level	3.20	0.55	2.14	0.38	17.89	21	< .001
Intellectual response	2.36	0.47	2.36	0.47			
General impression	3.41	0.48	2.34	0.58	8.59	21	< .001
Total score	45.6	4.2	39.2	4.2	11.04	21	< .001

Note: Bonferroni correction, $\alpha = .003$.

and touch; fear and nervousness; nonverbal communication; activity level; and general impression. In two items (activity level and general impression) an improvement higher than 25% was found.

The C-GAS and CGI-I scores at baseline and at the end of the study are reported in Table 13.1. The C-GAS score at baseline was 19.59 (SD 4.12) and at the end of the study was 27.86 (SD 5.61) ($t = -10.33$, $df = 21$, $p < .001$) (improvement 29.6%). None of the subjects worsened on the CGI-I during the study, 3 subjects were unchanged, 11 subjects were minimally improved, and 8 subjects (36.4%) were much or very much improved. These 8 subjects showed at least a 25% reduction of CPRS total score and were considered responders. Only these 8 subjects improved more than 15% on the CARS score. Ten subjects (41.6%) improved more than 50% on their C-GAS score.

Being a responder or nonresponder was not affected by age, risperidone dosage, severity at baseline (CARS and CPRS total score and C-GAS), or weight gain (Table 13.4). Severity of mental retardation was not related to drug response.

The most severe and troublesome side effects that induced suspension of treatment in two subjects are described above. Other side effects are described in Table 13.1. Thirteen subjects (54.1%) did not report any side effects. In the other patients the most frequently reported side effect was disturbed appetite: in six children appetite increased and in three children it decreased. Subjects' mean weight increased from 20.18 kg (SD 4.07) to 21.31 kg (SD 4.4). Only

TABLE 13.4
Comparison Between Responders and Nonresponders to Risperidone Treatment

	Responders ($N = 8$)	Nonresponders ($N = 16$)	t Score	*df*	*p*
Age (yr, mo)	4.8 ± 0.9	4.7 ± 0.9	0.257	22	.800
Dosage (mg/day)	0.53 ± 0.09	0.47 ± 0.12	1.245	22	.226
CARS (baseline)	46.9 ± 4.3	44.8 ± 4.12	1.161	22	.258
CPRS (baseline)	53.2 ± 4.6	52.5 ± 4.65	0.349	22	.731
C-GAS (baseline)	19.5 ± 1.8	19.6 ± 5	−0.054	22	.957
Weight gain (kg)	1 ± 0.8	1.1 ± 0.7	−0.315	22	.756

Note: CARS = Childhood Autism Rating Scale; CPRS = Children's Psychiatric Rating Scale; C-GAS = Children's Global Assessment Scale.

three patients experienced a weight gain of more than 10%. The next most common adverse effects were modest agitation and enuresis. One child had suspected transitory dystonic episodes at the neck, reported by the child's parents in the first week, which did not require further medication. There were no changes in blood count or liver enzymes during the period of the study. No changes in ECG were noted in any of the subjects.

DISCUSSION

The aim of this study was to assess the efficacy and safety of risperidone monotherapy in children with PDD. The age range (3.6 to 6.6 years) and mean age (4.6 ± 0.8 years) of these patients is significantly lower than in previous case series. Rating scales including multiple items were used in this study (CPRS and CARS), and both total score and individual item scores were considered. Although multiple statistical analyses, in the search for the treatment effect, required a high statistical price in Bonferroni corrections (Arnold et al., 2000), changes in specific symptoms may determine a significant clinical improvement.

The improvement in the CPRS total score was 21%; the improvement in the CARS total score (14%) was lower. This last finding may be affected by the relatively brief period of time between CARS assessments, as this instrument may be less sensitive to changes in relatively short periods of time (Zuddas et al., 2000). Items that improved more than 25% on the CPRS were related to control of activity level (hyperactivity, fidgetiness, rhythmic motions), stability of affects (lability of affect, angry affect), and, to a lesser degree, the relationship with the external world (withdrawal). Hyperactivity and general impression items from the CARS were reduced by more than 25%.

General measures of functioning, such as the CGI-I and the C-GAS, also improved. According to the CGI-I, eight subjects scored 1 or 2 (very much improved or much improved). These eight subjects showed at least a 25% decrease of CPRS total score and were considered clinical responders. Global functioning, assessed with the C-GAS, improved about 30%, but 10 subjects (41.6%) were improved more than 50%. It was not possible to find predictors of clinical response to treatment.

Side effects (sedation and tachycardia) were responsible for the discontinuation of treatment in two children (8.3%). A transient increase in heart rate was reported in two of the six preschool autistic children described by Casaer et al. (1994), who considered these episodes as transitory and benign. Posey et al. (1999) reported tachycardia and QTc interval prolongation at the ECG, which resolved when risperidone was discontinued. In our study, effects on ECG during treatment were not reported. However, an ECG at baseline and as part of routine monitoring is recommended (Posey et al., 1999).

No severe side effects were noted in the children who completed the trial. Weight gain has been frequently reported during risperidone treatment in children and adolescents (Armenteros et al., 1997). Although increased appetite was found in six subjects, only three (12.5%) had a weight gain greater than 10%. The mean weight increase (1.100 kg) may be explained by normal developmental gain. Low dosage and slow titration may account for this finding. Alternatively, it may indicate a lower sensitivity of younger children to the effect of risperidone on appetite.

A negative effect of risperidone on liver function (Kumra et al., 1997b) was not confirmed in our study. Extrapyramidal symptoms related to rapid dosage escalation of risperidone have been reported (Mandocki, 1995). Only one of our patients had a slight and transitory episode of dystonia at the neck in the first week of treatment, reported by parents, which did not necessitate specific medication. The absence of significant effects on EEG is important, given the higher risk of seizures in PDD patients (Volkmar and Nelson, 1990).

Limitations

The first and most important limitation is the lack of a placebo control group. Even if the placebo effect is not properly studied in PDD patients, blind placebo-controlled studies are recommended because clinical improvement may be due to other factors, such as environmental variables or normal fluctuations of autistic symptoms or examiners' expectations.

Second, we used a low dosage of risperidone, compared with that used in studies of older children. Greater improvement and/or more side effects may have resulted if higher dosages had been used. However, in Anderson and Campbell's study (1989), the optimal dose of haloperidol in 45 autistic children was 0.8 mg/day. Third, reliance on only two ratings on baseline and posttreatment may preclude strong conclusions. Although patients' response to the treatment was monitored for efficacy and untoward effects with at least weekly contacts, standardized measures were conducted only after 4 months for practical reasons (long distance from our hospital) and to highlight more clear changes, particularly with the CARS, which needs longer periods of time between assessments (Zuddas et al., 2000). Inclusion of other objective rating scales for more relevant behaviors, such as the Ritvo-Freeman Real Life Rating Scale (Freeman et al., 1986), may have further improved the outcome measure.

Clinical Implications

Although these considerations may limit our findings with regard to efficacy, this study offers some contributions relative to the existing literature. Sparse data are available about pharmacological treatments in preschool children with PDD. Given the paucity of information about safety of atypical antipsychotics in very young patients, our study can introduce further research on short- and long-term efficacy and safety. Our results are encouraging in this regard. Risperidone was well tolerated and was effective in treating some aspects of autistic symptomatology. This finding is consistent with findings on risperidone efficacy in the short-term treatment of PDD in older children, adolescents, and adults (McDougle et al., 1997, 1998; Zuddas et al., 2000). It may be hypothesized that early treatment can allow for a greater improvement of social function in autistic children and may positively affect the natural history. This may enhance the ability of more severely disturbed children to benefit from educational and psychosocial intervention. Prospective studies with larger samples and controlled design are needed to confirm this hypothesis.

REFERENCES

American Academy of Pediatrics, Committee on Drugs (1996). Unapproved uses of approved drugs: the physician, the package insert, and the Food and Drug Administration: subject review. *Pediatrics* 98:143–145.

American Psychiatric Association (1994). *Diagnostic and Statistical Manual of Mental Disorders, 4th edition (DSM-IV)*. Washington, D.C.: American Psychiatric Association.

Anderson L, Campbell M (1989). The effects of haloperidol on discrimination learning and behavioral symptoms in autistic children. *J Autism Dev Disord* 19:227–239.

Armenteros JL, Whitaker AH, Welikson M, Stedge DJ, Gorman J (1997). Risperidone in adolescents with schizophrenia: an open pilot study. *J Am Acad Child Adolesc Psychiatry* 36:694–700.

Arnold LE, Aman MG, Martin A et al. (2000). Assessment in multisite randomized clinical trials of patients with autistic disorder: the Autism RUPP Network. *J Autism Dev Disord* 30:99–111.

Campbell M, Armenteros JL, Malone RP, Adams PB, Eisenberg ZW, Overall JE (1997). Neuroleptic-related dyskinesias in autistic children: a prospective, longitudinal study. *J Am Acad Child Adolesc Psychiatry* 36:835–843.

Campbell M, Palij M (1985). Behavioral and cognitive measures used in psychopharmacological studies of infantile autism. *Psychopharmacol Bull* 21:1047–1053.

Casaer P, Walleghem D, Vandenbussche I, Huang ML, De Smedt G (1994). Pharmacokinetics and safety of risperidone in autistic children (abstract). *Pediatr Neurol* 11:89.

Chouinard G, Jones B, Remington G et al., (1993). A Canadian multicenter placebo-controlled study of fixed doses of risperidone and haloperidol in the treatment of chronic schizophrenic patients. *J Clin Psychopharmacol* 13:25–40.

Corbett R, Hartman H, Kerman LL et al. (1993). Effects of atypical antipsychotic agents on social behavior in rodents. *Pharmacol Biochem Behav* 45:9–17.

DiLalla DL, Rogers SJ (1994). Domains of the Childhood Autism Rating Scale: relevance for diagnosis and treatment. *J Autism Dev Disord* 24:115–128.

Findling RL, Maxwell K, Wiznicker M (1997), An open clinical trial of risperidone monotherapy in young autistic children. *Psychopharmacol Bull* 33:155 -159.

Fish B (1985). Children's Psychiatric Rating Scale. *Psychopharmacol Bull* 21:753–764.

Fisman S, Steele M (1996). Use of risperidone in pervasive developmental disorders: a case series. *J Child Adolesc Psychopharmacol* 6:177–190.

Freeman BJ, Ritvo ER, Yokota A, Ritvo A (1986). A scale for rating symptoms of patients with the syndrome of autism in real life settings. *J Am Acad Child Psychiatry* 25:130–136.

Garfin DG, McCallon D, Cox R (1988). Validity and reliability of the Childhood Autism Rating Scale with autistic adolescents. *J Autism Dev Disord* 18:367–378.

Griffiths R (1970). *The Abilities of Young Children: A Comprehensive System of Measurement for the First Eight Years of Life*. London: Child Development Research Centre.

Guy W (1976). *ECDEU Assessment Manual for Psychopharmacology, Revised*. Rockville, MD: US Department of Health, Education and Welfare.

Jensen PS (1998). Ethical and pragmatic issues in the use of psychotropic agents in young children. *Can J Psychiatry* 43:585–588.

Jensen PS, Bhatara VS, Vitiello B, Hoagwood K, Feil M, Burke LB (1999). Psychoactive medication prescribing practices for US children: gaps between research and clinical practice. *J Am Acad Child Adolesc Psychiatry* 38:557–565.

Kumra S, Frazier JA, Jacobsen LK et al., (1997a). Childhood-onset schizophrenia: a double-blind clozapine-haloperidol comparison. *Arch Gen Psychiatry* 53:1090–1097.

Kumra S, Herion D, Jacobsen LK, Briguglia C, Grothe D (1997b). Case study: risperidone-induced hepatotoxicity in pediatric patients. *J Am Acad Child Adolesc Psychiatry* 36:701–705.

Leiter RG (1979). *Leiter International Performance Scale*. Chicago: Stoelting.

Locascio J, Malone R, Small A et al. (1991). Factors related to haloperidol response and dyskinesias in autistic children. *Psychopharmacol Bull* 27:119–126.

Mandocki MW (1995). Risperidone treatment of children and adolescents: increased risk of extrapyramidal side effects. *J Child Adolesc Psychopharmacol* 5:69–79.

Masi G, Cosenza A, Mucci M, De Vito G (2001). Risperidone monotherapy in preschool children with autistic disorder. *J Child Neurol* 16:395–400.

McDougle CJ, Holmes JP, Bronson MR et al. (1997). Risperidone treatment of children and adolescents with pervasive developmental disorder: a prospective, open-label study. *J Am Acad Child Adolesc Psychiatry* 36:685–693.

McDougle CJ, Holmes JP, Carlson DC, Pelton GH, Cohen DJ, Price LH (1998). A double-blind, placebo-controlled study of risperidone in adults with autistic disorder and other pervasive developmental disorders. *Arch Gen Psychiatry* 55:633–641.

McDougle CJ, Lawrence S, McCracken JT et al. (2000). Research Units on Pediatric Psychopharmacology (RUPP)-Autism Network: background and rationale for an initial controlled study of risperidone. *Child Adolesc Psychiatr Clin N Am* 9:201–224.

Mesibov GB, Schopler E, Schaffer B, Michal N (1989). Use of the Childhood Autism Rating Scale with adolescents and adults. *J Am Acad Child Adolesc Psychiatry* 28:538–541.

Nicolson R, Awad G, Sloman L (1998). An open trial af risperidone in young autistic children. *J Am Acad Child Adolesc Psychiatry* 37:372–376.

Overall JE, Campbell M (1988). Behavioral assessment of psychopathology in children: infantile autism. *J Clin Psychol* 44:708–716.

Perry R, Campbell M, Adams P et al., (1989). Long-term efficacy of haloperidol in autistic children: continuous versus discontinuous drug administration. *J Am Acad Child Adolesc Psychiatry* 28:87–92.

Perry R, Pataki C, Munoz-Silva DM, Armenteros J, Silva RR (1997). Risperidone in children and adolescents with pervasive developmental disorder: pilot trial and follow-up. *J Child Adolesc Psychopharmacol* 7:167–179.

Posey DJ, Walsh KH, Wilson GA, McDougle CJ (1999). Risperidone in the treatment of two very young children with autism. *J Child Adolesc Psychopharmacol* 9:273–276.

Rogers SJ, Lewis H (1989). An effective day treatment model for young children with pervasive developmental disorders. *J Am Acad Child Adolesc* Psychiatry 28:207–214.

Schopler E, Reichler R, DeViellis R, Daly K (1980). Towards objective classification of childhood autism: Childhood Autism Rating Scale (CARS). *J Autism Dev Disord* 10:91–103.

Shaffer D, Gould M, Brasic J et al. (1983). A children's global assessment scale (CGAS). *Arch Gen Psychiatry* 40:1228–1231.

Vitiello B (1998). Pediatric psychopharmacology and the interaction between drugs and the developing brain. *Can J Psychiatry* 43:582–584.

Vitiello B, Jensen PS (1995). Developmental perspectives in pediatric psychopharmacology. *Psychopharmacol Bull* 31:75–81.

Volkmar FR, Klin A, Marans W, Cohen DJ (1996). The pervasive developmental disorders: diagnosis and assessment. *Child Adolesc Psychiatr Clin N Am* 5:963–978.

Volkmar FR, Nelson DS (1990). Seizure disorders in autism. *J Am Acad Child Adolesc Psychiatry* 29:127–129.

Zuddas A, Di Martino A, Muglia P, Cianchetti C (2000). Long-term risperidone for pervasive developmental disorder: efficacy, tolerability and discontinuation. *J Child Adolesc Psychopharmacol* 10:79–90.

14

Two-Year Prediction of Children's Firesetting in Clinically Referred and Nonreferred Samples

David J. Kolko, Brian T. Day, Jeffrey A. Bridge, and Alan E. Kazdin

This study provides the first prospective evaluation of the course and predictors of children's involvement with fire over a 2-year period in 268 nonpatient and patient children (ages 6 to 13 years). Selected predictor variables obtained at initial (intake) assessment, which included firespecific and general psychosocial measures, were examined in each sample using hierarchical logistic regression. Both samples reported heightened involvement in matchplay and firesetting at follow-up, though the frequency of each behavior was nearly four times higher in patients than in nonpatients. Fifty per cent and 59% of the initial firesetters in the nonpatient and patient samples, respectively, became recidivists. In the nonpatient sample, the child's initial involvement in firesetting and level of covert antisocial behavior were the only psychosocial predictors of follow-up firesetting that added incremental variance beyond demographics. In the patient sample, the child's initial involvement in fire-related acts and level of covert antisocial behavior were the only predictors of follow-up firesetting beyond any initial involvement in matchplay. The findings highlight somewhat different risk factors for subsequent firesetting in nonpatient and patient children, especially prior firesetting and matchplay, respectively, and bear implications for the prevention of firesetting recidivism.

Firesetting among children and adolescents is a prevalent and serious problem (Grolnick, Cole, Laurenitis, & Schwartzman, 1990). In 1995, children playing with fire caused 96,020 fires reported to fire departments, $286.7 billion in property damages, 2,528 civilian injuries, and 304 fatalities (Hall, 1997). Fireplay was the most common cause of death among preschoolers. Several features of firesetting children (e.g., curiosity, aggression) and their parents and families (e.g., poor parental monitoring, family discord) have been identified in empirical studies (see Kolko, 1996). Unfortunately, firesetters who exhibit heightened psychopathology may not receive referrals for mental health treatment (Pierce & Hardesty, 1997).

Little is known about the course of firesetting in children and youth. Retrospective and anecdotal data have documented variable rates of recidivism as reported on admission among outpatient or inpatient children and their parents (52% to 72%; Kolko & Kazdin, 1988b) and following participation in fire department programs (1% to 6%; Kolko, 1988). A few prospective studies have yielded lower though variable recidivism rates in community (3%, Cole et al. 1986), clinic (23%, Stewart & Culver, 1982; 9%, Strachan, 1981), and forensic samples (15%, Repo & Virkkunen, 1997). These rates vary due to differences in patient composition of samples, whether treatment was provided, and whose reports were used to determine recidivism, among other variables. Prospective studies are needed to understand the course of firesetting and to identify variables that predict subsequent involvement with matchplay or firesetting, which may alter the course of firesetting when targeted by intervention (Kolko, Watson, & Faust, 1991).

Theory and research have suggested some of the factors that may contribute to the continuation of firesetting. In patient samples, recidivism has been associated with serious antisocial and noncompliant behavior and parental psychiatric disturbances (Stewart & Culver, 1982) Other variables, such as anger or revenge toward caretakers, sexual conflicts or excitement regarding fire-impulsivity and poor social judgement, and limited empathy toward others have been found related to the *repetition* of firesetting among disturbed youth (Sakheim & Osborn, 1994). An early study of community children found recidivism to be associated with severe family problems and contact with social services (Cole et al., 1986). Our prospective study of 138 children (100 community nonpatients, 38 outpatients) and their parents identified similar types of child, parent, and family problems associated with recidivism (Kolko & Kazdin, 1992). For example, recidivism was related to the child's firesetting interest and involvement (e.g., greater involvement in fire-related activities), child psychopathology or antisocial behavior (e.g., greater hostility), and family dysfunction (e.g., high conflict, limited family affiliation). Despite this progress, however, there are few studies in this area and only one was prospective.

These initial studies suggest that certain fire-specific variables and more general psychosocial functioning measures have predicted the continuation of firesetting. Certainly, additional information is needed regarding recidivism rates for and predictors of follow-up matchplay and firesetting behavior. However, studies must extend this initial work in several important ways. First, predictors of follow-up firesetting have never been examined in separate analyses of children with or without a recent history of treatment. For example, clinically referred and nonreferred children were combined in our prior follow-up study (Kolko & Kazdin, 1992) and virtually all of our other studies, even though these samples have differed in demographics (e.g., gender, age, single-parent, income, SES: see Kolko & Kazdin, 1989a, 1991a,b), prevalence rates for firesetting (Cole, Laurenitis, McAndrews, McKeever, & Schwartzman, 1983; Kolko & Kazdin, 1992), fire-risk factors (Kolko & Kazdin, 1989a,b), and measures of child psychopathology (e.g., antisocial behavior, internalizing symptoms) and parent/family dysfunction (e.g., depression, poor parenting practices) (Kolko & Kazdin, 1991b). Thus, it is plausible that patients and non-patients may have distinct predictors of firesetting behavior. Studies with patients alone show very different findings (Sakheim & Osborne, 1994) from those with just community cases (Showers & Pickrell, 1987). Accordingly, predictors among patients may be most related to heightened individual and family dysfunction, whereas predictors in nonpatients may be most related to the child's firesetting interest and exposure to fire-related models/materials. Separate analyses may bear implications for the unique risks and psychological characteristics associated with increased rates of firesetting and matchplay in each sample. Specifically, identifying predictors in nonpatients may help to understand ways to prevent involvement in firesetting, whereas documenting predictors in patients may highlight variables that need to be considered in treatment with known firesetters.

A second methodological advance is the need to examine concurrently several important variables from multiple domains (see Kolko & Kazdin, 1986). Surprisingly, the child's prior firesetting and matchplay have never been examined as predictors of subsequent fire involvement, even though they are the most likely predictors of follow-up matchplay and firesetting. Thus, we hypothesize that matchplay and firesetting at intake will predict firesetting at follow-up. Beyond these prior behaviors, other important constructs (see Cole, Grolnick, & Schwartzman, 1993; Kolko, 1996; Sakheim & Osborn, 1994) reflect firesetting risk factors (e.g., curiosity, fire exposure, fire competence), the child's level of dysfunction and social competence (e.g., externalizing behavior, social competence), parental practices and distress (e.g., positive parenting, parental distress), and family dysfunction/stress (e.g., positive relationships, family violence). These domains were examined using a set of new, higher-order aggregate constructs based on the combination of several variables. The domains were tested in a hierarchical model that began with general demographic and fire history variables before evaluating the incremental benefit of more complex clinical variables. By developing and testing these variables empirically in both the patient and nonpatient samples, this study incorporates a broad range of potential predictors that reflect the child's fire history and child, parent, and family dysfunction.

Other aspects of the current sample and methodology differ from those reported in prior studies. In this study, we examine predictors of follow-up firesetting, rather than recidivism as reported in our prior study (Kolko & Kazdin, 1992). It is certainly possible that different variables predict each of these two behaviors. The present study also includes an additional sample of 140 cases to the 128 cases reported in our previous study (Kolko & Kazdin, 1992) and employs a 2-year follow-up interval to establish the children's fire history. This is important to document because changes in the status of the children since their 1-year follow-up assessment could significantly alter the findings. To our knowledge, no study of childhood firesetters has included a 2-year follow-up.

The purpose of this study is to identify predictors of firesetting at 2-year follow-up and to determine the incremental variance of psychosocial dysfunction beyond initial fire history in predicting these outcomes. Child, parent, and family predictors of firesetting and matchplay are being examined separately for patients and nonpatients. A secondary purpose of the study is to document for the first time 2-year recidivism rates for firesetting and matchplay in each sample. The study has three primary hypotheses. First, recent (current year) and past (more than a year ago) firesetting and matchplay will serve as predictors of their respective follow-up behaviors (matchplay, firesetting) in both of the samples. This hypothesis will reflect the documentation of considerable continuity in a child's involvement with fire. Second, both fire-specific risk factors and more general clinical characteristics in the aforementioned child, parent, and family domains will add to the prediction of follow-up fire involvement beyond the child's initial fire history. Third, the types of predictors identified in this second step will differ, to some extent, by sample, with fire-risk variables being more salient in nonpatients and clinical variables being more salient in patients.

METHOD

Participants

Firesetting and nonfiresetting children (ages 6 to 13 years) and their parents/guardians were recruited from a longitudinal study of firesetting and antisocial behavior conducted in Pittsburgh. Community cases with no history of treatment within the past 12 months (nonpatients) were recruited through the Pittsburgh Public School System, while outpatients were recruited after their assessment in an outpatient clinic serving children and youth, and their families at Western Psychiatric Institute and Clinic. The community sample was recruited through a mailing of 4,360 postcards randomly selected from a list of names of all children within the designated age range. Parents who contacted the project office were invited to participate in the study and scheduled for an initial assessment· The outpatient sample represented a near-consecutive sample of children within the designated age range whose parents agreed to be contacted for research purposes and who later agreed to participate in the assessment for this study. All eligible firesetters were recruited, whereas only one of every two eligible nonfiresetters was recruited in random order for this study.

At initial assessment, 462 nonpatients and outpatients and their caregivers participated in assessment interviews. To assure adequate numbers of firesetters and given limited resources to conduct follow-up with all cases, efforts were made to recruit 75% of this sample at follow-up ($N = 347$). Of these 347 cases, 79 families could not be located or declined to participate, which left a total of 268 (78%) children who participated in the follow-up assessment. Slightly less than half of these cases were included in our 1-year follow-up report (Kolko & Kazdin, 1992).

The study sample consisted of 162 (60%) community nonpatients and 106 (40%) outpatients who were primarily male (62%) and young (mean age = 9.5, $SD = 1.9$). Fifty-one percent of the children were African American; 49% were Caucasian. Forty percent of the children lived with both of their biological parents. Most of the families were small in size (mean = 4.1 persons; SD = 1.4) and fell in the lower two of five socioeconomic classes (58%; Hollingshead & Redlich, 1958). Fifty-six percent of the families received public assistance. Background characteristics of the nonpatient and patient samples are shown in Table 14.1. Briefly, the two samples were similar in age, gender, race, family size, and contact with Children and Youth Services. The patient sample had a lower proportion of families containing both biological parents, a higher proportion of families with lower SES, and a greater history of any treatment by follow-up.

Procedures and Sample Comparisons

Parents and children were interviewed separately by research assistants at initial and 2-year follow-up assessments. Both informants provided written informed consent using forms approved by the University's Institutional Review Board. Firesetting-related measures were administered first, followed by the remaining measures. Audiotapes of randomly selected interviews were evaluated by a supervisor and the project director to monitor assessment integrity. Families received $35 for their participation at initial assessment and $40 at follow-up. During the follow-up period, newsletters were sent 6 months and 1 week prior to the follow-up interval, and periodic phone calls made to facilitate retention in the project. Five separate attempts were made to contact each family. Families that could not be contacted were sent letters describing the follow-up assessment.

TABLE 14.1
Demographic Characteristics of the Nonpatient and Patient Samples

	Nonpatients		Patients		
Characteristics	*N*	%	*N*	%	Group comparisons t/χ^2
Age (Mean, SD)	9.37	2.02	9.80	2.14	t (244) = 0.87, n.s.
Gender–Male	93	58.10	51	59.30	χ^2 (1, N = 246) = 0.03, n.s.
Race–African American	87	54.40	43	50.00	t (246) = 1.07, n.s.
Family size (Mean, SD)	3.96	1.26	3.81	1.32	t (241) = 0.88, n.s.
Custody					
Both parents	74	46.80	25	29.10	χ^2 (1, N = 244) = 7.29**
Biological mother	36	44.30	50	58.10	
Other	14	8.90	11	22.80	
Family SES class					
I–II	82	53.90	58	69.80	χ^2 (1, N = 235) = 5.66*
III–IV	70	46.10	25	30.20	
CYS contact	22	13.80	19	22.10	χ^2 (1, N = 246) = 2.8 1, n.s.
Any treatment by follow-up	13	9.56	62	68.89	χ^2 (1, N = 226) = 85.98***

SES = Socioeconomic status; CYS = Children and Youth Services. *N*s vary due to missing data.
*$p < .05$; **$p < .01$; ***$p < .001$.

To determine any differences in the characteristics of the follow-up sample due to attrition, children who were included in this follow-up study were compared to those from the larger sample who participated only in the initial assessment (Time 1) on several demographic and clinical variables. There were no sample differences in age, gender, racial/ethnic background, or SES class. The sample that was followed was characterized by a higher proportion of nonpatient (vs. patient) cases due to the exclusion of inpatients at follow-up (70% vs. 30%), χ^2 (2, N = 462) = 26.48, $p < .001$, and of two-parent (vs. single-parent) families (52% vs. 48%), χ^2 (2, N = 457) = 10.23, $p < .001$. In terms of clinical characteristics, parent reports indicated that the two samples were comparable in the proportion of children who set fires or who played with matches, and in overall levels of family stress, parental psychological distress, and child externalizing and internalizing behavior. Child reports also revealed comparability in the proportion of children who set fires or who played with matches, and in levels of child externalizing and internalizing behavior.

Comparisons of the two subsamples of firesetters (i.e., followed vs. nonfollowed firesetters) likewise showed that the two subsamples were comparable on all of the same 12 demographic and clinical background variables, with the one exception that there was a higher proportion of nonpatients (vs. outpatients) in the followed sample, χ^2 (2, N = 190) = 14.21, $p < .001$. These findings suggest that the followed sample was generally representative of the full sample of children included in the study at initial assessment.

Documentation of Firesetting History

Firesetting History Screen (FHS). The child's firesetting status was assessed based on child and parent responses to the Firesetting History Screen (FHS) (see Kolko & Kazdin, 1988a,b). These questions evaluated the children's interest in fire, frequency of matchplay and firesetting, and, if applicable, the severity of firesetting. This was the only instrument used to evaluate the frequency of matchplay and firesetting behavior, and thus it did not overlap with any of the other measures.

At initial assessment, these questions were administered to reflect the child's firesetting history in two separate time periods: the current or recent year (i.e., in the last 12 months) and the past (i.e., more than 12 months ago). At 2-year follow-up, these questions were readministered to assess the child's firesetting history since the initial assessment. Thus, three time periods were sampled on two separate occasions.

Parent–child agreement as to the presence/absence of firesetting or matchplay was calculated using Cohen's kappa. The overall kappas for firesetting and matchplay were .51 and .46 for the current year, and .61 and .33 for prior years (past period), respectively. The kappas for firesetting were generally similar to that obtained in our earlier prospective study (.41) (Kolko & Kazdin, 1992) in which moderate overall agreement (.51) was found as to the child's overall classification into firesetter or nonfiresetter groups. There is also moderate-to-high agreement over a 2-week test-retest interval for firesetting and matchplay based on the current (.86, .66) and past periods (.63, 43). Consistent with the agreement data reported for other covert behaviors (see Loeber, Farrington, Stouthamer-Loeber, & Van Kammen, 1998), these data suggest the benefit of obtaining reports from both sources to document a child's involvement in firesetting or matchplay.

Patterns of firesetting across time. Children were classified as firesetters if they were involved in burning some type of property or setting a fire as acknowledged by themselves *or* their parents, a definition that has been used in prior studies (Kolko Kazdin, 1988b, 1989a,b; Kolko, Kazdin, & Meyer, 1985). This definition included any act in which an object was burned or set on fire, such as small objects, personal property, furniture, or a residence or structure. Children were classified as nonfiresetters if *both* sources agreed about the absence of firesetting. Children were classified as nonfiresetters if their fireplay was limited to matchplay only (e.g., playing with candles, striking matches). Across both periods, children were classified into one of four mutually exclusive firesetting history patterns based on both informants' reports (see Kolko & Kazdin, 1992); these subgroups parallel those used to classify cases based on other antisocial behaviors (Loeber et al., 1989). Among children with no initial history of firesetting, those who did vs. did not exhibit firesetting by follow-up were described as Late-starters and Controls, respectively. Among children with an initial history of firesetting, those who did vs. did not exhibit firesetting by follow-up were described as Recidivists and Desistors, respectively.

Data Reduction: Measures and Constructs

At initial assessment, several measures were administered evaluating variables in primary domains that have been related empirically to firesetting behavior (see Cole et al., 1986, 1993; Gaynor & Hatcher, 1987; Kolko & Kazdin, 1989a; Kolko et al., 1991). Given the large number of assessment instruments, an effort was made to reduce the number of individual variables into constructs that reflected key aspects of child, parent, and family domains of functioning, as has been done effectively in prior work on child antisocial behavior (e.g., Vuchinich, Bank, & Patterson, 1992). As summarized by Kolko (1996), these variables fall into two general categories. The first reflects fire involvement, interest, and awareness and the various conditions that support the use of fire (e.g., firesetting history, curiosity, skill) and the second reflects the child's overall behavioral dysfunction. The latter category includes conditions that support the use of aggression and other aspects of the child's dysfunction (e.g., covert behavior, poor social skills), parental practices/dysfunction (e.g., distress, monitoring and discipline practices), and family dysfunction/stress (e.g., positive relationships, violence).

The constructs were developed to reflect the aforementioned variables found in our prior work (Kolko, 1989; Kolko & Kazdin, 1992), the psychological and family characteristics of firesetting youth (Cole et al., 1986, 1993; Showers & Pickrell, 1987), and prior conceptualizations of firesetting or descriptive studies of firesetters (e.g., Sakheim & Osborne, 1994; Stewart & Culver, 1982), with some constructs (e.g., parent practices) figuring prominently in general formulations of child conduct problems (see Loeber et al., 1998).[1] In all, three multivariable constructs and eight 2-item constructs were so identified. Five individual variables were included that evaluated specific characteristics (e.g., parental distress, social service involvement) that were reflected by a single factor score or item rating.

[1]A principal components factor analysis with varimax rotation was conducted to document the underlying dimensions associated with this array of variables. However, the results yielded numerous factors with a small number of variables that were difficult to interpret.

After all variables were converted to *z*-scores, Cronbach's alphas (multiple-variable constructs) or Pearson correlations (two-item constructs) were computed for each subsample. Overall, 16 variables showed acceptable internal consistency ($\alpha > .60$ in at least one sample) and had minimal missing data. Inspection of the construct intercorrelations in each sample revealed only two intercorrelations above .60. In the nonpatient sample, only five intercorrelations were above .50, most were small (.15 to .20), and the range was from –.47 to .63. The highest correlation was between complaints about fire/general behavior and covert antisocial behavior/traits. In the patient sample, only four intercorrelations were above .50, the majority were small (.10 to .15), and the range was from –.57 to .58. The highest correlation was between positive family relationships and child acceptance. One of the constructs (fire competence; see next section) had a low number of cases. Descriptions of the content of these variables are listed in the following sections, with alphas or correlations for the two respective subsamples (nonpatients, patients) noted in parentheses.

Fire-specific risk. Four constructs related to fire-specific risk factors were evaluated. First, curiosity about fire was composed of the curiosity subscales of the parent-reported Firesetting Risk Interview (FRI) (Kolko & Kazdin, 1989a) and the child-reported Children's Firesetting Interview (CFI) (Kolko & Kazdin, 1989b; $r(154.) = .16, p < .05$; $r(87) = .24, p < .03$). Curiosity about fire has been found to differentiate firesetters from nonfiresetters. Second, exposure to fire-related models/materials was composed of the FRI peer/family exposure and the CFI exposure to models/materials subscales, $r(109) = .40$; $p < .001$; $r(54) = .38, p < .004$. Exposure is a correlate of the onset of firesetting and may predict its continuation. Third, involvement with fire-related activities was composed of the FRI and CFI involvement in fire-related acts subscales, $r(153) = .31, p < .001$; $r(91) = .23, p < .02$. Because the distribution of this variable was highly skewed in the patient sample only, scores on this subscale were dichotomized (none vs. any). Fourth, the FRI complaints about fire/general behavior subscale (αs = .74, .81) was included to examine community reports of children's fire contact, as firesetters may be in contact with incendiary materials over time.

Child dysfunction/social competence. Four constructs were evaluated in this child-related domain. Child externalizing behavior consisted of the combination of the T-scores for the Child Behavior Checklist (CBCL) (Achenbach & Edelbrock, 1983) and Youth Self-Report (YSR) (Achenbach & Edelbrock, 1989) externalizing behavior scales, $r(162) = .42, p < .001$: $r(93) = .22, p < .04$. Behavioral dysfunction has generally characterized firesetters across studies. Second, child hostility reflected the child and parent hostility factors of the Children's Hostility Inventory (CHI) (Kazdin, Rodgers, Colbus, & Siegel,

1987): $r(154)$ .24, $p < .02$; $r(80) = .12$, $p < .29$. Hostility is an important motive (Kolko & Kazdin, 1991c) and may help to understand the emergence of firesetting. Third, covert antisocial behavior and antisocial traits was composed of scores from the Covert Problem Behavior Scale (CPBS) (Loeber, Stouthamer-Loeber, Van Kammen & Farrington, 1989; αs = .86, .86). Items in each factor (e.g., lying, property destruction, careless, secretive) are rated along 3-point frequency scales (e.g., 0 = not true, 2 = very or often true) and relate to follow-up involvement in delinquent activities and police contacts. Covert behavior may be related to firesetting beyond the child's involvement in overt antisocial or aggressive acts, especially as it may relate to the commission of other property offenses. Fourth, social competence consisted of the CBCL social competence factor that consisted of three subscale scores (i.e., skill, school, social skill), since children did not complete the corresponding section in the YSR. Heightened social skills deficits have been documented among firesetters (Kolko & Kazdin, 1991a).

Parental practices/dysfunction. Five constructs were evaluated in this domain. Positive parenting practices was composed on the monitoring and discipline subscales from the Child Rearing Interview (CR1) (Stouthamer-Loeber & Loeber, 1985) minus the scores from the tax control (e.g., nonenforcement factor from the Parenting Behavior Inventory [PBI] (Schaefar, 1965; overall αs = .56, .59). The PBI evaluates child-rearing practices and child–parent interactions in the home. Prior studies of similar constructs have-documented their relationship to child antisocial behavior (e.g., Loeber et al. 1998) and other formulations suggest their association with the continuation of firesetting (Kolko, 1989). Second, psychological control consists of reports on the psychological control subscales (e.g., instilling anxiety) of the Child's Report of Parental Behavior Inventory (CRPBI) and the PBI, $r(161) = .24$, $p < .003$; $r(95) = .24$, $p < .02$. Because parents of firesetters have been characterized by the use of harsh punishment, it was of interest to determine if they would be less likely to use psychological control methods.

Third, mild (appropriate) punishment consisted of the sum of the frequency and efficacy of mild punishment subscales of the FRI (Kolko & Kazdin, 1989a); $r(153) = .67$, $p < .001$; $r(92) = .63$, $p < .001$. Parents of firesetters have been noted to report less use of routine forms of punishment (Kolko & Kazdin, 1991a; Showers & Pickrell, 1987). Fourth, harsh punishment consisted of parent reports on the FRI efficacy of harsh punishment subscale (αs = .60, .52). Excessive physical or harsh punishment has been reported for parents of firesetters (Kolko & Kazdin, 1991a; Showers & Pickrell, 1987). Finally, parental psychological distress reflected the overall score on the Hopkins Symptom Checklist (SCL-90), which provides a measure of general psychological distress (Derogatis, Lipman, & Covi, 1973). Parents of firesetters have reported high levels of personal distress (Kolko & Kazdin, 1991b).

Family functioning/stress. There were three constructs in this domain.[2] Family sociability was composed of the sociability and affiliation subscales of the Home Environment Questionnaire (HEQ) (Laing & Sines, 1982); $r(61) = .24, p < .003$; $r(81) = .12, p < .27$. Limited family involvement in social activities may be a contributor to the firesetting child's own social effectiveness difficulties. Second, positive relationships included scores from the cohesion, conflict (reversed), and expressiveness subscales of the Family Environment Scale (FES) (Moos, Insel, & Humphrey, 1974; overall αs = .65, .67). Heightened family discord and lowered cohesion have been reported as correlates of both the onset and recurrence of firesetting (Kolko & Kazdin, 1991a, 1992). Finally, involvement with the Allegheny County Children and Youth Service was documented and coded by time period for five specific reasons (e.g., child physical or sexual abuse, neglect, extent of family child protective services involvement, child dependency). Prior research suggests that similar social service contact relates to the emergence or repetition of firesetting (Cole et al., 1983, 1986; Showers & Pickrell, 1987; Wooden & Berkey, 1984).

RESULTS

Demographic Backgrounds of Cases with vs. Those without Any Subsequent Firesetting

Cases who did vs. those who did not report any follow-up involvement with fire (firesetting, matchplay) within each sample were compared for initial differences on baseline demographics. In the nonpatient sample, the firesetters and nonfiresetters who participated at follow-up were comparable in child age, family constellation, size, and SES, and history of social service involvement. However, a higher proportion of the firesetters (vs. nonfiresetters) who were followed in the nonpatient sample were males (77% vs. 52%), $\chi^2(1, N = 160) = 7.49, p < .01$, were African American (74% vs. 51%); $\chi^2(1, N = 160) = 6.43, p < .01$, and had received any treatment during the follow-up interval (31% vs. 14%); $\chi^2(1, N = 151) = 5.20, p < .02$. There were no differences between those with vs. those without any follow-up firesetting in the patient sample on any of these variables. Further, there were no significant group differences as a function of follow-up matchplay status in either of these samples.

[2]A fourth variable (family violence) was deemed important to include given that physical mistreatment has been described in the histories of firesetting children (Kolko, 1996), but the Ns for this factor were too low for inclusion in these analyses. Family violence consisted of parent reports for the verbal aggression and physical violence subscales of the Conflict Tactics Scales (CTS) (Straus, 1990; αs = .81, .78). Scores on each subscale were summed for the two primary dyadic patterns (e.g., child-to-mother, mother-to-child).

History of Firesetting and Matchplay in Each Sample

Rates at each time period. Table 14.2 shows the firesetting histories of the nonpatient and patient samples based on an aggregate of child and parent reports. Nearly one third of the nonpatient sample and half of the patients had set at least one fire within the current year and many of the children in both samples had also played with matches within the current year. There was also considerable involvement in matchplay and firesetting reported retrospectively for the past period. It can be seen that most of the cases in both samples reported an incident of firesetting by follow-up, especially in the nonpatient sample, where nearly three quarters of the cases had engaged in matchplay and firesetting behavior. On average, nonpatients had engaged in approximately one additional incident of matchplay and firesetting at follow-up. Patients had engaged in an average of about four incidents of matchplay and three incidents of firesetting. In both samples, there was considerable variability in the number of incidents reported.[3] As displayed in Table 14.2, a comparison of the fire histories of the two samples indicated that a higher proportion of patients evidenced a past history interest and firesetting; current fire interest, matchplay, and firesetting; and follow-up interest, matchplay, and firesetting. The frequency of matchplay incidents was also higher in patients than nonpatients.

Case classification at each time period. Information from this assessment was used to classify cases into one of three categories in order to determine how many children engaged in firesetting or matchplay only. Based on the aggregated reports for the current year, there were 50 firesetters (31.3%), 15 matchplayers only (9.4%), and 95 nonfiresetters (59.4%) in the nonpatient sample; similar percentages of firesetters (24.4%, or 39), matchplayers only (20.0%, or 32), and nonfiresetters (55.6%, or 89) were found for the follow-up period. In the patient sample, there were 44 firesetters (51.2%), 10 matchplayers only (11.6%), and 32 nonfiresetters (37.2%); likewise, similar percentages of firesetters (43.3%, or 37), matchplayers only (12.8%, or 11), and nonfiresetters (44.2% or 38) were found for the follow-up period.

Cases also were classified into different subgroups based on their firesetting history at both assessments. The number of nonpatient cases in each mutually exclusive group was as follows: (1) Nonfiresetters ($N = 96$; fire at neither time); (2) Late-starters ($N = 14$; fire at follow-up only); (3) Desistors ($N = 25$; fire at initial assessment only); and (4) Recidivists ($N = 25$; fire at both times). The number of patient cases in each of the same mutually exclusive groups was as follows: (1) Nonfiresetters ($N = 31$); (2) Late-starters ($N = 11$); (3) Desistors ($N = 18$); and (4) Recidivists ($N = 26$). Thus, 13% and

[3]One outlier in each sample was removed because the reported incident frequencies of firesetting were substantial in the nonpatient (325) and patient samples (352).

TABLE 14.2
Firesetting Histories of the Nonpatient and Patients Samples (*Aggregated Reports*)

Behavior	Nonpatients %	Nonpatients *N*	Patients %	Patients *N*	Group comparisons t/χ^2
Past period					
Interest in fire	30.3	47	48.8	39	$\chi^2(1, N = 235) = 7.72^{**}$
Matchplay	42.8	65	52.0	39	$\chi^2(1, N = 227) = 1.72$, n.s.
Firesetting	26.9	43	45.8	38	$\chi^2(1, N = 243) = 8.79^{**}$
Current (initial) year					
Interest in fire	25.6	40	42.3	33	$\chi^2(1, N = 234) = 6.73^{**}$
Matchplay	42.8	65	63.3	50	$\chi^2(1, N = 231) = 8.76^{**}$
Firesetting	31.3	50	51.2	44	$\chi^2(1, N = 246) = 9.39^{**}$
2-year follow-up					
Interest in fire	23.8	38	40.0	34	$\chi^2(1, N = 245) = 7.06^{**}$
Matchplay	35.6	57	50.6	43	$\chi^2(1, N = 245) = 5.15^{*}$
No. of incidents (Mean, SD)	1.1	2.8	4.2	11.2	$t(86.4) = -2.54^{**}$
Firesetting	24.4	39	43.5	37	$\chi^2(1, N = 245) = 9.52^{**}$
No. of incidents (Mean, SD)	0.9	4.3	3.1	13.7	$t(241) = -1.40$, n.s.

Percentages reflect the number of cases reporting each individual behavior within each time period.
$^*p < .05$; $^{**}p < .01$.

26% of these two respective samples were late-starters, and 50% and 59% of these samples were recidivists.

Inter-relationships among Fire-status Measures

We examined the degree of overlap among the three primary fire history measures, namely, current firesetting, current matchplay, and past firesetting. Chi-square tests examined the relationship between each pair of variables separately for patients and nonpatients. In the patient sample, the only significant inter-relationship was found for current or recent year firesetting and matchplay, $\chi^2(1, N = 79) = 40.81$, $p < .0001$. In the nonpatient sample, significant inter-relationships (all *p*s < .0001) were found between past and current year firesetting, $\chi^2(1, N = 157) = 28.46$, current year firesetting and matchplay, $\chi^2(1, N = 154) = 56.75$, and past firesetting and current year matchplay, $\chi^2(1, N = 79) = 35.29$.

Prediction of Any Firesetting at Follow-up

Full sample. We sought to first identify which of the initial predictor variables in each domain were significantly associated with follow-up firesetting in an effort to reduce the number of predictors to be tested in a final predictive model. In each sample, logistic regression analyses were computed for each of the four primary assessment domains, as well as two other general background domains (demographics, fires history). Variables were retained for subsequent model testing if they survived both forward ($p < .10$) and backward ($p < .05$) selection criteria. A total of seven and six variables were retained in the nonpatient and patient samples, respectively.

Once these variables were identified, they were entered into a series of hierarchical regression analyses designed to evaluate general background variables before testing more complex psychosocial or clinical variables in each sample separately (Hosmer & Lemeshow, 1989). Accordingly, the survivors in each domain were entered in the following order: demographics, fire history, firespecific risk, child dysfunction/social competence, parental practices/functioning, and family functioning/stress. Demographic variables were entered first in the patient sample only because there were demographic differences between follow-up firesetters and nonfiresetters, and because these are among the most commonly available background characteristics of children.

Each hierarchical logistic regression was conducted using only those cases who had all of the data across the full range of covariates in order to avoid having any attrition of cases across steps in the analysis. We also conducted separate logistic regression models with the full number of cases that had any of these data for comparison purposes. In both instances, the results of the two analyses were similar; to maximize interpretation of the Likelihood Ratio Statistic (LRS) in these analyses, we chose to report in the table the results for those cases who had all of the data.

Table 14.3 shows the results of these hierarchical regression analyses for the nonpatient sample, including the odds ratios (ORs) for each predictor and the LRS for each individual block (domain). The findings revealed that two demographic variables (male gender, African American ethnicity) contributed to the prediction of follow-up firesetting and generally maintained their high ORs as other variables were added to this prediction. The child's history of firesetting in the current year was the next predictor of follow-up firesetting. Current firesetting had a large OR (6.13) after adjusting for the demographic variables and continued to have a large OR as other variables were entered in subsequent analyses.

One variable from the fire-risk domain, namely the extent to which complaints were received about the child's fire behavior, was associated with follow-up firesetting in the univariate analyses, but the relative contribution of

TABLE 14.3
Adjusted Odds Ratios (OR) and 95% Confidence Intervals (CI) from Hierarchical Logistic Regression Analysis Predicting Any Firesetting at 2-year Follow-up: Nonpatients

	Demographic		Fire history		Fire risk		Child		Parent		Family	
Variables	OR	CI	OR	CI	OR	CI	OR	CI	OR	CI	OR	CI
Demographic												
Race–African-Amer.	3.66	1.55–9.48	3.78	1.51–10.44	3.87	1.53–10.87	3.38	1.49–10.92	3.18	1.18–9.37	3.16	1.16–9.43
Gender–Male	3.54	1.50–9.17	2.46	0.97–6.70	2.40	0.94–6.59	2.76	1.04–7.97	2.58	0.96–7.47	2.65	0.98–7.78
LRS (*df*) for block	17.00 (2)	0.0002										
Fire history												
Current firesetting			6.13	2.55–15.40	5.60	2.11–15.49	4.65	1.69–13.19	4.87	1.76–13 94	5.00	1.80–14.42
LRS (*df*) for block			16.60 (1)	0.0001								
Fire-specific risk												
Complaints about child behavior					1.42	0.27–7.32	0.45	0.05–3.41	0.32	0.03–2.53	0.26	0.03–2.15
LRS (*df*) for block					0.17 (1)	0.68						
Child dysfunction/competence												
Covert antisocial acts							1.08	1.00–1.17	1.08	1.00–1.17	1.06	0.98–1.16
LRS (*df*) for block							3.70 (1)	0.06				
Parental practices/functioning												
Psychological control									1.03	0.99–1.08	1.03	0.99–1.08
LRS (*df*) for block									1.96 (1)	0.18		
Family functioning/stress											0.95	0.87–1.04
Positive family relats.											1.36 (1)	0.25
LRS (*df*) for block												
Full model H-L GOF	7.70 (2)	$p < .26$	3.68 (6)	$p < .60$	7.96 (7)	$p < .34$	2.02 (8)	$p < .98$	8.28 (8)	$p < .41$	11.93 (8)	$p < .15$

N select for all steps was 147; H-L GOF = Hosmer-Lemeshow Goodness-of-Fit test.

this variable was minimal when other covariates were included in the model. The one variable retained from the child dysfunction/social competence domain (covert antisocial behavior) was found to be a modest predictor of recidivism. One variable in the parental practices/functioning domain, namely parental use of psychological control techniques, contributed very little to the prediction of follow-up firesetting after adjusting for other covariates. Similarly, the one variable that was evaluated from the final family dysfunction domain (positive family relationships) contributed minimally to the prediction of follow-up firesetting. The Hosmer-Lemeshow Goodness-of-Fit (GOF) test for each domain indicated adequate fit for the models. The overall correct classification rate for these seven predictor variables was 80.3%. Inspection of the ability of these variables to classify all of the nonpatient cases found that there was greater accuracy in classifying nonfiresetters (102/112, or 91.1%) than firesetters (16/35, or 45.7%).

The hierarchical regressions computed for the patient sample are shown in Table 14.4. The analyses revealed that the child's current history of matchplay was a substantial initial predictor of follow-up firesetting. Interestingly, however, the magnitude of the OR for this variable showed a substantial decline as other variables were added to the prediction. Specifically, when covert antisocial acts were added to the model, this variable showed the greatest decline and was no longer a significant contributor. Two fire-specific risk variables—whether the child had any involvement in fire-related acts and the level of the child's fire safety competency—were then added to the model. Whereas fire competency did not contribute to the prediction of follow-up firesetting, it bears noting that the OR for the child's involvement in fire-related acts increased modestly as other variables were added to the prediction equation.

One variable from the child dysfunction/social competence domain, reflecting the child's level of involvement in covert antisocial behavior, was significantly associated with follow-up firesetting. This association remained unchanged by the addition of other covariates in subsequent models. Although one variable each in the parental practices/dysfunction and family functioning/stress domains was examined in the hierarchical model, neither of these variables was a significant contributor to the prediction of follow-up firesetting. The Hosmer-Lemeshow GOF test for each domain indicated adequate fit for the models. The overall correct classification rate for these six predictor variables was 72.9%, with greater accuracy found in classifying nonfiresetters (28/35, or 80.0%) than firesetters (15/24, or 62.5%).

Subsample replication. In order to assess the stability of the regression analyses (Tabachnick & Fidell, 1989), separate hierarchical logistic regression models were calculated on a random 50% of the sample using the RANUNI function in SAS (*SAS Programming,* 1992). Because the patient sample size

TABLE 14.4

Adjusted ORs and 95% CIs from Hierarchical Logistic Regression Analysis Predicting Any Firesetting at 2-year Follow-up: Patients

	Fire history		Fire risk		Child		Patient		Family	
Variables	OR	CI	OR	CI	OR	CI	OR	CI	OR	CI
Fire history										
Current matchplay	8.31	2.33–39.92	6.24	1.65–0.92	4.07	0.98–21.17	4.10	0.96–21.97	4.02	0.91–22.18
LRS *(df) for* block	11.59 (1)	0.0007								
Fire-specific risk										
Any involvement in fire acts			3.26	0.85–14.03	4.56	1.07–23.62	4.56	1.07–23.61	4.68	1.08–24.83
Fire competency			0.92	0.81–1.03	0.91	0.79–1.02	0.90	0.79–1.02	0.92	0.80–1.04
LRS *(df)* for block			4.32 (2)	0.17						
Child dysfunction/competence										
Covert antisocial acts					1.10	1.01–1.21	1.10	1.01–1.21	1.09	1.01–1.21
LRS *(df)* for block					4.71 (1)	0.03				
Parental practices/functioning										
Psychological control							1.00	0.94–1.06	0.99	0.93–1.06
LRS *(df) for* block							0.02 (1)	0.96		
Family functioning/stress										
Positive family relations									0.93	0.81–1.04
LRS *(df)* for block										
Full model									1.75 (1)	0.19
H-L GOF			5.01 (7)	$p < .66$	4.09 (8)	$p < .85$	4.09 (8)	$p < .85$	2.60 (8)	$p < 0.96$

N select for all steps was 59; H-L GOF = Hosmer-Lemeshow Goodness-of-Fit test.

was small ($N = 59$) relative to the number of predictors ($k = 6$) (Kleinbaum et al., 1988), these cross-validation analyses were restricted to the nonpatient sample. Odds ratios, 95% confidence intervals, and classification rates were compared. A high degree of consistency was found using this classification scheme. For example, for the cross-validation cases there was an 83% correct classification rate, comparable to the 78% correct classification rate found in the full sample. Moreover, for both the full and split samples, there was greater accuracy in classifying nonfiresetters (86 % for each sample) than firesetters (53 for full, 88% and 64% for split samples).

DISCUSSION

The course and prediction of children's involvement with fire were documented among 268 patient and nonpatient children and their parents over a 2-year period. Both informants completed structured fire history interviews that documented the presence and frequency of firesetting and matchplay, and self-reports evaluating fire-related risk factors and child, parent, and family dysfunction based on prior research (e.g., Kolko & Kazdin, 1989a,b; 1991a,b). A novelty of this study is that predictors of follow-up firesetting were reported separately for each sample, and they included both matchplay and firesetting, among other psychosocial functioning measures.

Aggregate data from the two informants revealed that a high percentage of children had engaged in firesetting and matchplay at follow-up. Specifically, almost half of the patients had exhibited both behaviors, whereas a third and a quarter of the nonpatient sample had exhibited firesetting and matchplay, respectively. On average, nonpatients reported one follow-up incident of firesetting and matchplay; patients reported three and four of these incidents, respectively. The high percentage of nonpatients for whom any matchplay was reported is, in part, due to having oversampled for firesetters on a 2:1 basis at the outset of the study and the fact that only the patient sample, by definition, had received psychiatric services likely to impact the severity of their behavior problems. Still, this prospective study found that a majority of the two samples were involved in both firerelated behaviors upon follow-up in the community.

In terms of the course of firesetting in the two samples, 13% and 26% of the nonpatient and patient nonfiresetters at initial assessment became late-starters by 2-year follow-up, respectively, whereas 50% and 59% of the firesetters in these two respective samples became recidivists. These recidivism rates, which may be the first figures based on a 2-year follow-up interval, are somewhat higher than those described in prospective studies (Cole et al., 1986; Stewart & Culver, 1982; Strachan, 1981), retrospective program evaluations (Kolko, 1988), or our 1-year follow-up study (Kolko & Kazdin, 1992), due, in part, to the use of a longer interval and variations in sample characteristics, definitions, and measures. Further, only this study conducted structured, prospective fire history interviews, and included both children and their parents. One implication of these findings is that *approximately half* of a sample of firesetters will set at least one additional fire and that a modest percentage of children will become firesetters for the first time within a 2-year period, regardless of their patient status.

The predictive relationship between selected constructs in several domains obtained at intake and the children's involvement in firesetting 2 years later was examined in each sample. In the nonpatient sample, the hierarchical model began with an examination of two child demographics, namely, male gender and African American background. Beyond these two background variables, involvement in firesetting at initial assessment was a substantial predictor of follow-up firesetting. This variable continued to serve as a significant contributor even when subsequent variables were added to the model. In contrast, other variables that entered the model were weak predictors of later firesetting, such as complaints about the child's fire behavior, parental use of psychological control, and positive family relationships. The only additional contributor was the level of the child's involvement in covert antisocial behavior. This combination of seven variables predicted nonfiresetters with high accuracy, but was relatively inaccurate in predicting firesetters. Prior studies in this area have not evaluated the predictive significance of ethnicity, so the generality of this variable and its interpretation are difficult to determine. Thus, for children without a recent history of clinical referral, two demographic variables and fire setting reported at initial assessment, rather than parent or family dysfunction, contributed to the prediction of subsequent firesetting behavior.

In the patient sample, the hierarchical model that was tested did not include any initial demographic characteristics. Involvement in matchplay at initial assessment was a substantial contributor to the prediction of follow-up firesetting behavior and this association was maintained even after other variables were entered into the model. Of the two fire-risk variables that were next examined, only the variable that reflected any involvement in fire-related acts was found to be a contributor of later firesetting. The child's level of covert antisocial behavior contributed incremental variance to the prediction. In contrast, neither of the parent nor the family variables that were examined contributed to the model. Although social service contact was a significant predictor in another study (Cole et al., 1986), it did not meet the criteria for evaluation as a predictor of follow-up firesetting in this study. That follow-up firesetting was predicted by child-related variables, but not heightened parent or family problems, conveys further support for the importance of evaluating the child's firesetting history and behavioral repertoire among clinic cases.

Relative to the percentages found for nonpatients, classification of patients tended to be somewhat higher for firesetters but lower for nonfiresetters.

These individual fire history models highlight both similarities and differences in the predictors of follow-up firesetting in the nonpatient and patient samples. Demographics were related to later firesetting in nonpatients only; likewise, follow-up firesetting was predicted by a history of firesetting at initial assessment in nonpatients but a history of matchplay at initial assessment in patients. Even the rates of follow-up firesetting and matchplay were nearly four times as high in patients as nonpatients. However, parent and family measures failed to contribute incremental variance to the model in both samples. Further, the child's level of covert antisocial behavior was a predictor found in both samples. In addition, certain predictors in the two samples were firespecific variables (e.g., fire competence), whereas others were general psychosocial characteristics. Given some empirical support for both types of variables reported in our prior study, this combination of variables should be considered in assessing the potential determinants of firesetting activity (see Kolko, 1999). The study of specific subgroups of children whose patterns of firesetting behavior or, for that matter, other antisocial acts, vary is important in order to document their natural history or course, and long-term prognoses (Loeber et al., 1998).

The absence of other predictors that reflect firesetting risk factors and individual or family psychosocial characteristics in either sample stands in contrast to the identification of several predictors of recidivism in our 1-year follow-up study, which combined patient and nonpatient samples in all analyses (Kolko & Kazdin, 1992). It is important to note that other studies of antisocial children have found that predictors and risk factors assessed at a given point in time do not always emerge as significant when later follow-up assessments are conducted (Farrington & Hawkins, 1991; Offord, Boyle, & Racine, 1991). Similar inconsistencies have been reported in replication studies with firesetters (Sakheim & Osborne, 1994). Variations in the expression of different problem behaviors support the importance of longitudinal assessments of the developmental course of children's deviant behaviors (see Loeber et al., 1993).

A few methodological issues and limitations also deserve mention. Our definition of firesetting at follow-up included any fire set between study intake and 2-year follow-up; the inclusion of reports from prior or subsequent time periods in this definition may have changed their final classification. This classification is complicated by the uncertain status or placement of matchplaying children who, in this study, were classified as nonfiresetters because no property was damaged. This decision clearly impacts on the findings. Unfortunately, the small number of matchplayers precluded independent analysis of the unique role of this subgroup and its relationship to follow-up outcomes. Second, although the intercorrelations used to develop certain constructs were generally significant, the magnitudes were sometimes low and suggest some heterogeneity within these constructs. Finally, this sample of patients was limited to outpatients, whereas our prior studies included inpatients as well. The absence of inpatients may have restricted the ranges on certain variables and, possibly, attenuated the number of predictors identified.

These limitations notwithstanding, our findings lend support to the need to examine individual acts of firesetting and matchplay, and bear implications for hypotheses about the determinants of subsequent firesetting involvement. Recent work by Loeber et al. (1993) shows the importance of evaluating individual behaviors over time and documenting key sequences in which these behaviors emerge. A similar type of analysis may highlight different patterns in which firesetting or another antisocial act emerges. Our findings show somewhat different predictors for patients and nonpatients, but in both cases fire-related behaviors obtained at initial assessment were primary predictors of later firesetting. Although this relationship is hardly surprising, careful assessment of children's firesetting history is not always conducted. In the absence of an assessment of a past history, the continuity of the firesetting exhibited by the two samples would not have been as accurately identified. Studies of adult arsonists have confirmed the predictive significance of early childhood firesetting (Rice & Harris, 1991).

Of course, other variables may contribute to an understanding of children's involvement in firesetting, such as attraction to fire and individual motives for the fire. Perhaps greater attention to some of the predictor variables identified in this study, such as the child's involvement in matchplay and covert antisocial behavior, may help to expand both the scope and impact of existing intervention programs. Additional studies that examine novel assessment measures are needed to enhance our understanding of a child's involvement with fire (Kolko, 1999). Understanding the role of these variables may stimulate new research designed to prevent firesetting among community cases and to intervene more effectively with children whose firesetting histories necessitate clinical referral for services.

ACKNOWLEDGMENTS

This study was supported by a Grant (MH-39976) to the first two authors, a Research Scientist Award (MH-00353) to the second author, and a Center Grant (MH-55123; David Brent, PI), all from the National Institute of Mental Health. The authors appreciate the editorial assistance of Rachelle Parks and technical assistance of Dana Young, Amy Van Dyke, Marcia Bonder Warren, and the other associates of the Child Firesetting Project. Brian Day is now with the National Institute of Occupational Safety and Health, Morgantown, WV.

REFERENCES

Achenbach, T. M., & Edelbrock, C. (1983). *Manual for the Child Behavior Checklist and Revised Child Behavior Profile.* Burlington, VT: Queen City Publishers.

Achenbach, T. M., & Edelbrock, C. (1989). *Manual for the Youth Self-Report.* Burlington, VT: University of Vermont, Department of Psychiatry.

Cole, R. E., Grolnick, W. S., Laurenitis, L. R., McAndrews, M. M., Matkoski, K. M., & Schwartzman, P. I. (1986). *Children and fire: Rochester Fire-Related Youth Program Project.* Rochester, NY: University of Rochester.

Cole, R. E., Grolnick, W. S., & Schwartzman, P. I. (1993). Fire setting. In R. T. Ammerman, C. Last, & M. Hersen (Eds.), *Handbook of prescriptive treatments for children and adolescents.* Boston, MA: Allyn & Bacon.

Cole, R. E., Laurenitis, L. R., McAndrews, M. M., McKeever, J. M., & Schwartzman, P. I. (1983). *Juvenile firesetter intervention: Report of the Rochester Fire-Related Youth Program Project.* Rochester, NY: University of Rochester.

Derogatis, L. R., Lipman, R. S., & Covi, L. (1973). SCL-90: An outpatient psychiatric rating scale: preliminary report. *Psychopharmacology Bulletin, 24,* 454–464.

Farrington, D. P., & Hawkins, J. D. (1991). Predicting participation, early onset and later persistence in officially recorded offending. *Criminal Behavior and Mental Health, 1,* 1–33.

Gaynor, J., & Hatcher, C. (1987). *The psychology of child firesetting: detection and intervention.* New York: Brunner/Mazel.

Grolnick, W. S., Cole, R. E., Laurenitis. L., & Schwartzman, P. I. (1990). Playing with fire: a developmental assessment of children's fire understanding and experience. *Journal of Clinical Child Psychology, 19,* 128–135.

Hall, J. R. (1997). *Children playing with fire: U. S. experience.* 1980–1995. Quincy, MA: National Fire Protection Association.

Hollingshead, A. B., & Redlich, F. C. (1958). *Social class and mental illness.* New York: Wiley.

Hosmer, D. W., & Lemeshow, S. (1989). *Applied logistic regression.* New York: Wiley.

Kazdin, A. E., Rodgers, A., Colbus, D., & Siegel, T. (1987). Children's Hostility Inventory: measurement of aggression and hostility in psychiatric-inpatient children. *Journal of Clinical Child Psychology, 16,* 320–328.

Kolko, D. J. (1988). Community interventions for juvenile firesetters: a survey of two national programs. *Hospital and Community Psychiatry, 39,* 973–979.

Kolko, D. J. (1989). Fire setting and pyromania. In C. G. Last & M. Hersen (Eds.), *Handbook of child psychiatric diagnosis* (pp. 443–459). New York: Wiley.

Kolko, D. J. (1996). Education and counseling for child firesetters: a comparison of skills training programs with standard practice. In E. D. Hibbs & P. S. Jensen (Eds.), *Psychosocial treatments for child and adolescent disorders: empirically based strategies for clinical practice* (pp. 409–433). Washington, D.C.: American Psychological Association.

Kolko, D. J. (1999). Firesetting in children and youth. In M. Hersen & V. V. Hasselt (Eds.), *Handbook of psychological approaches with violent criminal offenders: contemporary strategies and issues.* New York: Plenum Press.

Kolko, D. J., & Kazdin, A. E. (1986). A conceptualization of firesetting in children and adolescents. *Journal of Abnormal Child Psychology, 14,* 49–62.

Kolko. D. J., & Kazdin, A. E. (1988a). Parent-child correspondence in identification of firesetting among child psychiatric patients. *Journal of Child Psychology and Psychiatry, 29,* 175–184.

Kolko, D. J., & Kazdin, A. E. (1988b). Prevalence of firesetting and related behaviors in child psychiatric inpatients. *Journal of Consulting and Clinical Psychology, 56,* 628–630.

Kolko, D. J., & Kazdin, A. E. (1989a). Assessment of dimensions of childhood firesetting among patients and nonpatients: the Firesetting Risk Interview. *Journal of Abnormal Child Psychology, 17,* 157–176.

Kolko, D. J., & Kazdin, A. E. (1989b). The Children's Firesetting Interview with psychiatrically referred and nonreferred children. *Journal of Abnormal Child Psychology, 17,* 609–624.

Kolko, D. J., & Kazdin, A. E. (1991a). Matchplaying and firesetting in children: relationship to parent, marital, and family dysfunction. *Journal of Clinical Child Psychology. 19,* 229–238.

Kolko, D. J., & Kazdin, A. E. (1991b). Aggression and psychopathology in matchplaying and firesetting children: a replication and extension. *Journal of Clinical Child Psychology, 20,* 191–201.

Kolko, D. J., & Kazdin, A. E. (1991c). Motives of childhood firesetters: firesetting characteristics and psychological correlates. *Journal of Child Psychology and Psychiatry, 32,* 535–550.

Kolko, D. J., & Kazdin, A. E. (1992). The emergence and recurrence of childhood firesetting: one-year prospective study. *Journal of Abnormal Child Psychology, 20,* 17–37.

Kolko, D. J., Kazdin, A. E., & Meyer, E. C. (1985). Aggression and psychopathology in childhood firesetters: parent and child reports. *Journal of Consulting and Clinical Psychology, 53,* 377–385.

Kolko, D. J., Watson, S., & Faust, J. (1991). Fire safety/prevention skills training to reduce involvement with fire in young psychiatric inpatients: preliminary findings. *Behavior Therapy, 22,* 269–284.

Laing, J. A., & Sines, J. O. (1982). The Home Environment Questionnaire: an instrument of assessing several behaviorally relevant dimensions of children's environments. *Journal of Pediatric Psychology, 7,* 425–449.

Loeber, R., Farrington, D. P., Stouthamer-Loeber, M., & Van Kammen, W. (1998). *Antisocial behavior and mental health problems: explanatory factors in childhood and adolescence.* Mahwah, NJ: Lawrence Erlbaum.

Loeber, R., Stouthamer-Loeber, M., Van Kammen, W. B., & Farrington, D. P. (1989). Development of a new measure of self report antisocial behavior in young children: prevalence and reliability. In M. W. Klein (Ed.), *Self-report methodology in criminological research* (pp. 203–225). Boston: Kluwer-Nijhoff.

Loeber, R., Wung, P., Keenan, K., Giroux, B., Stouthamer Loeber, M., Van Kammen, W. B., & Maughan, B. (1993). Developmental pathways in disruptive child behavior. *Development and Psychopathology, 5,* 103–133.

Moos, R. H., Insel, P. M., & Humphrey, B. (1974). *Family, work and group environment scales.* Palo Alto, CA: Consulting Psychologists Press.

Offord, D. R., Boyle, M. H., & Racine, Y. A. (1991). The epidemiology of antisocial behavior. In D. J. Pepler & K. H. Rubin (Eds.), *The development and treatment of childhood aggression* (pp. 31–54). Hillsdale, NJ: Lawrence Erlbaum.

Pierce, J. L., & Hardesty, V. A. (1997). Non-referral of psychopathological child firesetters to mental health services. *Journal of Clinical Psychology, 53,* 349–350.

Repo, E., & Virkkunen, M. (1997). Young arsonists: history of conduct disorder, psychiatric diagnoses and criminal recidivism, *The Journal of Forensic Psychiatry, 8,* 311–320.

Rice, M. E., & Harris, G. T. (1991). Firesetters admitted to a maximum-security psychiatric institution: offenders and offenses. *Journal of Interpersonal Violence, 6,* 461–475.

Sakheim, G. A., & Osborn, E. (1994). *Firesetting children: risk assessment and treatment.* Washington. DC: Child Welfare League of America.

SAS Programming. (1992). Cary, NC: SAS Institute Inc.

Schaefer, E. S. (1965). Children's reports of parental behavior: an inventory. *Child Development, 36,* 413–424.

Showers, J., & Pickrell, E. P. (1987). Child firesetters: a study of three populations. *Hospital and Community Psychiatry, 38,* 495–501.

Stewart, M. A., & Culver. K. W. (1982). Children who set fires: the clinical picture and a follow-up. *British Journal of Psychiatry, 140,* 357–363.

Stouthamer-Loeber, M., & Loeber, R. (1985). *Child Rearing Practices—Pilot version.* Unpublished instrument. Pittsburgh Youth Study, University of Pittsburgh. Western Psychiatric Institute and Clinic, Pittsburgh, PA.

Strachan, J. C. (1981). Conspicuous firesetting in children. *British Journal of Psychiatry, 138,* 26–29.

Straus, M. A. (1990). Measuring intrafamily conflict and violence: the Conflicts Tactics (CT) Scales. In M. A. Straus & R. J. Gelles (Eds.). *Physical violence in American families: risk factors and adaptations to violence in 8145 families* (pp. 29–47). New Brunswick, NJ: Transaction.

Vuchinich, S., Bank, L., & Patterson. G. R. (1992). Parenting, peers, and the stability of antisocial behavior in preadolescent boys. *Developmental Psychology, 28,* 510–521.

Wooden, W., & Berkey, M. L. (1984). *Children and arson. America's middle-class nightmare. New* York: Plenum Press.

15

Predictors of Later Schizophrenia and Affective Psychosis Among Attendees at a Child Psychiatry Department

Mary Cannon, Elizabeth Walsh, Christopher Hollis, Maresc Kargin, Eric Taylor, Robin M. Murray, and Peter B. Jones

Background: *Schizophrenia has been linked with psychological problems in childhood but there is little information on precursors of affective psychosis.* ***Aims:*** *To compare childhood psychological antecedents of adult schizophrenia and affective psychosis.* ***Method:*** *Childhood item sheets, which give standardized information on signs and symptoms of mental illness in the year preceding assessment are completed for all attendees at the children's department of the Maudsley and Bethlem Royal Hospital. We examined item sheet data on individuals with an adult diagnosis of schizophrenia (N = 59) or affective psychosis (N = 27) and a comparison group with no adult mental illness (N = 86) (all had attended the department).* ***Results:*** *Abnormal suspiciousness or sensitivity and relationship difficulties with peers are associated with later schizophrenia. In contrast, affective psychosis is associated with childhood hysterical symptoms and disturbances in eating.* ***Conclusions****: Childhood psychological precursors for schizophrenia and affective psychosis differ and do not simply reflect nonspecific psychiatric disturbance in adolescence.*

INTRODUCTION

Longitudinal research shows that many mental disorders do not arise *de novo* in adult life but have roots further back in childhood (Rutter, 1984; Caspi et al., 1996). Schizophrenia is associated with significant impairments in childhood, but little work has yet been carried out on affective psychosis. Longitudinal prospective studies are an ideal way to study childhood precursors of adult psychotic illness, but the length of the follow-up period and the large sample sizes required make this a prohibitively costly exercise. One approach is to use existing general population birth cohorts (Done et al., 1994; Jones et al., 1994), but although such samples have the advantage of an epidemiological design, they usually have few data on psychological symptoms in childhood, and have low statistical power to study relatively rare disorders such as schizophrenia. Data collected from attendees at child psychiatric clinics can overcome both of these difficulties. We have utilized a valuable resource of standardized psychological data collected over many years from a large child psychiatric service to examine predictors of later psychosis.

METHOD

Childhood Information

Since 1968 the Children's and Adolescents' Department of the Maudsley and Bethlem Royal Hospital has used a computer-based system of clinical data gathering, storage and retrieval (Thorley, 1982). This system uses a structured data recording sheet called an item sheet that employs Likert-type scales and is completed in addition to the usual medical file. The first part of the item sheet covers clinical symptoms and signs that have occurred within the previous 12 months, and is completed by the assessing psychiatrist within 2 weeks of the child's initial assessment (which comprises a mental state examination and a parental interview).

Each symptom on the item sheet is rated by the clinician as absent ('0'), minimal or dubious ('1') or definitely present ('2'). The list of symptoms and sociodemographic variables recorded on the item sheets comprises the following.

Emotional symptoms: abnormal suspiciousness or 'sensitivity'; morbid anxiety; morbid depression; specific phobias; obsessions/compulsions/ruminations; suicidal ideas or attempts; hypochondriasis; morbid irritability; school refusal; abnormally elevated mood/hypomania; depersonalization; derealization; conversion hysterical symptoms.

Somatic symptoms: disturbance of eating (pica, faddiness, refusal); disturbance of sleeping; pains of mental origin; encopresis; enuresis; non-epileptic disturbance of consciousness.

Disturbance of relationships: overt disturbance of: child–mother relationship; child–father relationship; relationship with other adults (e.g. teacher); patient–sibling relationship; relationships with other children (isolation, failure to make friends); autism/social withdrawal; social disinhibition.

Speech and language: disorder of rhythm; disorder of articulation; disorder of comprehension, disorder of production; elective mutism.

Motor disturbance: tics; other abnormal repetitive movements; clumsiness or poor coordination; restlessness or fidgetiness; gross overactivity; hypoactivity; habitual manipulations (thumb-sucking, rocking, etc.).

Antisocial behavior: defiance or lying; stealing; destructiveness; truancy; running away; sexual misbehavior, fighting/bullying, etc; violent assault; taking drugs; other substance misuse; cruelty to animals; other antisocial behavior.

Sociodemographic and administrative variables: main referral agency; duration of child's psychiatric disorder; patient status at time of admission; school attended; special school/day unit attended; special educational needs; employment; legal status; current parental situation; number of children under 17 years in the household; ordinal position; twin; seen by psychiatrist previously; seen by paediatrician for psychological disorder; brought before juvenile court previously; place of residence; country of birth of mother; country of birth of father; country of birth of child; occupation of father or main breadwinner.

Cases

All discharge summaries from the Maudsley Hospital Adult Psychiatric Service up to 1993 were searched for a unique identifying code signifying that patients had previously attended the Children's and Adolescents' Department of the Maudsley and Bethlem Royal Hospital between 1968 and 1989. Discharge summaries with a diagnosis of psychosis were entered into the OPCRIT system (version 3.2) (McGuffin et al., 1991) to give ICD-10 diagnoses (World Health Organization, 1992). In total, 56 cases fulfilling ICD-10 criteria for schizophrenia and 24 fulfilling ICD-10 criteria for affective psychosis (defined as bipolar affective disorder or severe depression with psychotic symptoms) were identified.

Comparison Group

The next four children, of the same age and gender, who were registered at the clinic after the index psychosis case were taken as the initial "raw" comparison group. We then undertook a follow-up study in order to identify a final comparison group who had no mental illness in adulthood, and to identify those individuals who later developed psychosis and had been treated elsewhere. Tracing was carried out in three stages:

1. names and dates of birth of the "raw" comparison group were matched against the National Health Service Central Register at the Office of

Population Censuses and Surveys (now the Office for National Statistics), which gave the name of the relevant Family Health Service Authority (FHSA) for each subject;
2. each FHSA was contacted to request the names of the general practitioner for each subject;
3. we then wrote to each general practitioner requesting information on the adult psychiatric history of the subject who was registered with them, enclosing a questionnaire.

Using these methods, we located general practitioners for 256 subjects. The general practitioners for 203 subjects agreed to participate in the study. From this group we identified 86 individuals who had never suffered any mental illness in adulthood, and these were taken as the "final" comparison group. Nine individuals were found to have an adult diagnosis of schizophrenia and four had a diagnosis of affective psychosis. In order to increase statistical power, we decided to add these individuals to our original case group. The remainder of the traced comparison group had suffered nonpsychotic psychiatric disorders in adulthood.

Final Sample

We identified 65 childhood attendees with an adult diagnosis of schizophrenia and 28 childhood attendees with an adult diagnosis of affective psychosis, comprising 20 cases with bipolar disorder and 8 cases with psychotic depression. Our comparison group comprised 86 childhood attendees who had not suffered mental illness in adulthood. We could not locate childhood item sheets for six subjects with schizophrenia and one subject with affective psychosis. The final sample available for analysis thus comprised: 59 subjects with schizophrenia; 27 subjects with affective psychosis; 86 controls.

Statistical Analysis

We included only variables rated as "definite" (score = 2) on the item sheets in our analysis. Odds ratios and confidence intervals were calculated to measure the association between each variable from the item sheet separately with later schizophrenia or affective psychosis. Items that were associated significantly with schizophrenia or affective psychosis at the 5% level on the univariate analysis. Stepwise logistic regression was used to identify those variables that were independently associated with later schizophrenia or affective psychosis. Analyses were performed using STATA v.5 (Stata Corporation, 1995).

RESULTS

Sample Characteristics

Table 15.1 presents the sociodemographic characteristics for the three groups of subjects: schizophrenia, affective psychosis and comparison. There were no significant overall differences between the groups on gender, socioeconomic group (defined by parental occupation) (Goldthorpe & Hope, 1974) or referral status (tertiary or local). Subjects were assessed at the children's department when they were aged between 13 and 14 years on average, so were, strictly speaking, in early adolescence rather than childhood at that time. Their assessments usually occurred some 3 to 5 years before a diagnosis of schizophrenia or affective psychosis. However, 12 of the schizophrenia group (20%) and 12 of the affective psychosis group (44%) were already diagnosed with psychosis while attending the children's department. These are called the "early-onset" cases (onset before age 17 years) and analyses are carried out both with and without these cases.

Univariate analysis

Variables from the item sheets that were associated significantly with later schizophrenia are presented in Table 15.2. Fifteen variables (nine symptom variables and six sociodemographic variables) were associated significantly with later schizophrenia on univariate analysis. Odds ratios could not be

TABLE 15.1
Sociodemographic Characteristics of Subjects with Childhood Item Sheet Data[1]

Variable	Schizophrenia ($N = 59$) No. %	Affective Psychosis ($N = 27$) No. %	Comparison group ($N = 86$) No. %	Test statistic[2] (d. f.)	p value
Male	37 (62.7)	11 (40.7)	50 (58.1)	4.6 (2)	0.1
SEG I, II	9 (20.0)	8 (44.4)	18 (26.6)	5.4 (2)	0.2
SEG III, IV, V	36 (80)	10 (55)	50 (73.4)		
Tertiary referrals	8 (13.5)	2 (7.3)	14 (16.3)	1.4 (2)	0.5
Mean age at assessment (s.d.)	14.1 (2.7)	13.8 (2.5)	13.4 (3.05)	1.13 (2, 170)	0.3
Mean age at diagnosis (s.d.)	19.4 (4.3)	17.0 (3.6)	N/A		

Note: SEG = socioeconomic group.
[1]Values are missing for 32 subjects (5 schizophrenia, 9 affective psychosis, 18 comparison).
[2]For categorical variables, the χ^2-test was used; for continuous variables, F-test was used.

TABLE 15.2
Association Between Item Sheet Variables and Schizophrenia

Item sheet variable	Odds ratio (95% CI)	Schizophrenia % Reporting variable	Schizophrenia No.[1]	Comparison group % Reporting variable	Comparison group No.[1]
Symptoms or signs in the past year					
Abnormal suspiciousness or sensitivity	9.86 (3.4–28.6)	43	51	7.1	70
Autism/social withdrawl	5.21 (1.6–17.3)	24	50	5.7	70
Morbid irritability/ temper tantrums	3.32 (1.4–7.7)	32.7	58	12.8	86
Disturbance of relationship with peers	2.97 (1.5–5.9)	53.4	58	27.9	86
Disturbance of sleeping	2.63 (1.2–6.0)	30.5	59	14.3	84
Morbid depression	2.48 (1.2–5.2)	39.6	58	20.9	86
Disturbance of relationships with other adults	2.12 (1.1–4.4)	41.1	56	24.7	85
Elective mutism	—	7.8	51	0.0	70
Hypoactivity	—	3.9	51	0.0	70
Sociodemographic variables					
Family psychiatic history (parent or sibling)	3.99 (1.7–9.2)	46.8	47	18.1	72
Past psychiatric history (child)	3.73 (1.1–13.2)	65	55	37.4	83
Currently in institution or children's home	2.69 (1.0–7.5)	19.3	57	8.1	86
Parent born in Caribbean or Africa	2.63 (1.1–6.1)	39	49	19.4	67
Twin	—	5.2	58	0.0	86
In-patient status on referral	—	17.5	57	0.0	86

[1]Number with available data on item sheet.

calculated for four variables (elective mutism, hypoactivity, in-patient status on referral and twin) because they did not occur in the comparison group. The strongest univariate association was between the symptom of abnormal suspiciousness or sensitivity and later schizophrenia, with an odds ratio of about 10. Three symptom variables (disturbance of relationship with other adults, disturbance of relationship with peers, and autism/social withdrawal) that were concerned with aspects of interpersonal relationships (outside the family) were associated significantly with later schizophrenia. Because the three variables were felt to be describing the same underlying phenomenon, they were combined into one variable called "relationship difficulties (extrafamilial)" for the multivariate analysis. Other symptom variables associated with later schizophrenia were: morbid depression, morbid irritability/temper tantrums, and disturbance, of sleeping. There was no association with speech and language disturbance (apart from elective mutism), motor disturbance, or antisocial behavior. Among the socio-demographic variables, family psychiatric history, previous psychiatric assessment, residing in a children's home or other type of institution, or parent born in the Caribbean or Africa were associated significantly with later schizophrenia.

Symptoms associated with affective psychosis on the univariate analysis are presented in Table 15.3. The strongest associations were with hysterical symptoms (which, because of low base rates of endorsement, was a combination variable comprising depersonalization, conversion hysterical symptoms and non-epileptic disturbance of consciousness) and gross overactivity, with odds ratios of about 20. Morbid depression, hypochondriasis and disturbance of eating also were associated significantly with affective psychosis. Among the antisocial behaviors there was a positive association with violent assault, but stealing was significantly less likely to occur than among the comparison group. There were no associations with speech and language disturbance. Among the sociodemographic variables, family psychiatric history and referral by another psychiatrist were associated positively with affective psychosis. Odds ratios could not be calculated for the symptoms of hypomania and hypoactivity or for the sociodemographic variable in-patient on referral because they did not occur in the comparison group.

Multivariate Analysis

All variables that were associated significantly with schizophrenia or affective psychosis on univariate analysis were entered into multivariate analyses. Table 15.4 shows the variables that were associated independently with schizophrenia and affective psychosis after logistic regression. The final model for schizophrenia comprised two symptom variables ('abnormal suspiciousness or sensitivity' and "relationship difficulties") and two sociodemographic variables ("family psychiatric history" and "past psychiatric contact"). The positive predictive power of the model for this sample of child psychiatric clinic attenders was 81.2% (26/32 cases correctly classified) and the model sensitivity was 65%. Adjusting for gender made no difference to the model. When we examined the Maudsley cases only, the associations did not change.

TABLE 15.3
Association Between Item Sheet Variables and Affective Psychosis

Item sheet variable	Odds ratio (95% CI)	Schizophrenia % Reporting variable	Schizophrenia No.[1]	Comparison group % Reporting variable	Comparison group No.[1]
Symptoms or signs in the past year					
Hysterical symptoms[2]	24.2 (2.6–224)	26.3	19	1.5	69
Gross overactivity	19.3 (2.1–173)	18.5	27	1.2	86
Hypochondriasis	10.6 (1.1–107)	11.1	27	1.2	86
Disturbance of eating	4.7 (1.4–15.4)	25.9	27	6.9	86
Violent assault	4.9 (1.2–19.8)	19.2	26	4.6	86
Morbid depression	2.5 (1.02–6.1)	48.0	27	27.1	85
Stealing	0.2 (0.04–0.9)	7.7	26	29.1	86
Hypomania	—	21.1	19	0.0	70
Hypoactivity	—	5.3	19	0.0	70
Sociodemographic variables					
Family psychiatric history (parent or sibling)	6.12 (2.2–17.2)	54.2	24	18.1	72
Referral by another psychiatrist	3.61 (1.3–10.1)	34.6	26	12.8	86
In-patient status on referral	—	15.4	26	0.0	86

[1]Number with available data on item sheet.
[2]Include depersonalization, conversion hysterical symptoms, and non-epileptic disturbance of consciousness.

When the early-onset cases were excluded, the association with relationship difficulties became stronger. The associations with past psychiatric history and family psychiatric history were no longer statistically significant, although the odds ratios remained above 2. The final model for affective psychosis comprised three variables: hysterical symptoms, disturbance of eating and family psychiatric history. The positive predictive power of the model for this sample was 63.6% (7/11 cases correctly classified) and the model sensitivity was 43.8%. The likelihood ratio test showed that gender made a significant difference to the model, so the odds ratios are presented after adjustment for gender. The wide confidence intervals for hysterical symptoms reflect the loss of precision due to the 25 missing values in the comparison group. After excluding the early-onset cases, the association with family psychiatric history became stronger but the associations with hysterical symptoms and disturbance of eating were no longer significant.

TABLE 15.4
Independent Association between Schizophrenia, Affective Psychosis, and Item Sheet Variables: Final Models

Item sheet variable	Odds ratio (95% CI) for all cases	Odds ratio (95% CI) for adult-onset cases only (>17 years)
Schizophrenia	*N* = 59	*N* = 47
Abnormal suspiciousness or sensitivity	21.5 (4.9–94.8)	12.4 (2.6–59.8)
Family psychiatric history (parent or sibling)	4.68 (1.4–15.6)	3.46 (0.9–12.1)
Past contact with psychiatrist	3.54 (1.1–11.4)	2.67 (0.8–8.9)
Relationship difficulties (extrafamilial)	3.34 (1.04–10.7)	4.22 (1.2–14.7)
Affective psychosis	*N* = 27	*N* = 15
Hysterical symptoms	26.24 (2.03–339)[1]	22.4 (0.96–520)[1]
Disturbance of eating	15.67 (1.9–124)[1]	19.5 (0.85–447)[1]
Family psychiatric history (parent or sibling)	5.54 (1.3–24.13)[1]	25.7 (2.4–274.0)[1]

[1]Adjusted for confounding by gender.

DISCUSSION

Strengths of the Study Design

The main strength of this study was the availability of standardized ratings, made on first assessment at a child psychiatric clinic, which cover most aspects of childhood psychopathology. The content validity and reliability of the item sheet data has been shown to be very high (Thorley, 1987; Goodman & Simonoff, 1991). Although the data were collected for other reasons and cannot encompass all the questions that one would possibly wish to address, it is rare to find such a detailed source of psychological data covering a large sample of children on whom information is available for adult outcome. Our study is unique in including a relatively large group of children who develop affective psychosis in adulthood, because previous studies have either not studied such children or had very small numbers (Pritchard & Graham, 1966; Zeitlin, 1986). Another strength of the study design is the follow-up strategy to determine the adult psychiatric status of the comparison group, which increases the sensitivity of the associations reported in this paper.

Limitations

A limitation of this study design is the possible lack of representativeness of our findings. Our sample represents adults who were sufficiently disturbed as children to be seen in a child psychiatric clinic that accepted both local and tertiary referrals. Strictly speaking, therefore, our results apply only to prediction of later psychosis among children who attend child psychiatric clinics. However, we will discuss the similarity of our results to findings from epidemiological general population samples, and show that there may be a wider application for our findings. In addition, by choosing as the comparison group children who had not suffered from mental illness in adulthood we hoped to find a comparison group as close as possible to a general population control group. Another limitation of this study is that some of the children were diagnosed with psychosis while still in the children's department. However, such diagnoses would have been made, in most cases, after a period of inpatient evaluation and not on the initial assessment, and the assessing psychiatrist would not have distinguished between schizophrenia and affective psychosis at that time. In addition, when we conducted our analysis without these early-onset cases, it made little difference to the findings. We feel, therefore, that we have identified precursors for psychosis rather than prodromes.

Comparison with Previous Work on Schizophrenia

The two childhood symptoms independently associated with later schizophrenia in this study were "abnormal suspiciousness or sensitivity" and "relationship difficulties (extrafamilial)". Relationship difficulties and social withdrawal in childhood and adolescence have long been known to be risk factors for schizophrenia and have been found in previous work on precursors of schizophrenia among child psychiatric clinic attendees (Offord & Cross, 1969; Hartman et al., 1984; Ambelas, 1992). Indeed, a review of this literature revealed so much evidence of pervasive social isolation that Garmezy (1974) deemed it "the fundamental dimension that is most integral in the developmental histories of schizophrenics." Our study had the power to distinguish between different types of relationship and found that familial relationships in childhood were not disturbed to the same extent as relationships with peers and other adults (usually teachers). Findings of relationship difficulties preceding schizophrenia are not confined to child psychiatric clinic samples. Two large cohort studies of male conscripts have found that poor social functioning at ages 16 to 18 years was the strongest predictor of later schizophrenia (Malmberg et al., 1998; Davidson et al., 1999). General population birth cohort studies have found problems with socialization at even earlier ages: in the 1946 British birth cohort (National Survey of Health and Development), a preference for solitary play was apparent by 4 years of age among children who later developed schizophrenia (Jones et al., 1994). However, the inability to relate effectively with peers during childhood is probably a nonspecific predictor of psychiatric and social morbidity, and we cannot determine the degree to which peer rejection contributes to this morbidity or is merely a marker of risk (Brown & Dodge, 1997; Hollis & Taylor, 1997).

The strongest risk factor for schizophrenia in this study was abnormal suspiciousness or sensitivity in childhood and adolescence, and this was independent of relationship difficulties. Few studies have examined this symptom separately, and it may have been incorporated into many of the earlier reports of relationship difficulties. One exception is the Swedish conscript study (Malmberg et al., 1998) mentioned above, which found that reporting oneself as "more sensitive than others" at age 18 years was a risk factor for schizophrenia, and conscripts who endorsed this symptom, in combination with having fewer than two close friends, preferring to socialize in small groups and not having a steady girlfriend, were 30 times more likely to develop schizophrenia than their peers. Accumulation of exposure to these four variables was associated with a linear increase in the risk of developing schizophrenia: a dose–response relationship (Malmberg et al., 1998). Reports of childhood experiences by patients with schizophrenia also describe hypersensitivity as a prominent feature (Wagner, 1996). Investigation of the neuro-psychological basis of this symptom in childhood may give insight into the development of psychotic phenomena.

Comparison with Previous Work on Affective Psychosis

The literature regarding childhood precursors of affective psychosis is less clear than for schizophrenia. There is evidence for premorbid social impairment although to a lesser degree than in schizophrenia (Cannon et al., 1997). In the 1958 British birth cohort study (National Child Development Study), boys who later developed affective psychosis were rated as more hostile to other children and more restless at age 7 years but these differences had disappeared by age 11 years and otherwise they were very similar to the control group (Done et al., 1994; Crow et al., 1995). This is the first study to demonstrate that childhood hysterical symptoms and eating problems can precede adult affective psychosis, but these associations have wide confidence intervals, are based on small numbers of cases, and need replication in other samples.

Genetic Risk Factors

It is well known that both schizophrenia and affective psychosis have substantial genetic components; having a first-degree relative who suffers from bipolar disorder or schizophrenia increases the risk for the illness in probands by 6 to 10-fold (Sham, 1995). We found that children who developed either schizophrenia or affective psychosis were more likely to have a family history of psychiatric illness in a first-degree relative, but we had no information about the exact nature of the psychiatric illness in the relatives. A previous study of Maudsley Child Psychiatric Clinic attendees found that the presence of any psychiatric illness in relatives was a significant predictor of early-onset affective disorder (Guth et al., 1993).

Disagreement with Previous Studies

The schizophrenia group was more likely to have been seen by a psychologist or psychiatrist previously, emphasizing that psychological difficulties began at a very early age. We were initially surprised to find no evidence for motor or language developmental impairments in our prepsychosis sample (apart from elective mutism, which was noted in about 8% of the schizophrenia group but did not occur in the comparison group). Our explanation is that the item sheets only rated symptoms or signs occurring over the past 12 months, and would therefore not detect very early developmental impairments. Previous studies of child psychiatric clinic populations that have found such impairments have examined early-onset patients only or have used maternal interview information recorded in case notes (Guth et al., 1993; Hollis, 1995; Sigurdsson et al., 1999).

Implications of Our Findings

Our findings suggest that the premorbid precursors for schizophrenia and affective psychosis differ and do not simply reflect nonspecific psychiatric disturbance in adolescence. There appear to be separate tracks leading from suspiciousness, sensitivity, and social difficulties to schizophrenia, and from eating disorders/hysterical symptoms to affective psychosis. An interesting question (which we cannot answer from our data) is whether these childhood problems are markers of the neurocognitive substrate of schizophrenia or affective psychosis, or are independent risk factors for the disorder. At a general population level, the predictive power of individual childhood symptoms is low (social difficulties are common and schizophrenia is rare) (Malmberg et al., 1998). However, within the context of a child psychiatric clinic the predictive power of our model was relatively high. Our study demonstrates the benefits of moving from a risk factor approach to a risk model approach to the prediction of adult psychosis, including not just symptoms but also measures of genetic risk, psychiatric history, and demographic variables.

CLINICAL IMPLICATIONS AND LIMITATIONS

Clinical Implications

- Symptoms detected on routine childhood psychological assessment can predict adult psychotic illness.
- There appear to be separate childhood precursors for schizophrenia and affective psychosis.
- Information on family psychiatric history, in combination with childhood psychological symptoms, can increase the power of predictive models for later psychosis.

Limitations

- Our results, strictly speaking, apply only to children who attend a child psychiatry service.
- Predictive power of childhood symptoms is generally low in the general population, owing to the high prevalence of childhood difficulties and the rarity of adult psychotic outcomes.

Symptom precursors of affective psychosis found in this study will need replication in other, larger samples.

ACKNOWLEDGMENTS

This study was funded in part by the Theodore and Vada Stanley Foundation. M.C. and E.W. were supported by Wellcome Trust Training Fellowships in Clinical Epidemiology. We thank John Harris and the staff of the medical records department of the Maudsley Hospital for their help in identifying the cases. We acknowledge the work carried out by the Office for National Statistics in tracing the comparison group, and we thank the general practitioners who participated in the study.

REFERENCES

Ambelas, A. (1992). Preschizophrenics: adding to the evidence, sharpening the focus. *British Journal of Psychiatry, 160,* 401–404.

Brown, J. & Dodge, K. A. (1997). Early peer relations and child psychiatry. In *Handbook of Child and Adolescent Psychiatry*, vol. I (eds S. Greenspan, S. Weider & J. Osofksy), pp. 304–319. New York: John Wiley & Sons.

Cannon, M., Jones, P., Gilvarry, C., et al. (1997). Premorbid social functioning in schizophrenia and bipolar disorder: similarities and differences. *American Journal of Psychiatry, 154,* 1544–1550.

Caspi, A., Moffitt, T.E., Newman, D.L., et al. (1996). Behavioural observations at age 3 years predict adult psychiatric disorders. *Archives of General Psychiatry, 53,* 1033–1039.

Crow, T.J., Done, D.J. & Sacker, A. (1995). Childhood precursors of psychosis as clues to its evolutionary origin. *European Archives of Psychiatry and Clinical Neuroscience, 245,* 61–69.

Davidson, M., Reichenberg, A., Rainowitz, J., et al. (1999). Behavioural and intellectual markers for schizophrenia in apparently healthy males. *American Journal of Psychiatry, 156,* 1328–1335.

Done, D.J., Crow, T.J., Johnstone, E.C., et al. (1994). Childhood antecedents of schizophrenia and affective illness: social adjustment at ages 7 and 11. *British Medical Journal, 309,* 699–703.

Garmezy, N. (1974). Child at risk: the search for the antecedents of schizophrenia. *Schizophrenia Bulletin, 8,* 13–90.

Goldthorpe, J. H. & Hope, K. (1974). *The Social Grading of Occupations—A New Approach and Scale.* Oxford: Clarendon Press.

Goodman, R. & Simonoff, E. (1991). Reliability of clinical ratings by trainee child psychiatrists: a research note. *Journal of Child Psychology and Psychiatry, 32,* 551–555.

Guth, C., Jones, P. & Murray, R. (1993). Familial psychiatric illness and obstetric complications in early-onset affective disorder. A case–control study. *British Journal of Psychiatry, 163,* 492–498.

Hartman, E., Milofsky, E. & Vaillant, G. (1984). Vulnerability to schizophrenia: prediction of adult schizophrenia using childhood information. *Archives of General Psychiatry, 41,* 1050–1056.

Hollis, C. (1995). Child and adolescent (juvenile onset) schizophrenia: a case control study of premorbid developmental impairments. *British Journal of Psychiatry, 166,* 489–495.

Hollis, C. & Taylor, E. (1997). Schizophrenia: a critique from the developmental psychopathology perspective. In *Neurodevelopment and Adult Psychopathology,* pp. 213–233. Cambridge: Cambridge University Press.

Jones, P. B., Rodgers, B., Murray, R. M., et al. (1994). Child developmental risk factors for adult schizophrenia in the 1946 British birth cohort. *Lancet, 344,* 1398–1402.

Malmberg, A., Lewis, G., David, A., et al. (1998). Premorbid adjustment and personality in people with schizophrenia. *British Journal of Psychiatry, 172,* 308–313.

McGuffin, P., Farmer, A. & Harvey, I. (1991). A polydiagnostic application of operational criteria in studies of psychotic illness: development and reliability of the OPCRIT system. *Archives of General Psychiatry, 48,* 764–770.

Offord, D. R. & Cross, L. A. (1969). Behavioural antecedents of adult schizophrenia. *Archives of General Psychiatry, 21,* 267–283.

Pritchard, M. & Graham, P. (1966). An investigation of a group of patients who have attended both the child and adult departments of the same psychiatric hospital. *British Journal of Psychiatry, 112,* 603–612.

Rutter, M. (1984). Psychopathology and development. I: Childhood antecedents of adult psychiatric disorder. *Australian and New Zealand Journal of Psychiatry, 18*, 225–234.

Sham, P. (1995).Genetic epidemiology. *British Medical Bulletin*, *52*, 408–433.

Sigurdsson, E., Fombonne, E., Sayal, K., et al. (1999). Neurodevelopmental antecedents of early-onset bipolar affective disorder. *British Journal of Psychiatry, 174*, 121–127.

Stata Corporation (1995). *Stata Statistical Software Release 5.0.* College Station, TX: Stata Corporation.

Thorley, G. (1982). The Bethlem Royal and Maudsley hospitals' clinical data register for children and adolescents. *Journal of Adolescence*, *5*, 179–189.

Thorley, G. (1987). Factor study of a psychiatric clinic child rating scale. Based on ratings made by clinicians on child and adolescent clinic attenders. *British Journal of Psychiatry, 150*, 49–59.

Wagner, P. S. (1996). First person account: a voice from another closet. *Schizophrenia Bulletin*, *22*, 399–401.

World Health Organization (1992). *Tenth Revision of the International Classification of Diseases and Related Health Problems* (ICD-10). Geneva: WHO.

Zeitlin, H. (1986). *The Natural History of Psychiatric Disorder in Children.* Oxford: Oxford University Press.

16

A Further Look at the Prognostic Power of Young Children's Reports of Depressed Mood and Feelings

Nicholas S. Ialongo, Gail Edelsohn, and Sheppard G. Kellam

A primary objective of the present study was to determine the validity of first graders' self-reports of depressed mood and feelings. To that end, the prognostic power of first-grade self-reports of depressed mood and feelings was examined with respect to later psychopathology and adaptive functioning in a population of urban school children (N = 946). First-grade self-reports of depressed mood predicted later child academic functioning, the need for and use of mental health services, suicidal ideation, and a diagnosis of major depressive disorder by age 14. The prognostic power of these early self-reports suggests that children as young as 5 or 6 years of age are capable of providing valid reports of depressed mood and feelings.

INTRODUCTION

After decades of debate (Digdon & Gotlib, 1985; Kovacs, 1986; Lefkowitz & Burton, 1978), there appears to be a growing consensus that children as young as 8 or 9 years of age do experience depressive syndromes similar to those seen in adults in terms of social and cognitive impairment and symptom presentation. Moreover, there appears to be general agreement that by the middle to late elementary school years, children can provide reliable and valid reports of their symptoms (Weisz, Weiss, Wasserman, & Rintoul, 1987). Debate continues, however, as to whether children as young as 5 or 6 years of age can experience such depressive phenomena, or reliably and validly report on depressed mood and feelings (Digdon & Gotlib, 1985; Edelsohn, Ialongo, Werthamer-Larsson, Crockett, & Kellam 1992; Ialongo, Edelsohn, Werthamer-Larsson, Crockett, & Kellam, 1993). Those who question the ability of young children to experience or report on adultlike depressive phenomena typically point to putative developmental constraints on the young child's ability to understand, recall, and label emotional states or to experience the debilitating cognitive features of adultlike mood disorders, including poor self-worth, guilt, hopelessness, and helplessness. The latter either represent integral features of current definitions of mood disorders in adults (American Psychiatric Association, 1994) or are at the core of prominent cognitive and cognitive/social learning-based theories of depression (Abramson, Seligman, & Teasdale, 1978; Beck, 1974).

Among the findings that have caused some to question the reliability and validity of young children's reports of depressed mood are those of Edelbrock, Costello, Dukau, Kalas, and Conover (1985), who found young children were relatively unreliable reporters of depressed mood on a structured diagnostic interview. Moreover, the literature on social cognitive development appears to provide some support for the contention that young children may be developmentally constrained from experiencing the debilitating cognitive features of adultlike depressive syndromes and disorders. For example, Harter (1986) argues that younger children, especially in the preschool and early elementary school years, are more likely to overrate their competence; they report what they wish they were like, rather than what they are really like. Harter (1986) suggests that, in general, it is not before third grade that children appear able to discriminate between the real and ideal self and to report more realistic perceptions of competence. Relatedly, Cowan (1978) contends that awareness of the discrepancies between the real and ideal self is a necessary precursor to guilt. Given that, according to Harter (1986), children typically don't achieve this discrimination until the middle to late elementary school years, it seems reasonable to believe that children would not experience decrements in self-worth or guilt before this time. Also consistent with Harter's (1986) contention that young children tend to overrate their competence, Weisz (1986) reports that before the middle to late elementary school years, children appear highly susceptible to "illusory contingency" and, as such, are more resistant to experiencing "learned helplessness."

Despite such findings, there appears to be a number of reasons to question the contention that young children can neither reliably nor validly report on depressive phenomena. In terms of the ability of young children to provide reliable reports of past events, Friedman (1991) found that children as young as 6 years of age can localize a past event 7 weeks prior by the time of day, day of the week, month, and season. Indeed, the 6-year-olds were able to recall the time of the event to within 15 minutes of the time of day it occurred. Even 4-year-olds were able to recall the time of day of the event, although they had difficulty in localizing the event with respect to the day of the week, month, and season. Nevertheless, they could accurately judge the relative recency of two events, one 7 weeks prior and the other 1 week prior. Of note, in contrast to Edelbrock et al. (1985), Silverman and Eisen (1992) reported that in a study of the reliability of parent and child reports of child anxious symptomatology using a structured interview (Anxiety Disorders Interview Schedule for Children) (Silverman & Nelles, 1988), 6- to 11-year-olds' self-reports appeared to be reasonably reliable over a 10- to 14-day test–retest interval for affective disorder, $r = .61$. Complementing the findings of Silverman and Nelles (1992) are those of Edelsohn et al. (1992) and Ialongo et al. (1993). These investigators found first graders' self-reports of depressive symptoms to be relatively stable over intervals of 2 weeks (.60) and 4 months (.44). The level of stability was particularly impressive for first graders initially in the highest quartile of depressive symptoms, all of whom remained in the highest quartile at retest 4 months later.

With respect to those who have questioned the ability of young children to label and understand the emotional states typically associated with depressive phenomena, Russell (1990) found that as early as the preschool years children were able to understand the causes and consequences of a wide range of emotions including fear, anger, sadness, happiness, and surprise. Moreover, preschoolers proved able to verbally label the emotions and explain their causes and consequences. In addition, Beizer-Seidner, Stipek, and Deitch-Feshbach (1985) found that children as young as age 5 years understood the feelings of pride and embarrassment and could give examples of each.

As to the young child's ability to experience the debilitating cognitive features of depression seen in older children and adults (such as helplessness and hopelessness), the authors of the present study argue that the age at which a particular cognitive milestone is reached may vary considerably across children. Indeed, consistent with Hergenrather and Rabinowitz's (1991) theorizing on children's knowledge and conceptualization of physical illness, and Byrnes and Wasik's (1991) work on the interplay of conceptual and procedural knowledge, children's cognitive developmental trajectories may vary within specific domains as a function of their experience and accumulation and organization of knowledge within that domain. As more knowledge is accumulated and operated upon, the greater is the likelihood of improved reasoning and problem solving and the learning of skills within a particular domain. Given the role experiential factors appear to play in children's development of knowledge structures in specific domains (e.g., Byrnes & Wasik, 1991; Hergenrather & Rabinowitz, 1991), it may be that children's reactions to uncontrollable events will vary as a function of their experience with such events and not the domain-general logic available to them vis-à-vis Piagetian stages. Importantly, one might expect that the earlier is the exposure to significant and uncontrollable life events the earlier is the development of the concepts of helplessness and hopelessness—integral features of depressive syndromes seen in older children and adults.

The findings of Edelsohn et al. (1992) and Ialongo et al. (1993) also bear upon the question of whether young children are capable of validly reporting on depressed mood and feelings. These investigators found that self-reports of depressed mood and feelings were significantly related to the negotiation of a number of salient developmental tasks at entrance to first grade, including academic achievement and peer relations. Perhaps the most impressive finding to come out of these studies was that self-reports of depressed mood in first grade strongly predicted standardized achievement scores at fourth and fifth grade, even after controlling for first-grade achievement scores.

In the present study, the authors sought to extend their previous findings on the concurrent (Edelsohn et al., 1992) and predictive validity (Ialongo et al., 1993) of first graders' reports of depressed mood to a wider and more distal set of social adaptational and mental health outcomes. To that end, the degree to which children's reports of depressed mood and feelings in first grade predict their adaptive functioning—special education service use, referral for special education evaluation, grade retention, and overall grade point average (GPA)—in sixth grade and suicidal ideation and major depressive disorder at age 14 years was examined. Also assessed was whether these first- grade self-reports of depressed mood predict parent report of child mental health service use and teacher report of the need for mental health services in sixth grade. Finally, the prognostic power of children's reports of depressed mood was contrasted with parent reports. Given that reliable and cost-efficient methods and measures are available for obtaining parent reports of child depressed mood (e.g., Mood and Feelings Questionnaire) (Angold, Costello, Pickles, Winder, & Silver 1987), it would be important to know whether child reports provide unique information in terms of the prediction of later mental health outcomes and adaptive functioning. If they do not, the cost and burden of collecting child reports of depressed mood in large-scale epidemiologic field studies would be unnecessary.

METHOD

Participants

Participants were 1,197 first-grade children from 19 public elementary schools in the eastern catchment area of the city of Baltimore, Maryland. With respect to ethnicity, 66.1% were African American, 32.1% were European American, and the remaining 1.8% were made up of Native Americans, Asian Americans, and Hispanic Americans. Just over 49% (49.1%) were boys. Nearly 70% of the children were receiving free lunch, which the school system made available to children from families at or below federal poverty levels. The children were originally recruited for participation in two school-based, preventive intervention trials targeting early learning and aggression (Kellam & Rebok, 1992). Three to four schools—closely matched in terms of school size, achievement levels, promotion rates, and a variety of sociodemographic variables—were selected from each of five sociodemographically distinct areas in eastern Baltimore. Schools were randomly assigned to either an intervention or control condition within a geographic area. Children had been randomly assigned to classrooms before assignment of classrooms to intervention conditions. The interventions were universal in that they were provided to all the children in the intervention classrooms. They were in place throughout the course of first and second grade—and only during those grades. Intervention classroom teachers were trained in either an enhanced Mastery Learning curriculum, which targeted reading achievement, or a classroom contingency management procedure, which targeted aggression and social participation.

The five geographic areas in which the participating schools were located were defined by census tract data and vital statistics obtained from the Baltimore City Planning Office. These areas varied by ethnicity, type of housing, family structure, income, unemployment, violent crime, suicide, and school dropout rates. Of the 1,197 children who were available for participation in the fall of first grade, parental consent was obtained for 1,030 children, or 86.05% of the eligible population. Chi-square analyses revealed that consent rates varied as a function of geographic area, $\chi^2(4, N = 1{,}197) = 13.66$, $p < .01$. The lowest rates of parental consent were in Areas 1 and 4, which were made up primarily of middle-income, two-parent families living in well-maintained row or detached homes.

Assessment Design

Data for this report were gathered in the fall of first grade and the spring of fourth, sixth, and eighth grades. First-grade assessments were carried out before the initiation of the interventions. The data gathered in the first-grade assessments included children's self-reports of depressed mood and feelings, intervention condition, free lunch status, and standardized achievement scores. Parent reports of child depressed mood were obtained in fourth grade, along with data on family structure (the number of adult caregivers in the household and their relationship to the target child) and years of education for each of the adults in the household. Parent reports of child mental health service use were obtained in fourth and sixth grades. Teacher reports of the need for child mental health service use were obtained in sixth grade. Grades and special education services use were also obtained in sixth grade from school records, along with grade retentions. Finally, child self-reports of depressive symptoms (including suicidal ideation and behavior) were obtained in eighth grade.

Measures

Children's Depression Inventory. The Children's Depression Inventory (CDI) (Kovacs, 1983) was used in first grade to obtain child self-reports of depressed mood and feelings. It consists of 27 items designed to assess affective, cognitive, and behavioral symptoms associated with depression. For each item, one of three sentences (rated on a scale from 0 to 2) that best describes the child over the past 2 weeks is endorsed. The CDI is among the most widely used children's self-report measures of depression. Saylor, Finch, Spirito, and Bennett (1984) report an α coefficient of .84 and test–retest correlations of .87 over a 1-week interval and .59 over a 5-week interval in a population of emotionally disturbed children. Some modifications in the CDI in terms of the content of the scale and administration format were made for the first-grade assessment. A decision was made to delete three items that focused specifically on social adaptational status rather than psychological well-being (school work inhibition, lack of enjoyment at school, poor school performance), which left 24 items. In addition, the CDI administration format was changed so that the instrument could be given on a classroom-wide basis and would require no reading skills on the children's part. All items were read aloud twice to the class by a member of the assessment team, while a second team member circulated through the classroom maintaining classroom order and assisting children who were having difficulties. To further obviate the need for reading skills, pictures of common objects (e.g., a ball, apple, etc.) were used to represent the items and the answer choices in the booklets in which the children recorded their answers. The score used in the logistic analyses described later was the mean of the 24 items making up the CDI as revised for this study. That is, a total score was computed by simply summing the 24 items and then dividing the sum by 24. Scores for the population studied ranged from 0 to 2.

The California Achievement Test. The California Achievement Test (CAT, Forms E and F) represents one of the most frequently used standardized achievement batteries (Wardrop, 1989). Subtests in CAT Forms E and F cover both verbal (reading, spelling, and language) and quantitative (computation, concepts, and applications) topics. The CAT was standardized on a nationally representative sample of 300,000 children. Internal consistency coefficients for virtually all of the subscales exceed .90. Alternate form reliability coefficients are generally in the .80 range (Wardrop, 1989). Scale scores on the CAT Total Reading scale ranged from 142 to 445 for the study population.

School records. Free lunch status (used as a proxy for family income) was obtained from school records in first grade, whereas special education services use was obtained in sixth grade, along with sixth-grade overall GPA and history of grade retention.

Parent reports of child mental health service use for depressed mood. In the fourth and sixth years of the study, parents were asked to report on the child's lifetime use of mental health services for depressed mood and feelings ("Has your child ever been to someone to get help for depression or being sad or unhappy?" "Yes?" or "No?"; "Where did s/he go and whom did s/he see about this?"). Use was defined as being seen for mental health services for depressed mood at least once by a health professional, including a psychologist, social worker, psychiatrist, school counselor, psychiatric nurse, or primary care physician, in either an out- or inpatient setting. The data on parent report of child mental health service use for depressed mood from fourth and sixth grades were combined for analytic purposes. That is, if a parent reported service use at either time, or both times, service use was coded as 1; otherwise it was coded as 0, because the parent did not report service use at either time.

Mood and Feelings Questionnaire–Parent Short Form. The Mood and Feelings Questionnaire–Parent Short Form (MFQ-PS) (Angold et al., 1987) is a 12-item questionnaire developed for use as a first-stage, or screening, measure in epidemiological studies of depression in children and adolescents. The items are keyed to the symptom areas described in the *DSM-III-R* (American Psychiatric Association, 1987) for depression in children and adolescents. The MFQ consists of statements that require a response on a 3-point scale ("True," "Sometimes true," and "Not true"). The MFQ was scored in general accord with the symptom criteria used in the *DSM-III-R* for determining major depressive disorder. Children were assigned a score of 1 if their caregiver endorsed as "true" either of the two items, "didn't enjoy anything" or "felt miserable or unhappy," and rated four or more MFQ items (symptoms) as "sometimes true" or "true." All other children were assigned a score of 0.

Family demographic characteristics. In addition to obtaining parent reports of child depressed mood and child mental health service use in fourth grade, data on the years of education for each adult caregiver in the household and family structure (the number of adult caregivers in the household and their relationship to the target child) were also collected. For analytic purposes, the family structure data were recoded into single- (coded 1) versus dual-parent household (coded 0). Given that the majority of households consisted of single-parent families and few parents had more than a high school education, the parent education variable used in our analyses was coded as 1 if there was at least one adult caregiver with a high school education or greater in the household or 0 if there were no adult caregivers with at least a high school education in the household.

Teacher reports of the need for child mental health services for emotional and behavioral problems. In the sixth year of the study, teachers were asked to report on their perception of the child's need for mental health services for behavioral and emotional problems within the last year. Teachers were instructed to answer the question regardless of whether they knew the child was currently receiving mental health services in, or outside of, the school setting. The specific questions asked were: "Does this child need treatment or counseling for emotional or psychological problems?," "Yes?" or "No?"; and "Does this child need medication for hyperactivity/attention problems?," "Yes?" or "No?" A Yes response was coded as 1, and a No response was coded as 0. The teachers' responses to these two questions were combined for analytic purposes. That is, if a teacher reported service need in response to either question, or both, service need was coded as a 1; otherwise it was coded as 0, since the teacher did not report any need for service.

Composite International Diagnostic Interview–University of Michigan Version. In eighth grade, the Composite International Diagnostic Interview-University of Michigan Version (CIDI-UM) (Kessler et al., 1994) was used to determine the past year occurrence of Major Depressive Disorder (MDD) on the basis of youth's self-report. The diagnosis was derived in accordance with *DSM-III-R* criteria by using the scoring algorithm developed by Kessler et al. (1994). The CIDI-UM was also used to determine whether there was at least one lifetime episode of 2 weeks or more of suicidal ideation or behavior, including one or more of the following: "... thought about death...," "... wanted to die ...," "... thought about hurting yourself...," or "... tried to hurt yourself." The CIDI-UM is a fully structured psychiatric interview that specifies the exact wording and sequence of questions and provides a complete set of categories for classifying respondents' replies. The highly structured format is intended to minimize clinical judgment in eliciting diagnostic information and recording responses. The CIDI-UM is designed to be administered by lay interviewers and was successfully employed in the National Co-Morbidity Study (Kessler et al., 1994) with children as young as 15 years of age. In the present study, the CIDI was administered by young adult, lay interviewers as part of a larger, standardized interview that took place in a confidential location at the youth's school. The interviewers received approximately 50 hours of training in the use of the larger interview, of which about 16 hours were dedicated to training on the CIDI-UM MDD module. The training included practice interviews with adolescent volunteers. These interviews were observed by the supervisory staff, who provided corrective feedback. Only those trainees who proved competent in the administration of the interview were sent into the field. Interviewers were deemed competent once they demonstrated that they could (1) read aloud the interview questions as written in a fluent and a conversational manner, (2) engage and maintain the respondent's interest and attention to the interview, (3) avoid being sidetracked by tangential responses on the part of the respondent, (4) correctly probe ambiguous responses on the part of the respondent, (5) follow the appropriate skip patterns, (6) ask sensitive questions in a neutral manner, and (7) respond in a neutral manner to the respondent's answers to such questions. Daily debriefing sessions were held throughout the fielding period along with spot checks of interviewers in the field.

RESULTS

Analytic Plan

Logistic regression analysis was used to examine the prognostic value of first graders' reports of depressed mood and feelings with respect to later indicators of adaptive functioning, depressed mood, and mental health service need and use. The decision to use logistic regression was based on the fact that most of the outcomes of interest were categorical in nature, and the few interval-level dependent variables (as well as a number of the independent variables) had highly skewed distributions. In each analysis, the background and predictor variables (child or parent report of child depressed mood) were entered simultaneously. The background variables included free lunch status, ethnicity, intervention condition, family structure, and parent education. All analyses were conducted separately by gender.

Missing Data and the Number of Subjects Available for Analysis at Each Time Point

Self-reports of depressed mood were obtained from 946 of the 1,130 children with parental consent. There were no differences in terms of geographic area, intervention condition, free lunch status, or ethnicity between those 946 children and the 84 children with parental consent who were missing data in first grade. In the spring of fourth grade, 742 children were available for analysis with complete data (i.e., parent report of child depressed mood, intervention condition, ethnicity, parent education, family structure, fall of first-grade child self-report of depressed mood, and free lunch status), whereas 625 of these 742 children were available for analysis and had complete data in the spring of sixth grade; and 494 in the spring of eighth grade. Complete data in sixth grade included parent report of child mental health service use for depressed mood at both fourth and sixth grades, school records, teacher report of the need for child mental health service use for emotional and psychological problems, family and child background variables, and fall of first grade child self-report of depressed mood. The eighth-grade data included child self-report of depressive symptoms and suicidal ideation on the CIDI, along with complete data at first, fourth, and sixth grades. Table 16.1 characterizes the children with complete data at the fourth, sixth, and eighth grades in terms of ethnicity, free lunch status, intervention condition, gender, fall of first grade child self-reports of depressed mood, and CAT standardized achievement scores. Data on family structure and parent education are presented for the fourth, sixth, and eighth grades. As can be seen in Table 16.1, from grade 4 on there were few differences in terms of the characteristics of the children with complete data.

Those children with complete data at fourth grade (i.e., parent report of child depressed mood, family and child background characteristics, and fall of first-grade child self-reports of depressed mood) were contrasted with those with missing data at fourth grade. The dependent variables in these

TABLE 16.1
Characteristics of Children with Complete Data at Grades 1, 4, 6, and 8

	Grade 1	Grade 4	Grade 6	Grade 8
Ethnicity				
African American	66.4%	70.8%	75.8%	78.5%
European American[a]	33.6%	29.4%	24.1%	21.3%
% Receiving free lunch	69.6%	75.1%	78.4%	78.3%
Gender (% boys)	50.6%	51.6%	51.0%	48.8%
Intervention design (% controls)	56.1%	55.6%	56.0%	53.3%
First-grade child self-report of depressed mood—CDI	12.87 (8.03)	13.12 (8.16)	13.23 (8.02)	13.29 (7.92)
Standardized achievement in grade 1—CAT	261.09 (36.59)	260.88 (36.04)	259.41 (35.80)	260.28 (36.56)
Family structure: % single-parent families		62.9%	61.2%	61.8%
Parent education (presence of an adult in the household with a high school education or greater)		73.6%	72.8%	74.4%

Note: Standard deviations are in parentheses. CDI = Children's Depression Inventory; CAT = California Achievement Test.
[a] European American or other.

contrasts were the following first-grade variables: free lunch status, ethnicity, child self-reports of depressed mood, standardized achievement scores, gender, and intervention condition. No differences were found between those children with missing data and those with complete data in terms of first-grade self-reports of depressed mood, standardized achievement scores, gender, and intervention condition. There were, however, significant differences between those with missing versus complete data in terms of ethnicity. Children with complete data were significantly more likely to be African American and to have received free lunch in first grade. That is, whereas 70.8% of the children with complete data were African American, only little more than half (52.0%) of those with missing data at fourth, sixth, or eighth grades were African American. Similarly, 75.1% of the children with complete data received free lunch in first grade, but only 50.2% of the children with missing data received free lunch.

Contrasts between children with complete data and those with missing data were also carried out at the sixth and eighth grades, respectively, by using the same set of first-grade dependent variables. As with the fourth-grade analyses, the only significant differences found were for free lunch status. Once again, children with complete data were significantly more likely to be African American and to have received free lunch in first grade. In a final set of missing data analyses, no differences were found in terms of family structure or years of parent education between the children with complete data and those with missing data at the sixth and eighth grades, respectively.

Prevalences of the Outcomes of Interest

The prevalence for each of the outcomes of interest is presented in Table 16.2. Because there are few studies of urban, African American children of a similar age with which to compare this study's rates of MDD, suicidal ideation, and service use, comparisons with studies of largely European American populations had to be used. Perhaps the closest in age to this study's population is the population described by Garrison, Addy, Jackson, McKeown, and Waller (1992) of 12- to 14-year-olds in the southeastern United States, wherein the rate of an episode of a MDD in the last year of the study was 9.04% for boys and 8.90% for girls. Thus, the rates reported in the present study were roughly commensurate with Garrison et al. (boys: 7.1% vs. 9.04%, girls: 12.0% vs. 8.90%). The rate of suicidal ideation reported by the Centers for Disease Control and Prevention (Kann et al., 1997) for a nationwide sample of students in grades 9 through 12 was 20.5%. Ideation was defined as having seriously considered attempting suicide within the last year, with female students nearly twice as likely to report suicidal ideation as males (27.1% vs. 15.1%). Of note, the somewhat higher prevalence found in

TABLE 16.2
Prevalences of Outcomes of Interest

	Prevalence	
	Males	Females
CIDI MDD diagnosis last year, grade 8	7.1	12.3
CIDI suicidal ideation lifetime, grade 8	26.6	31.2
Mental health services for depression—parent report, grades 4 and 6	10.7	8.5
Need for mental health services for behavioral & emotional problems—teacher report, grade 6	27.9	15.4
Received special education services, grade 6	28.0	14.1
Evaluation for special education services, grade 6	23.8	12.1
Grade retention	27.0	31.7
GPA of C or worse, grade 6	83.6	68.8
Parent report of child depressed mood and feelings in grade 4—MFQ	3.1	3.1

Note: CIDI MDD = Composite International Diagnostic Interview, Major Depressive Disorder; GPA = grade point average; MFQ = Mood and Feelings Questionnaire.

the present study may be due to the use of a broader definition of ideation and the use of a lifetime framework as opposed to the past year. With respect to the rates of mental health service use for depressed mood, Leaf et al. (1996), using data from the Methods for the Epidemiology of Child and Adolescent Mental Disorders study (MECA), found that 20.9% of children between the ages of 12 and 17 were seen for mental health services during the prior year. The rates of parent-reported service use in the present study were generally commensurate with those of Leaf et al. (1996). The percentage of children rated as in need of child mental health services by their sixth-grade teacher was also in line with Garrison et al.'s (1992) reported prevalence rate of 22.77% for any mental disorder.

Predictive Validity Analyses

Table 16.3 contains the results of the logistic regression analyses using child self-reports and parent report of child of depressed mood in first grade to predict academic and mental health outcomes at the fourth, sixth, and eighth grades, or ages 10, 12, and 14, respectively. Both the odds ratios (OR) and their 95% confidence intervals (CI) are presented. In the case of continuous predictor variables, the (OR) translated into the change in the odds of the occurrence of the dependent variable given a 1-unit change in the independent variable. The sixth-grade GPA variable was dichotomized into those children with a GPA deemed by the school system to fall in the good-to-excellent range (80 to 100) versus those whose GPA fell into the failing, barely passing, or passing range (60 to 79). The traditional letter-grade equivalents for the latter group were F, D, and C, respectively.

As can be seen in Table 16.3, for each 1-unit increase in boys' first-grade self-reports of depressed mood and feelings, there was a statistically significant increase in the odds of an episode of MDD within the last year, a report of suicidal ideation, having received mental health services on the basis of parent report, being perceived as in need of mental health services by the sixth-grade teacher, and experiencing five or more depressive symptoms during a 2-week period in fourth grade according to parent report on the MFQ. A similar pattern emerged for girls. In contrast to boys, however, no significant relation was found between girls' reports of depressed mood in first grade and parent report of child depressed mood in fourth grade or parent report of child mental health service use. Nor was a significant relationship found between

TABLE 16.3
Analyses of the Predictive Validity of Child and Parent Reports of Depressed Mood When Analyzed Separately

	Child Report				Parent Report			
	Males		Females		Males		Females	
	OR	95% CI	OR	95% CI	OR	95% CI	OR	95% CI
CIDI MDD diagnosis last year, grade 8	4.39	1.02–18.89	3.50	1.05–11.65	.64	.09–4.81	1.95	.57–6.76
CIDI suicidal ideation lifetime, grade 8	2.80	1.23–6.34	3.58	1.54–8.30	1.21	.44–3.35	2.40	1.63–5.57
Need for mental health services for behavioral & emotional problems—teacher report, grade 6	2.11	1.03–4.33	1.99	.76–5.24	4.06	1.62–1.64	1.55	.56–4.31
Mental health services for depression—parent report	3.47	1.38–8.73	1.20	.41–3.56	12.57	4.99–39.53	2.47	.83–7.29
Received special education, grade 6	2.21	1.08–4.54	4.39	1.59–12.20	3.92	1.57–9.79	2.29	.89–5.87
Evaluation for special education, grade 6	3.02	1.39–6.54	6.74	2.23–20.33	2.78	1.08–7.13	1.75	.63–4.88
Grade retention	2.09	1.02–4.27	1.04	.48–2.25	1.19	.47–3.01	.78	.34–1.80
GPA of C or worse, grade 6	5.71	1.95–16.65	3.16	1.32–7.55	8.31	1.68–41.11	.90	.37–2.19

Note: CI = confidence interval; CIDI MDD = Composite International Diagnostic Interview, Major Depressive Disorder; GPA = grade point average; OR = odds ratio.

girls' self-report of depressed mood in first grade and teacher-reported need for child mental health service use in sixth grade. With respect to the academic outcomes, a statistically significant relation was found between first-grade depressed mood and each of the academic outcomes for both boys and girls, with the exception of grade retention for girls. Each of the significant relations for girls remained significant once first-grade achievement was controlled for (Special Education: OR = 3.47, 95% CI 1.20–10.01; Received Evaluation for Special Education: OR = 5.33, 95% CI 1.70–16.75; GPA: OR = 2.47, 95% CI 1.02–5.97). For boys, both GPA (OR = 4.22, 95% CI 1.41–12.67) and grade retention (OR = 2.32, 95% CI 1.10–4.88) remained significant after adjusting for first-grade achievement.

Predictive Validity of Child Versus Parent Reports of Depressed Mood

Table 16.3 also contains the results of the analyses examining the relation between parent perceptions of child depressed mood in fourth grade and the sixth- and eighth-grade outcomes. Child report of depressed mood in first grade was not included in these analyses. Once again, however, ethnicity, free lunch status, intervention condition, parent education, and family structure were included as covariates in each analysis. With respect to boys' academic outcomes, significant relations were found between caregiver perceptions of child mood and sixth-grade GPA, the receipt of special education services, and having been evaluated for special education services. This held true when first-grade standardized achievement was included as a covariate (GPA: OR = 10.31, 95% CI 1.97–54.10; Special Education: OR = 6.10, 95% CI 2.25–16.49; Received Evaluation for Special Education: OR = 4.41, 95% CI, 1.57–12.44). In contrast, the analyses involving girls' academic outcomes yielded no significant results. With respect to mental health outcomes, no significant relations were found between parent perceptions of child depressed mood in fourth grade and a diagnosis of MDD or suicidal ideation in eighth grade for boys. A significant relation was found, however, between parent perceptions of child mood and girls' report of suicidal ideation. Moreover, parent report of child mood significantly predicted boys' mental health service use and teachers' perceptions of the child's need for such services.

Overall, each of the eight comparable prognostic relations (i.e., receipt of special education services, receipt of an evaluation for special education, a GPA of C or worse, grade retention, a diagnosis of MDD, suicidal ideation, parent report of child mental health service use, and teacher perception of the child's need for mental health services) were significant for boys' self-reports of depressed mood, whereas five of eight reached significance for parent reports. For girls, only one of the eight prognostic relations proved significant for parent reports, whereas five of eight reached significance for girls' self-reports of depressed mood in first grade.

Examining the Overlap in the Predictive Validity of Child and Parent Reports of Depressed Mood

Table 16.4 contains the results of those predictive validity analyses, wherein both child- and parent-reported depressed mood were included as predictors of the sixth- and eighth-grade outcomes. The rationale for these analyses is that they provide a means of assessing the overlap between parent and child report in terms of predictive power. If a previously significant relation between child-reported depressed mood and one of the study

TABLE 16.4
Analyses of the Predictive Validity of Child and Parent Reports of Depressed Mood When Child and Parent Reports Are Entered into the Same Model

	Child Report				Parent Report			
	Males		Females		Males		Females	
	OR	95% CI	OR	95% CI	OR	95% CI	OR	95% CI
CIDI MDD diagnosis last year, grade 8	4.41	1.03–18.99	3.32	.98–11.24	.61	.80–4.72	1.65	.47–5.87
CIDI suicidal ideation lifetime, grade 8	2.81	1.24–6.37	3.45	1.48–8.07	1.23	.44–3.43	2.25	.96–5.29
Mental health services for depression—parent report	3.00	1.04–8.69	.89	.24–3.30	12.75	4.07–39.98	2.48	.84–7.34
Need for mental health services for emotional problems—teacher report, grade 6	2.17	1.04–4.53	1.94	.73–5.13	4.10	1.64–10.23	1.47	.52–4.12
Received special education services, grade 6	3.41	1.17–9.91	4.33	1.55–12.16	3.98	1.59–9.96	2.19	.84–5.73
Received evaluation for special education, grade 6	3.09	1.41–6.77	6.68	2.20–20.28	2.84	1.10–7.42	1.66	.57–4.80
Grade retention	2.09	1.03–4.28	1.06	.49–2.29	1.21	.48–3.04	.77	.33–1.79
GPA of C or worse, grade 6	5.68	1.95–16.53	3.19	1.34–7.64	9.14	1.69–49.36	.84	.34–2.05

Note: CI = confidence interval; CIDI MDD = Composite International Diagnostic Interview, Major Depressive Disorder; GPA = grade point average; OR = odds ratio.

outcomes fell to nonsignificance when parent-reported depressed mood was entered into the equation, it would then be concluded that the child reports did not make a unique contribution to the prediction of the outcome of interest. In only one instance did a significant relation fall to nonsignificance upon entering parent reports of child mood into the equation (a diagnosis of MDD for girls). The change in the significance level and the size of the odds ratio was quite small, however.

DISCUSSION

In a series of studies, we have assessed the test–retest reliability and internal consistency of young children's reports of depressed mood and feelings (Edelsohn et al., 1992; Ialongo et al., 1993). We have also examined the extent to which these self-reports predict concurrent and later indices of adaptive functioning. The purpose in doing so has been to shed further light on the question of whether young children are reliable and valid reporters of their moods and feelings. The answer to this question is particularly relevant to psychiatric epidemiologists interested in estimating the prevalence of mood disorders among young children, and who are aware of the limitations of parent reports of depressed mood and feelings in older children and adolescents. That is, whereas parent reports tend to be highly specific, they tend to be less sensitive than child and adolescent self-reports (Angold, 1988).

Our previous reports demonstrated that self-reports of depressed mood and feelings by young children (i.e., 5- to 6-year-olds) were reasonably stable over 10- to 14-day intervals and that they were related to concurrent and future indices of adaptive functioning. In this report, besides examining the extent to which first graders' self-reports of depressed mood predict later indices of adaptive functioning, the prognostic power of these early self-reports with respect to parent report of child depressed mood, mental health service use, suicidal ideation, and a diagnosis of major depressive disorder by age 14 years was also studied. In addition to finding consistent relations between first-grade self-reports of depressed mood and later academic functioning, substantial evidence of the prognostic power of these first grade self-reports with respect to mental health outcomes in fourth, sixth, and eighth grades was found.

These findings attest to the prognostic power of young children's reports of depressed mood and feelings. Furthermore, although the relations between first-grade self-reports of depressed mood and academic outcomes in middle school were attenuated for boys when first-grade standardized achievement scores were added to the model, first-grade boys' self-reports of depressed mood still made a significant and unique contribution to GPA and grade retention at age 12 years. The degree of prognostic power found is even more remarkable given the group administration procedure used. Greater reliability and prognostic validity might have been attained had an individually administered assessment battery been employed. A one-on-one administration in a confidential location might have allowed the children to be more trusting of the assessment team, and they may, therefore, have been more likely to divulge feelings of depressed mood. A one-on-one assessment may also have allowed the assessors to more carefully probe children's responses and to answer children's questions about the meaning of the items employed. The benefits of a semistructured interview done one-on-one are highlighted by Silverman and Nelles' (1992) results with respect to the short-term test–retest reliability of the MDD module of the Anxiety Disorders Interview for Children. In line with Valla, Bergeron, Berube, Gaudet, and St. Georges (1994), pictorial representations of the feeling states assessed may have further increased reliability and predictive validity.

In and of themselves, these findings on prognostic power do not suggest a causal relation between a depressed mood in first grade and later mental health and academic outcomes. Indeed, the findings may simply reflect the fact that children who fail to meet the academic challenges of first grade are likely to experience emotional distress as a result. In line with Kellam and Rebok's (1992) life course/social field framework, these early academic failures may set the stage for subsequent failures and, thus, increased punishment and reductions in reinforcement from parents, teachers, and peers. This chronic history of failure may result in sustained emotional distress and the risk of MDD. Alternatively, it may be the case that a third variable—such as a chronically poor caregiving environment—may explain both the social adaptational failures and the decrements in psychological well-being. Nevertheless, the prognostic power of these early self-reports suggests that children as young as 5 or 6 years of age are capable of providing valid reports of depressed mood and feelings.

As pointed out earlier, a question that child psychiatric epidemiologists are often faced with is whether to simply rely on parent reports in large field studies of mental disorders in young children. Evidence from Edelbrock et al. (1985) suggests that parent reports are more stable than child reports. Moreover, in the present study, parent reports of child depressed mood were more consistently related to parent- and teacher-reported mental health service need and utilization. Nevertheless, as indicated above, whereas five of eight of the prognostic relations proved significant in the present study for first-grade girls' self-reports of depressed mood, only one of eight proved significant for parent reports. Since the mental health service utilization data were collected in fourth and sixth grades, parents were at a decided advantage in terms of the length of the prognostic interval. Consequently, these data may underestimate the prognostic power of child self-reports relative to parent report of child depressed mood.

A few caveats are in order. First, as was found in Ialongo et al. (1993), the stability of children's self-reports of depressed mood does increase with age. Moreover, as indicated previously, parent reports show considerably more stability than young children's reports. Third, these results should not be construed as evidence that structured interviews like the Diagnostic Interview Schedule for Children (DISC 2.1) (Shaffer, Fisher, Piacentini, Schwab-Stone, & Wicks, 1991) can be used successfully with young children. Relative to structured diagnostic interviews such as the DISC, the demands the CDI (used in our studies) places on children's recall of symptoms, including their onset, offset, and co-occurrence, are minimal. The children in the present study were simply asked to report on whether they had experienced the "feelings" included in the CDI over the last 2 weeks. Moreover, the CDI item stems are relatively brief and simply worded as compared with the DISC. Recent studies of the test–retest reliability of the DISC suggest that the greater the length of the item, the greater the reduction in test–retest reliability (Fallon & Schwab-Stone, 1994; Perez, Ascaso, Domenech-Massons, & de la Osa Chaparro, 1998). This was also the case for those DISC items that required recall of onset and offset of symptoms and the temporal relations between the onset of symptoms and impairments in adaptive functioning (Perez et al., 1998). The CDI does not include any such items, nor does it make such demands on recall.

To summarize, first graders' reports of depressed mood and feelings appear to have considerable prognostic power with respect to academic performance, psychological well-being, and mental health service need and use in early adolescence. These data are consistent with the results of previous studies that suggest that children as young as 5 or 6 years of age can report with reasonable reliability and validity on their mood and feelings. Thus, these results contradict the prevailing wisdom that young children cannot be counted on to provide either reliable or valid reports of depressed mood and feelings in large-scale epidemiologic field studies of child development and psychopathology. As indicated previously, the suggestion is not being made that these results argue for the use of highly structured and cognitively demanding structured interviews such as the DISC with 5- or 6-year-olds. Nor are the considerable variations in the validity and reliability of young children's reports of depressed mood and feelings being disregarded. Rather, the contention is that reliable and valid reports of depressed mood and feelings can be obtained using scales such as the CDI, which contain items that are simply worded and short, and that place limited demands on memory.

Of course, the present study was not without limitations. First, it was not designed as a study of the reliability and validity of young children as reporters of depressed mood and feelings. For example, parent reports of a depressed mood were not obtained until fourth grade. Nor were there any measures of cognitive developmental level vis-à-vis Piagetian stages to study variation in reliability and validity as a function of a stage of development. Perhaps the most significant limitation was the degree of missing data, particularly at age 14 years. Given, however, that the results of the present study are consistent with those of Edelsohn et al. (1992) and Ialongo et al. (1993), confidence in the study's conclusions is justified. Certainly, there is room for future longitudinal work that builds on the work presented here and explores the extent and sources of variation in the reliability and validity of child reports of depressed mood and feelings. Also worthy of continued study is the use of pictorial representations of feeling states in measures of children's mood and feelings (Valla et al., 1994). Finally, further study is necessary to determine whether the relations between first graders' self-reports of depressed mood and later adaptation and psychological well-being is specific to depressed mood. Indeed, it may be the case that the relation found in the present study could be explained by a co-occurring mental disorder or syndrome that was not measured.

ACKNOWLEDGMENTS

This article was supported by National Institute of Mental Health grants 5 PO MH38725 and RO 1 MH57005-02A and National Institute on Drug Abuse grant ROl DA11796-01A1. The authors would like to thank the Baltimore City Public Schools for their continuing collaborative efforts and the parents, children, teachers, and principals who participated.

ADDRESSES AND AFFILIATIONS

Corresponding author: Nicholas S. Ialongo, Department of Mental Hygiene, School of Hygiene and Public Health, Johns Hopkins University, 624 North Broadway, Baltimore, MD 21205; e-mail: nialongo@jhsph.edu. Sheppard G. Kellam is also at Johns Hopkins University; and Gail Edelsohn is at Jefferson Medical College, Philadelphia, PA.

REFERENCES

Abramson, L., Seligman, M., & Teasdale, J. D. (1978). Learned helplessness in humans: critique and reformulation. *Journal of Abnormal Psychology, 37,* 49–74.

American Psychiatric Association. (1987). *Diagnostic and statistical manual of mental disorders* (3rd ed., rev.) Washington, D.C.: American Psychiatric Publishing.

American Psychiatric Association. (1994). *Diagnostic and statistical manual of mental disorders.* Washington, D.C.: American Psychiatric Publishing.

Angold, A. (1988). Childhood and adolescent depression: I. Epidemiological and aetiological aspects. *British Journal of Psychiatry, 152,* 601–617.

Angold, A., Costello, E. J., Pickles, A., Winder, F., & Silver, D. (1987). *The development of a questionnaire for use in epidemiological studies of depression in children and adolescents.* Unpublished manuscript, London University.

Beck, A. T. (1974). The development of depression: a cognitive model. In R. M. Friedman & M. M. Katz (Eds.), *The psychology of depression: contemporary theory and research.* New York: Wiley.

Beizer-Seidner, L., Stipek, D. J., & Deitch Feshbach, N. (1985). A developmental analysis of elementary school-aged children's concepts of pride and embarrassment. *Child Development, 59,* 367–377.

Byrnes, J., & Wasik, B. (1991). Role of conceptual knowledge in mathematical procedure learning. *Developmental Psychology, 27,* 777–786.

Cowan, P. (1978). *Piaget with feeling: cognitive, social and emotional dimensions.* New York: Holt, Rinehart, & Winston.

Digdon, N., & Gotlib, I. H. (1985). Developmental considerations in the study of childhood depression. *Developmental Review, 5,* 162–199.

Edelbrock, C., Costello, A. J., Dulcan, M. K., Kalas, R., & Conover, N. C. (1985). Age differences in the reliability of the psychiatric interview of the child. *Child Development, 56,* 265–275.

Edelsohn, G., Ialongo, N., Werthamer-Larsson, L., Crockett, L., & Kellam, S. (1992). Self-reported depressive symptoms in first grade children: developmentally transient phenomena? *Journal of the American Academy of Child and Adolescent Psychiatry, 31,* 282–290.

Fallon, T., & Schwab-Stone, M. (1994). Determinants of reliability in psychiatric surveys of children aged 6-12. *Journal of Child Psychology and Psychiatry, 35,* 1391–1408.

Friedman, W. J. (1991). The development of children's memory for past events. *Child Development, 62,* 139–155.

Garrison, C. Z., Addy, C. L., Jackson, K. L., McKeown, R. E., & Waller, J. L. (1992). Major depressive disorder and dysthymia in young adolescents. *American Journal of Epidemiology, 135,* 792–802.

Harter, S. (1986). Processes underlying the construction, maintenance, and enhancement of self-concept in children. In J. Suis & A. Greenwald (Eds.), *Psychological perspectives on the self* (pp. 137–181). Hillsdale, NJ: Erlbaum.

Hergenrather, J. R., & Rabinowitz, M. (1991). Age related differences in the organization of children's knowledge of illness. *Developmental Psychology, 27,* 952–959.

Ialongo, N., Edelsohn, G., Werthamer-Larsson, L., Crockett, L., & Kellam, S. (1993). Are self-reported depressive symptoms in first-grade children developmentally transient phenomena? A further look. *Development and Psychopathology, 5,* 431–455.

Kann, L., Kinchen S. A., Williams, B. I., Ross, J., Lowry, R., Hill, C., Grunbaum, J., Blumson, P. S., Collins, J., & Kolbe, J. (1998). Youth risk behavior surveillance—United States, 1997. *Morbidity and Mortality Weekly Report Surveillance Summary, 47* (SS-3), 1–89.

Kellam, S., & Rebok, G. (1992). Building developmental and etiological theory through epidemiologically based preventive intervention trials. In J. McCord &

R. E. Tremblay (Eds.), *Preventing antisocial behavior: interventions from birth through adolescence* (pp. 162–195). New York: Neale Watson Academic Publishers.

Kessler, R., McGonagle, K., Zhao, S., Nelson, C. B., Hughes, M., Eshleman, S., Wittchen, H., & Kendler, K. (1994). Lifetime and 12-month prevalence of DSM-III-R psychiatric disorders in the United States. *Archives of General Psychiatry, 51,* 8–19.

Kovacs, M. (1983). *The Children's Depression Inventory: a self-rated depression scale for school-age youngsters.* Unpublished manuscript, University of Pittsburgh.

Kovacs, M. (1986). A developmental perspective on methods and measures in the assessment of depressive disorders: the clinical interview. In M. Rutter, C. Izard, & P. Read (Eds.), *Depression in young people* (pp. 435–465). New York: Guilford Press.

Leaf, P., Alegria, M., Cohen, P., Goodman, S., Horwitz, S., Hoven, C., Narrow, W., Vaden-Kiernan, M., & Regier, D. (1996). Mental health service use in the community: results from the four community MECA study. *Journal of the American Academy of Child and Adolescent Psychiatry, 35,* 889–897.

Lefkowitz, M. M., & Burton, N. (1978). Childhood depression: a critique of the concept. *Psychological Bulletin, 87,* 191–194.

Perez, R. G., Ascaso, L. E., Domenech-Massons, J. M., & de la Osa Chaparro, N. (1998). Characteristics of the subject and interview influencing the test-retest reliability of the Diagnostic Interview for Children and Adolescents—Revised. *Journal of Child Psychology and Psychiatry, 39,* 963–972.

Russell, J. A. (1990). The preschooler's understanding of the causes and consequences of emotions. *Child Development, 61,* 1872–1881.

Saylor, C., Finch, A., Spirito, A., & Bennett, B. (1984). The children's depression inventory: a systematic evaluation of psychometric properties. *Journal of Consulting Clinical Psychology, 52,* 955–967.

Shaffer, D., Fisher, P., Piacentini, J., Schwab-Stone, M., & Wicks, J. (1991). *Diagnostic Interview Schedule for Children (DISC 2.25).* New York: New York State Psychiatric Institute.

Silverman, W. K., & Eisen, A. R. (1992). Age differences in the reliability of parent and child reports of child anxious symptomatology using a structured interview. *Journal of the American Academy of Child and Adolescent Psychiatry, 31,* 117–124.

Silverman, W. K., & Nelles W B. (1988). Anxiety Disorders Interview Schedule for Children. *Journal of the American Academy of Child and Adolescent Psychiatry, 27,* 772–778.

Valla, J., Bergeron, L., Berube, H., Gaudet, N., & St. Georges, M. (1994). A structured pictorial questionnaire to assess DSM-III-R based diagnoses in children (6–11 years): development, validity, and reliability. *Journal of Abnormal Child Psychology, 22,* 403–424.

Wardrop, J. L. (1989). Review of the California Achievement Tests, Forms E and F. In J. Close Conoley & J. Kramer (Eds.), *The tenth mental measurements yearbook* (pp. 128–133), Lincoln: University of Nebraska Press.

Weisz, J. R. (1986). Understanding the developing understanding of control. In M. Perlmutter (Ed.), *Cognitive perspectives on children's social and behavioral develop-*

ment: the Minnesota symposia on child psychology (Vol. 18, pp. 219–275). Hillsdale, NJ: Erlbaum.

Weisz, J. R., Weiss, B., Wasserman, A., & Rintoul, B. (1987). Control-related beliefs and depression among clinic-referred children and adolescents. *Journal of Abnormal Psychology, 96,* 58–63.

Part IV

CULTURE AND SOCIETY

17

Mothers' Functioning and Children's Symptoms 5 Years after a SCUD Missile Attack

Nathaniel Laor, Leo Wolmer, and Donald J. Cohen

Objective: *The authors assessed the long-term consequences of the SCUD missile attack in Israel on children as a function of their mothers' psychological functioning, family cohesion, and the event itself.* ***Method:*** *Five years after the Gulf War, the authors assessed the internalizing, externalizing, stress, and posttraumatic symptoms of 81 children aged 8 to 10 years whose homes were damaged in the SCUD missile attack, as well as general and posttraumatic symptoms, defensive style, and object relations in their mothers.* ***Results:*** *There was a significant decrease in severity in most symptom domains and an increase in avoidant symptoms in the children. Greater severity of symptoms was associated with being displaced, living in a family with inadequate cohesion, and having a mother with poor psychological functioning. The association between the symptoms of children and mothers was stronger among the younger children. Posttraumatic symptoms increased in one third of the children and decreased in one-third over the last 30 months of the study. Severe posttraumatic symptoms were reported in 8% of the children.* ***Conclusions:*** *Despite a continuous decrease in symptom severity, risk factors identified shortly after the Gulf War continued to exert their influence on children 5 years after the traumatic exposure.*

INTRODUCTION

Considerable knowledge has accumulated during the last decade concerning children's responses to disasters.[1–4] Mental health professionals are aware that children, even preschoolers,[5] may display specific posttraumatic symptoms, although they are somewhat different from those reported by adults.[6] Young age,[7] high degree of exposure,[8] poor parental functioning,[9,10] and loss of family member[11] are some of the risk factors that predict poorer psychological functioning. Posttraumatic symptoms tend to decrease with time,[12] although they may have a delayed onset.[13]

The long-term consequences of traumatic events may serve as a suitable research paradigm for the growing field of developmental psychopathology.[14] The present is our third investigation of a group of preschool children whose homes were damaged by SCUD missiles during the 1991 Gulf War. Some of them were displaced as a result. Our earlier studies were conducted 6[15] and 30 months[16] after the conflict, and the present one after 5 years. This longitudinal approach with very young children, seldom reported in the literature,[16] allowed us a unique perspective on the natural course of psychopathological responses in displaced and residentially stable children. Specifically, we made five major observations.

1. Stress symptoms decreased over time in residentially stable children, whereas increased posttraumatic responses persisted in displaced children.
2. The high correlation between the reactions of mothers and their very young children disappeared for older children.
3. Adequate family cohesion was very important for the well-being of the child.
4. Children displayed reasonably adaptive behavior despite the presence of psychological symptoms.
5. The mother's capacity to control mental images had a direct moderating effect on her symptoms and an indirect effect on her child's symptoms. At 30 months after the war, the symptoms of the displaced mothers remained high and predicted a significant amount of the children's symptom levels.

The present study took a closer look at the role of the mothers' psychological functioning 5 years after the war. We sought to answer two main questions: (1) what was the natural course of the general (internalizing, externalizing, and stress) and specific (intrusion, avoidance or numbing, and arousal) posttraumatic symptoms of displaced and residentially stable children? and (2) how did the mothers' symptoms, maturity of defenses, object relations, and cognitive capacity to control mental images, as well as family functioning, affect the long-term adaptation of their children? On the basis of previous findings, we hypothesized that both general and specific posttraumatic symptoms would decrease over time and that the children's symptoms were associated with poorer psychological functioning in their mothers and families.

METHOD

Subjects and Procedure

We requested the 107 families in the longitudinal cohort who were directly exposed to SCUD missile attacks 5 years earlier, during the Gulf War, to participate in a new interview session. A total of 81 families agreed to do so, 10 refused, and 16 could not be located. Multivariate comparisons between participating and nonparticipating families showed no significant differences in the previous symptoms of the children (internalizing, externalizing, stress, and posttraumatic stress disorder) ($F = 1.72$, $df = 4, 101$, $p > 0.05$) or their mothers (intrusion, avoidance, and total SCL-90-R score) ($F = 1.24$, $df = 3, 104$, $p > 0.05$).

All the families lived in the same neighborhood and had a low socioeconomic level. Forty families were displaced for a period of up to 6 months owing to the considerable damage inflicted on their homes by missiles, and 41 families remained residentially stable. At the first assessment, 30 children were aged 8 years, 29 were aged 9 years, and 22 were aged 10 years.[10,15] There were 24 boys and 57 girls. Experienced assistant researchers interviewed the children (for 1 hour) and the mothers (for 2 hours) individually in their homes. Written informed consent was obtained for all subjects after they received a complete description of the study.

Child Measures

The Child Behavior Checklist[17] covers two symptom domains, internalizing and externalizing. The Preschool Children's Assessment of Stress Scale (unpublished, Mayes and Cohen, Yale Child Study Center, New Haven, Conn.) assesses stress reactions (fear, anxiety, or sleep problems) after a traumatic event (Cronbach's alpha = 0.89). Scales from these two instruments went through factor analysis previously,[15] and three domains of symptoms were defined: internalizing (poor communication, depression, and somatic complaints), externalizing (aggression, delinquency, or hyperactivity), and stress (separation and sleep problems, mood changes, fears, and tension). The Child Posttraumatic Stress Reaction Index[8] is a 20-item, semistructured interview that covers the specific posttraumatic symptom domains of intrusion, avoidance or numbing, and arousal.

Maternal Measures

The Bell Object Relations Inventory[18] assesses four domains of object relations: alienation, egocentricity, insecure attachment, and social incompetence.

The Defense Style Questionnaire[19] provides information on three defense styles: immature, neurotic, and mature. The SCL-90-R[20] measures general symptom profiles with the Global Severity Index. The Impact of Event Scale[21] measures intrusive and avoidant symptoms. Richardson's revision[22] of the Gordon Test of Visual Imagery Control, a 12-item scale, measures the capacity to manipulate the mental image of "a car" (i.e., change its color, position, or movement). Image control has been found to correlate with the mature development of personality characteristics,[23] intelligence,[24] creativity,[25] cognitive performance,[26] and the affective regulation of psychophysiological responses after traumatic events.[27]

At the 30-month assessment, the mothers also completed the Family Adaptability and Cohesion Evaluation Scales.[28] This instrument assesses the capacity of the family to change its power structure, roles, and norms as a result of external pressures (adaptability) and the affective bonds between family members (cohesion). In the Family Adaptability and Cohesion Evaluation Scales, extreme scores reflect worse family functioning.

RESULTS

On the basis of their level of symptoms (SCL-90-R score), object relations (score on Bell Object Relations Inventory), and defense style (score on Defense Style Questionnaire's immature style), we divided the mothers into three categories of psychological functioning ($N = 27$ in each). Mothers with poor functioning had a score above the median on the SCL-90-R and the Defense Style Questionnaire's immature style and a score below the median on the Bell Object Relations Inventory. Mothers with moderate functioning had a score above the median on one or two of these measures and a score below the median on the other(s). Mothers with good functioning had a score below the median on the SCL-90-R and the Defense Style Questionnaire's immature style and a score above the median on the Bell Object Relations Inventory. The intercorrelations between these scores were as follows ($N = 81$): SCL-90-R and Bell Object Relations Inventory: $r = -0.53$; SCL-90-R and Defense Style Questionnaire: $r = 0.49$; Bell Object Relations Inventory and Defense Style Questionnaire: $r = -0.75$; all $p < 0.001$.

Children's Symptoms

Table 17.1 summarizes the symptom scores of the displaced and residentially stable groups of children at three time points: 6 months, 30 months, and 5 years after the missile attack. Multivariate analysis of variance (MANOVA) with repeated measures (group by mother's functioning by time) revealed that irrespective of the mother's functioning (good, moderate, or poor; $p > 0.05$ for

TABLE 17.1

Symptoms of Displaced and Residentially Stable Israeli Children at Three Time Points after the Gulf War

	Score												MANOVA					
	Displaced Children (N = 40)						Residentially Stable Children (N = 41)											
	At 6 Months		At 30 Months		At 5 Years		At 6 Months		At 30 Months		At 5 years		Time		Group		Time by Group	
Symptom Measure	Mean	SD	Mean	SD	Mean	SD	Mean	SD	Mean	SD	Mean	SD	F	df	F	df	F	df
Symptom domains[a]																		
Internalizing	0.88	1.11	0.83	0.73	0.88	0.90	0.64	0.85	0.60	0.66	0.57	0.42	0.13	2,77	3.33	1,78	0.07	2,77
Externalizing	2.73	2.11	2.51	1.83	2.12	2.03	2.33	1.88	2.17	1.86	1.71	1.09	7.32**	2,78	1.34	1,79	0.00	2,78
Stress	43.39	18.18	29.70	13.72	27.87	10.35	29.45	12.51	25.01	10.55	23.30	7.28	24.50**	2,75	11.35**	1,76	4.76*	2,75
Child Posttraumatic Stress Reaction Index[a,b]																		
Total			23.62	11.33	23.44	12.27			19.33	10.19	19.32	11.07	2.97	1,75	3.72	1,75	1.38	1,75
Intrusion			1.45	0.92	1.17	0.77			1.00	0.89	0.98	0.74	9.00**	1,75	5.51*	1,75	0.39	1,75
Avoidance			0.97	0.75	1.37	0.71			0.78	0.55	1.03	0.76	6.12*	1,75	0.48	1,75	2.78	1,75
Arousal			1.03	0.69	0.97	0.84			1.16	0.65	0.72	0.60						

[a]Resulting from factor analysis of scales from Child Behavior Checklist and Preschool Children's Assessment of Stress Scale.

[b]Not administered at 6 months.

*p < .05. ** p < .005.

all interactions), there was an overall significant decrease in the child's externalizing symptoms ($F = 7.62$, $df = 2, 74$, $p < 0.001$) and stress ($F = 20.60$, $df = 2, 71$, $p < 0.0001$) but not in internalizing symptoms ($p > 0.05$). The decrease in the externalizing of symptoms from 30 months to the present assessment was significant ($F = 7.24$, $df = 1, 78$, $p < 0.01$), but the decrease in stress symptoms was marginal ($F = 3.47$, $df = 1, 77$, $p = 0.07$). Also a group-by-time interaction revealed that the decrease in stress symptoms was more remarkable in displaced children ($F = 3.33$, $df = 2, 71$, $p < 0.05$).

With regard to the Child Posttraumatic Stress Reaction Index, analyses showed a significant decrease in arousal symptoms ($F = 4.07$, $df = 1, 71$, $p < 0.05$), no significant changes in intrusive symptoms ($p > 0.05$), and a significant increase in avoidance symptoms ($F = 7.89$, $df = 1, 71$, $p < 0.007$). These effects were independent of the child's group and the mother's category of functioning ($p > 0.05$ for all interactions).

Symptom Severity: Children

A group-by-sex-by-age MANOVA showed that at the last assessment, symptom scores were similar for boys and girls ($F = 0.48$, $df = 7, 68$, $p > 0.05$), as well as for 8-, 9-, and 10-year-olds ($F = 0.46$, $df = 14, 136$, $p > 0.05$). Therefore, age and sex were not considered in the remaining analyses. Displaced children had marginally higher symptom scores than residentially stable children ($F = 1.96$, $df = 7, 68$, $p < 0.08$). For univariate analyses, differences were significant for the internalizing ($F = 3.95$, $df = 1, 79$, $p < 0.05$), stress ($F = 5.36$, $df = 1, 79$, $p < 0.05$), and avoidance ($F = 4.19$, $df = 1, 75$, $p < 0.05$) domains.

Symptom Severity: Mothers

Displaced mothers reported significantly more symptoms than residentially stable mothers (MANOVA, $F = 8.61$, $df = 3, 77$, $p < 0.001$). This was true for scores on the SCL-90-R (mean = 152.7, SD = 64.9, and mean = 126.2, SD = 45.0, respectively) ($F = 4.63$, $df = 1, 79$, $p < 0.05$), Impact of Event Scale intrusive symptoms (mean = 17.4, SD = 7.2, and mean = 11.1, SD = 4.6) ($F = 22.01$, $df = 1, 79$, $p < 0.001$), and Impact of Event Scale avoidance symptoms (mean = 6.5, SD = 4.8, and mean = 14.6, SD = 3.6) ($F = 4.25$, $df = 1, 79$, $p < 0.05$).

Children and Mothers

Table 17.2 presents the correlations between the symptom domains of the children and the psychological functioning variables of the mothers in

TABLE 17.2
Relation of Children's Symptoms and Mothers' Psychological Functioning for 39 Displaced Israeli Families 5 Years After the Gulf War

Measure of Mothers' Functioning	Correlation (r) of Mother's Funtioning to Children's Symptoms			
	Symptom Domains[a]			Child Posttraumatic Stress Reaction Index
	Internalizing	Externalizing	Stress	
SCL-90-R	0.81**	0.40*	0.63**	0.12
Impact of Event Scale				
Intrusion	0.30	0.03	0.25	0.02
Avoidance	0.60**	0.26	0.40*	0.13
Bell Object Relations Inventory	–0.49**	–0.57**	–0.43*	–0.46**
Defense Style Questionnaire				
Mature	–0.16	0.07	-0.11	0.18
Neurotic	0.10	0.32	0.14	0.40*
Immature	0.54**	0.64**	0.52**	0.30

[a]Resulting from factor analysis of scales from Child Behavior Checklist and Preschool Children's Assessment of Stress Scale
*p < 0.005 **p < 0.001

displaced families. Increased symptoms in children were associated with poorer object relations, more immature defenses, and increased psychological symptoms in the mothers. A similar pattern, although with smaller coefficients and marginal statistical significance, appeared in residentially stable families.

MANOVAs were performed to examine differences in symptoms among children of mothers from the three maternal function groups 5 years after the war (Table 17.3). For general symptoms (internalizing, externalizing, and stress), significant differences were noted on multivariate ($F = 4.91$, $df = 6, 154$, $p < 0.0001$) and univariate (all $p < 0.005$) analyses. Duncan's post hoc tests revealed that children of mothers with poor functioning were characterized by greater symptom levels (in all three domains) than children of mothers with good functioning and that children of mothers with moderate functioning showed more internalizing symptoms than children of mothers with good functioning and fewer stress symptoms than children of mothers with poor functioning.

In the Child Posttraumatic Stress Reaction Index domains, multivariate analysis revealed no significant differences ($F = 1.09$, $df = 8, 144$, $p > .05$), but univariate analysis reached significance for the arousal domain ($F = 4.16$ $df = 2, 74$, $p < 0.02$). According to Duncan's post hoc tests, children of

TABLE 17.3
Symptoms of 81 Israeli Children 5 Years After the Gulf War, by Their Mothers' Level of Functioning[a]

	Score of Child[b]					
	Poor Maternal Functioning		Moderate Maternal Functioning		Good Maternal Functioning	
Children's Symptom	Mean	SD	Mean	SD	Mean	SD
Internalizing	1.06_a	0.92	0.70_b	0.62	$0.40_{a,b}$	0.31
Externalizing	2.94_a	2.08	1.62	1.13	1.18_a	0.80
Stress	$29.70_{a,b}$	10.81	26.19_a	6.41	19.83_b	4.22
Score on Child Posttraumatic Stress Reaction Index						
Total	23.51	10.79	21.82	9.87	20.33	12.51
Intrusion (N = 77)	1.17	0.73	1.05	0.77	1.01	0.79
Avoidance (N = 77)	1.39	0.87	1.21	0.60	0.99	0.75
Arousal (N = 77)	1.07_a	0.91	0.93	0.65	0.50_a	0.48

[a]Categorized by means of scores on the SCL-90-R, the intrusion and avoidance domains of the Impact of Event Scale, the Bell Object Relations Inventory, and the mature, neurotic, and immature dimensions of the Defense Style Questionnaire. See text for full explanation.
[b]Similar subscripts indicate a significant difference between groups according to Duncan test.

mothers with good functioning reported fewer arousal symptoms than children with mothers with moderate and poor functioning.

Posttraumatic Stress

On the basis of the guidelines proposed by Pynoos et al.,[29] children were classified as suffering from doubtful, mild, moderate, or severe posttraumatic symptoms 30 months and 5 years after the war. (No child met the criteria for the very severe category.)

Table 17.4 shows that 28 out of 77 children (36%) were classified in the same category at the two time points, whereas 26 children (34%) "advanced" one (N = 21, 27%) or two (N = 5, 6%) categories, and 23 children (30%) "receded" one (N = 18, 23%) or two (N = 5, 6%) categories.

Analysis of the "mobility" of the children across symptom categories by the functioning of the mothers yielded the following findings:

1. All children who were classified as having doubtful posttraumatic symptoms at 30 months and had mothers with poor functioning ($N = 4$) showed a deterioration in symptoms and had advanced one or two categories at 5 years.

2. All children classified as having mild posttraumatic symptoms at 30 months and severe symptoms at 5 years ($N = 3$) had mothers with poor functioning.
3. The two children who were characterized as having severe posttraumatic symptoms at 30 months and had mothers with good functioning had receded two or three categories at 5 years.
4. No child classified as having severe posttraumatic symptoms at 5 years had a mother with good functioning.

Family Functioning

In displaced families, Pearson's correlations between family functioning at 30 months and the child's symptoms 5 years after the war yielded an association between adequate cohesion and fewer symptoms of externalizing ($r = 0.59$, $df = 79$, $p < 0.001$), internalizing ($r = 0.65$, $df = 79$, $p < 0.001$), and stress ($r = 0.64$, $df = 79$, $p < 0.001$). Also, adequate adaptability was associated with fewer internalizing ($r = 0.40$, $df = 79$, $p < 0.01$) and stress ($r = 0.35$, $df = 79$, $p < .02$) symptoms. In residentially stable families, there was no association between family functioning and the child's symptoms (all $p > .05$).

Children's Ages

Pearson's correlations tested how the children's symptoms by age group related to the mothers' symptoms (per SCL-90-R scores) and object relations 5 years after the war. The highest correlations were found for the youngest group (median = 0.60, range = 0.32 to 0.76), whereas most of the lowest correlations appeared in the oldest group (median = 0.24, range = 0.06 to 0.64).

TABLE 17.4
Relation of Level of Posttraumatic Symptoms of 77 Israeli Children 30 Months after the Gulf War to Level at 5 Years

Posttraumatic Symptoms at 5 Years[a]	Number of Children with Posttraumatic Symptoms at 30 Months[a]			
	Doubtful	Mild	Moderate	Severe
Doubtful	7	7	2	1
Mild	11	12	9	2
Moderate	2	8	8	2
Severe	0	3	2	1

[a]Determined from score on Child Posttraumatic Stress Reaction Index.

Integrative Analyses

Finally, hierarchical regression analyses were performed with the children's symptom domains as the dependent variables. The children's age and sex made no significant contribution in the analyses. Inadequate family cohesion and the mother's symptoms contributed to the explained variance of internalizing ($F = 36.61$, $df = 2, 71$, $p < 0.0001$, $R = 0.71$), externalizing ($F = 19.34$, $df = 2, 71$, $p < 0.0001$, $R = 0.59$), and stress ($F = 29.51$, $df = 3, 70$, $p < 0.0001$, $R = 0.75$) symptoms of the child. The mother's capacity to control mental images (per score on Gordon Test of Visual Imagery Control) also contributed significantly to the statistical prediction of stress symptoms, and it was the only predictor of the child's specific posttraumatic symptoms ($F = 4.40$, $df = 1, 67$, $p < 0.05$, $R = 0.25$). Family's inadequate cohesion, mother's maturity of defenses, and length of the evacuation period after the missile attack explained about 60% of the variance in the mother's symptoms ($F = 24.20$, $df = 4, 67$, $p < 0.0001$, $R = 0.77$).

DISCUSSION

This 5-year follow-up is the third report on the natural course of symptoms of preschool children and their mothers exposed to a missile attack. It focused on the symptoms of the children and the mothers and the critical role of the mother's psychological functioning and the adequacy of family cohesion.

Children's Symptoms

Five years after the traumatic event, the children's symptom profiles, both general (externalizing and stress), as well as specific posttraumatic symptoms (arousal), showed a significant decrease, regardless of gender or age. At the same time, however, there was a significant increase in the symptoms of avoidance. This may reflect the construction of long-term coping mechanisms to contain the distress generated by reexperiencing the traumatic event.[30]

The present study replicated our original finding that displaced children show greater symptoms than residentially stable ones (see, also, reference 31). Here, the specific symptom domains involved were internalizing, stress, and avoidance but not externalizing, intrusion, and arousal. We speculate that in children, the long-term struggle with traumatic displacement is expressed in implosive symptoms (e.g., internalizing and avoidance) rather than in the more externally oriented explosive symptoms (e.g., externalizing, intrusion, and arousal). By contrast, the displaced mothers reported significantly more general—as well as posttraumatic—symptoms than the residentially stable mothers.

Children and Mothers

The association between increased symptoms in the child and poor psychological functioning in the mother was clear and robust. It should be stressed that the mothers' psychological profile was assessed by means of three intercorrelated domains: competence to relate securely (object relations), skill in coping with internal and external stress (defensive style), and behavioral expressions of psychological dysfunction (symptoms). We observed that mothers with the poorest functioning had children with the most symptoms, whereas those with the best functioning had children with the least symptoms. Furthermore, the mothers' psychological functioning seemed to have more of an effect on the "mobility" of the children across posttraumatic severity categories from the 30-month to the 5-year assessment than on the amount of posttraumatic symptoms per se. It appears that good functioning in the mothers helped the children "recede" from the severe categories, whereas their poor functioning resulted in their children "advancing" to the severe categories.

A total of 8% (6 out of 77) of the children reported having severe posttraumatic symptoms 30 months and 5 years after the war. However, half the children classified after 5 years as having severe symptoms had mild symptoms at the previous assessment. About one third of the children in our study group showed the same severity of symptoms at both assessments (e.g., mild to mild), one third showed a decrease in symptom severity (e.g., moderate to mild), and one third showed an increase in severity (e.g., moderate to severe). Overall, the severity category of about two thirds of the children was unstable. These data indicate that children might develop severe posttraumatic symptoms during the 5-year period after exposure to a traumatic event, even if symptoms were of moderate severity at a previous assessment (see, also, reference 13). In our children, this development was partly explained by poor psychological functioning in the mother.

Child's Age

Although the symptoms of the children in our group were not associated with age, the correlations between the symptoms of the mothers and the children were different for the 8-, 9-, and 10-year-olds; there were significantly higher correlations in the group with the youngest members (who were 3 years old during the war). This finding is in line with our assessments at 6 and 30 months[10,15] and its long-term and entrenched effect strengthens our suggestion that the potential impact of traumatic events on very young children is twofold—direct and indirect—through their effect on the caretaker. Furthermore, our longitudinal study supports the notion of a traumatic impact on the parent-child dyad, which, in younger children, is integral to the processing of the adverse experience.[32]

Family Functioning

Family functioning at 30 months exerted a long-term effect on the children's symptoms. This was true mainly for the displaced children, who experienced multiple traumas: the missile attacks, the destruction of their homes, and the physical displacement. (We could not differentiate among these traumas because all the displaced families lost their homes in the missile attacks. For the specific impact of the length of the evacuation, see the following.) Of the two family domains we assessed, family cohesion exerted the more powerful influence. Specifically, the combination of family displacement and a disengaged or enmeshed family style apparently induces a significant amount of stress in children, which not only jeopardizes their capacity to recover from the initial trauma but may also result in an increase in symptoms. Conversely, a displaced family characterized by adequate cohesion (not too loose or too tight) appears to provide a favorable environment for the child to work through the initial impact of the trauma and the consequent stressful reaction. In the residentially stable families, there was no association between family functioning and the children's symptoms. We conclude that only under the stressful condition of displacement leading to increased symptoms is family functioning correlated with general symptoms of distress 5 years after the traumatic event.

Integrative Analyses

Our integrative analyses showed how the long-term effect of trauma in children is maintained by the combination of variables from different sources: symptoms, defensive style, and capacity to control mental imagery in the mothers, cohesion in the family, and length of the evacuation period.

Different variables predicted different aspects of the children's symptoms. Internalizing and externalizing symptoms were directly predicted by the mothers' general symptoms (SCL-90-R score) and by their family's cohesion. The prediction of stress symptoms included also the mothers' capacity to control mental images, which was the only predictor of the specific posttraumatic symptoms. Moreover, about 60% of the symptoms of the mothers were explained by their defensive style (more immature and less mature defenses) and (poor) capacity to control mental imagery, taken with the (inadequate) cohesion of the family and the (longer) period of evacuation of the family.

The issue of evacuation and displacement deserves special attention. The displacement of traumatized families and their temporary relocation may lead to social disintegration, with deleterious effects on family functioning (e.g., loss of daily family routine, loss of jobs, and attrition from school). Dysfunctional families serve as poor holding environments for their members, particularly for very young children, who still depend on parental support. In the absence of communal reactivation, the longer the evacuation period, the worse the effects on families and children.

In our previous report (at 30 months after the war), we found that the specific posttraumatic symptoms of the children were predicted by the mothers' symptoms of avoidance. In turn, the latter were explained by the mothers' general symptoms, capacity for image control, cohesion of the family, and length of evacuation. Five years after the war, the mothers' specific symptoms lost their centrality, whereas their nonspecific symptoms predicted the children's symptoms.

Our success in predicting the children's posttraumatic symptoms was limited (only 6%). However, other variables related to the child (e.g., social support, IQ, and defense style) may have a significant effect in the long-term persistence of posttraumatic symptoms. As development proceeds, the child's strengths and weaknesses begin to play a more central role in the dynamic interplay that involves the event and the responses of the immediate and distant environment, leading to long-term adaptation to the trauma.[2] The increase in avoidance symptoms at this phase may reflect this interplay and demands further study.

Limitations

Although it was large enough to detect significant differences, our group size has decreased since the time of our previous report. A larger group would provide more statistical power for generalizing the results. This is especially true when we consider that the posttraumatic symptoms in our group were moderate. Second, we lack information on the fathers. These data could help us understand the symptomatic changes in some children over time (e.g., increase in avoidance symptoms). Third, we lack information on the coping behavior and intelligence level of the children. As development proceeds, these domains may take a more significant part in the process culminating in symptom expression.

Clinical Implications

Mental health professionals have little control over the occurrence of disasters. However, we have much to do to diminish their psychological consequences.

Our data may be important for clinicians designing therapeutic interventions after disasters, as well as for authorities responsible for displaced populations. On the clinical level, therapeutic interventions involving traumatized children should integrate modules focusing on the family, allowing it to reach an adequate degree of cohesion in which individuals have enough personal space in which to retreat and also allowing the family members to feel supportive of each other. Furthermore, symptomatic mothers, especially of younger children, should be identified and helped, because their short-term and long-term functioning is a powerful risk factor for the children's well-being. Finally, authorities should consider the psychological effects of displacement and shorten its duration as much as possible.

REFERENCES

1. Pfefferbaum B: Posttraumatic stress disorder in children: a review of the past 10 years. *J Am Acad Child Adolesc Psychiatry* 1997;36:1503–1511.
2. Pynoos RS, Steinberg AM, Wraith R: A developmental model of posttraumatic stress disorder in children and adolescents, in Developmental Psychopathology, vol 2. Edited by Cicchetti D, Cohen DJ. New York, John Wiley & Sons, 1995, pp. 72–95.
3. Vogel JM, Vernberg EM: Children's psychological responses to disasters. *J Clin Child Psychol* 1993;22:470–484.
4. Yule W, Williams RM: Post-traumatic stress reactions in children. *J Trauma Stress* 1990;3:279–295.
5. Scheeringa MS, Zeanah CH, Drell MJ, Larrieu JA: Two approaches to the diagnosis of posttraumatic stress disorder in infancy and early childhood. *J Am Acad Child Adolesc Psychiatry* 1995;34:191–200.
6. Terr LC: Psychic trauma in children and adolescents. *Psychiatr Clin North Am* 1985;8:815–835.
7. Green BL, Korol M, Grace MC, Vary MG, Leonard AC, Gleser GC, Smitson-Cohen S: Children and disaster: age, gender, and parental effects on PTSD symptoms. *J Am Acad Child Adolesc Psychiatry* 1991;30:945–951.
8. Pynoos RS, Frederick C, Nader K, Arroyo W, Steinberg A, Eth S, Nunez F, Fairbanks L: Life threat and post-traumatic stress in school-age children. *Arch Gen Psychiatry* 1987;44:1057–1063.
9. Korol M, Green BL, Gleser GC: Children's responses to a nuclear waste disaster: PTSD symptoms and outcome prediction. *J Am Acad Child Adolesc Psychiatry* 1999;38:368–375.
10. Laor N, Wolmer L, Mayes LC, Gershon A, Weizman R, Cohen DJ: Israeli preschoolers under Scuds: a 30-month follow-up. *J Am Acad Child Adolesc Psychiatry* 1997;36:349–356.
11. Pfefferbaum B, Nixon SJ, Tucker PM, Tivis RD, Moore VL, Gurwitch RH, Pynoos RS, Geis HK: Posttraumatic stress responses in bereaved children after the Oklahoma City bombing. *J Am Acad Child Adolesc Psychiatry* 1999;38:1372–1379.

12. Becker DF, Weine SM, Vojvoda D, McGlashan TH: Case series: PTSD symptoms in adolescent survivors of "ethnic cleansing": results from a 1-year follow-up study. *J Am Acad Child Adolesc Psychiatry* 1999;38:775–781.
13. Sack WH, Him C, Dickason D: Twelve-year follow-up study of Khmer youths who suffered massive war trauma as children. *J Am Acad Child Adolesc Psychiatry* 1999;38:1173–1179.
14. Cicchetti D, Cohen DJ (eds): *Developmental Psychopathology.* New York, John Wiley & Sons, 1995.
15. Laor N, Wolmer L, Mayes LC, Golomb A, Silverberg D, Weizman R, Cohen DJ: Israeli preschoolers under Scud missile attacks: a developmental perspective on risk-modifying factors. *Arch Gen Psychiatry* 1996;53:416–423.
16. Green BL, Grace MC, Vary MG, Kramer TL, Gleser GC, Leonard AC: Children of disaster in the second decade: a 17-year follow-up of Buffalo Creek survivors. *J Am Acad Child Adolesc Psychiatry* 1994;33:71–79.
17. Achenbach TM, Edelbrock C: Manual for the Child Behavior Checklist and Revised Child Behavior Profile. Burlington, University of Vermont, Department of Psychiatry, 1983.
18. Bell M, Billington R, Becker B: A scale for assessment of object relations: reliability, validity, and factorial invariance. *J Clin Psychol* 1985;42:733–741.
19. Andrews G, Singh M, Bond M: The Defense Style Questionnaire. *J Nerv Ment Dis* 1993;181:246–256.
20. Derogatis LR: SCL-90-R: Administration, Scoring, and Procedures Manual, I, for the Revised Version. Baltimore, Johns Hopkins University, Clinical Psychometrics Research Unit, 1977.
21. Horowitz MJ, Wilner N, Alvarez W: Impact of Event Scale: a measure of subjective stress. *Psychosom Med* 1979;41:209–218.
22. Richardson A: Mental Imagery. London, Routledge & Kegan Paul, 1969.
23. Kovach BE: Imagery, personality, and emotional response. *J Ment Imagery* 1988;12:63–74.
24. Tedford WH Jr, Penk ML: Intelligence and imagery in personality. *J Pers Assess* 1977;41:405–413.
25. Shaw GA, DeMers ST: The relationship of imagery to originality, flexibility, and fluency in creative thinking. *J Ment Imagery* 1986;10:65–74.
26. Lowrie T: The use of visual imagery as a problem-solving tool: classroom implementation. *J Ment Imagery* 1996;20:127–140.
27. Laor N, Wolmer L, Wiener Z, Reiss A, Muller U, Weizman R, Ron S: The function of image control in the psychophysiology of posttraumatic stress disorder. *J Trauma Stress* 1998;11:679–696.
28. Olson DH: Circumplex Model VII: validation studies and FACES III. *Fam Process* 1986;25:337–351.
29. Pynoos RS, Goenjian A, Tashjian M, Karakashian M, Manjikian R, Manoukian G, Steinberg AM, Fairbanks LA: Posttraumatic stress reactions in children after the 1988 Armenian earthquake. *Br J Psychiatry* 1993;163:239–247.
30. McFarlane AC: Avoidance and intrusion in posttraumatic stress disorder. *J Nerv Ment Dis* 1992;180:439–445.

31. Lonigan CJ, Shannon MP, Taylor CM, Finch AJ Jr, Sallee FR: Children exposed to disaster, II: risk factors for the development of post-traumatic symptomatology. *J Am Acad Child Adolesc Psychiatry* 1994;33:94–105.
32. Wolmer L, Laor N, Gershon A, Mayes L, Cohen DJ: The mother-child facing trauma: a developmental outlook. *J Nerv Ment Dis* 2000;188:409–415.

18

Effects of War and Organized Violence on Children: A Study of Bosnian Refugees in Sweden

Birgitta Angel, Anders Hjern, and David Ingleby

Data from 99 school-aged Bosnian refugee children living in Sweden were analyzed to reveal the patterns of war stress experienced and the relation between these stressors and current psychological problems. A significant pattern of associations emerged. When children had experienced much stress, talking about their experiences seemed to exacerbate their negative effects.

Over the last half-century, the incidence of armed conflict worldwide has increased relentlessly (Gantzel & Schwinghammer, 1995). Most of these conflicts are inside national boundaries and their victims are mainly civilians; inevitably, a substantial proportion of these are children. Though precise figures are impossible to establish, it is an inescapable fact that war and organized violence constitute a major threat to the well-being of a large and steadily increasing number of children in the world.

Even when children and their caregivers succeed in finding refuge in another country, substantial psychosocial problems may remain as a result of preflight experiences and the difficulties of resettlement. Many researchers have documented the psychological problems of refugee children and have attempted to identify their major needs. However, the literature contains substantial disagreements concerning these children's vulnerability and the nature of their problems.

The best way to deal with those problems is also at issue. Psychosocial components have been included in many recent public health programs in war situations (Summerfield, 1999). Many programs for refugee children are based on principles from psychodynamic psychotherapy. This approach presupposes that the main route to psychological health for these children is by "working through" their war experiences, either directly, by talking with adults or in groups, or indirectly, through drawing or drama (Almqvist & Brandell-Forsberg, 1997; Summerfield, 1999). However, as Pfeffenbaum (1997) has pointed out, evidence is still lacking for the efficacy of working-through therapy with children suffering from posttraumatic stress disorder (PTSD). Some authors (Stubbs & Soroya, 1996; Summerfield, 1999) have questioned the effectiveness and appropriateness of these therapeutic principles in programs for refugee children.

In recent years, the settlement of hundreds of thousands of refugee families in Scandinavia has prompted considerable research attention. Several studies of the mental health of newly settled children in families from the Middle East and Latin America have yielded broadly comparable results: that 35% to 50% of the children were suffering from poor mental health. These studies have also identified experiences of organized violence in the home country as an important risk factor for mental health problems in exile (Almqvist & Brandell-Forsberg, 1995; Hjern, Angel, & Jeppsson, 1998; Ljungberg-Miklos, 1989; Montgomery, 1998; Svedin, Back, & Wadsby, 1994). However, not all results are clear-cut; a study of Southeast Asian refugee children in Australia (Krupinski & Burrows, 1986), while confirming the impact of traumatic experiences, demonstrated a general level of mental health that was actually better than that of the general population of children in Australia.

Clearly, there is no simple one-to-one relationship between the experience of organized violence and the occurrence of psychological problems. The children's individual characteristics, among them age, sex, cognitive development, temperament, and specific life events, must also be taken into account. At another level, so must the influence of the immediate social environment (family, school, social network). Finally, the effects of more global social, political, cultural, and historical factors must not be overlooked—the politics of the home country, the situation of refugees and other migrants in the host country, and cultural norms concerning development and the expression of distress.

The heterogeneity of war stressors and their psychological sequelae also needs consideration. However, most studies in the field have focused on a single link—that between extreme events and PTSD—and have not looked for others. Stress, hardship, deprivation, loss, and terrifying incidents are all assimilated to the term "war trauma"; data are then collected on the recognized symptoms of PTSD and the link with war trauma is confirmed, thus perpetuating an essentially one-dimensional paradigm.

BOSNIAN WAR EXPERIENCES

The war in Bosnia-Herzegovina broke out suddenly, in 1992. Within months, hundreds of thousands of Bosnians were forced to leave their homes. Most remained in Bosnia or the neighboring ex-Yugoslavian republics, but several hundred thousand found their way to other countries in Europe. Seventy thousand applied for asylum in Sweden and were temporarily lodged in refugee camps all over the country. In the fall of 1993 the Swedish government granted permanent residence to those who had applied. At the same time it effectively closed its border to spontaneous refugees from Bosnia-Herzegovina by introducing a new visa policy giving priority to victims of the early phases of the war, many of whom were Muslims from areas in the northern and northeastern area of Bosnia, where the Bosnian Serbian republic of Srpska was first declared in 1992 (and internationally recognized in 1995).

The war brought with it a wide range of stressors (in the home country, during the flight, and in the host country) for the civilian population. Children's everyday lives—schooling, nutrition, social networks, play facilities, and health services—were disrupted, and they were plunged into an atmosphere of terror, threat, and uncertainty. Many experienced potentially traumatizing events, including loss of relatives or friends. Their flight was often grueling, and most families were forced to leave all their possessions behind. Though they were largely restored to material security in the host country, the children were left with a fragmented social world and the task of adapting to a strange culture and land.

The aim of this study was systematically to document the stressors that these families had experienced and to relate them to the children's current state of mental health. In doing so, it sought to move beyond the one-dimensional paradigm that links war trauma to PTSD symptoms. By attempting to isolate different dimensions of war stressors and their psychological after-effects, it sought to broaden the scope of the inquiry to other possible links. The study focused on Bosnian refugee families who had settled in the city of Växjö in southern Sweden during 1993–1994, an average of 18 months after they arrived in Sweden.

METHOD

Study Population

All the refugee families from Bosnia-Herzegovina with children born in the home country who had settled in Växjö between November 1993 and November 1994 were invited to participate in the study. Of these 107 families, 97 (91%) came to the first interview, and 92 (86%) to both interviews. Data are presented on the 99 children aged 6 to 16 years from 67 families, who were reported to be in good physical health (two, one with Down's syndrome the other in treatment for leukemia, were excluded from the study group). The children's mean age was 11.3 years, with a range of 6 to 16 years. Seven families came from Sarajevo, in the central part of Bosnia-Herzegovina, but most were refugees from cities in the north and northeast (currently part of the Serbian republic of Srpska). There were three mixed marriages and one Catholic family with a Croatian background; the rest were Muslim.

Most parents had received at least secondary (high school) education, and 20% had been to university. The majority had been skilled or white-collar workers. Correlations between educational level and employment of mothers and fathers were high (alpha = .83 for the four standardized variables), and this permitted the construction of a socioeconomic status (SES) scale for use in subsequent analyses. Comparing the SES scores of families from different locations in Bosnia revealed that those from rural areas scored much lower than the rest and those from the city of Banja Luka much higher.

In 56 (87%) of the families, both parents were present at the time of the interview; in two families, the biological mother and a step-father were present; one family had a single divorced mother, and three had single (war) widowed mothers; the children in one family were living with relatives because their parents had remained in Bosnia-Herzegovina. The number of children of all ages in the families varied little: 51 had two children, seven had three or four, and nine had one child. All but two families had their own apartment at the time of the interview, and all had received permanent residence in Sweden. Three fathers were working, the rest were either studying or in jobtraining, often both, in accordance with the introduction scheme of Växjö's state-funded refugee reception program at the time.

Interviews

The families were informed about the purpose of the study by their community social worker, and received an invitation written in their own language. They were also informed that they could discuss children's and adults' mental health problems with skilled mental health professionals at the interviews. These were conducted during two visits to the child psychiatric clinic in Växjö. Two interviewers, a nurse and a child psychologist/social worker, were always present. All interviewers were experienced members of the child psychiatric hospital staff, and the psychologists and social workers were also members of the refugee team at the clinic. The same nurse was present at all interviews and recorded all information in writing. The head of the clinic's refugee team conducted some of the interviews and gave guidance to the other two child psychologists and the social worker. All interviews were conducted with the help of the same Bosnian interpreter.

Interviews were carried out between March 1994 and February 1995. The first was with parents and children together; it took place about 6.3 months (range 2 to 10 months) after their settlement in Växjö and 18 months (range 2 to 27 months) after they had arrived in Sweden. The interview included structured questions about the family's social background, events during the escape to Sweden, the physical health of each family member, and the present social situation of the family.

During approximately 90 minutes, the interviewers could also observe the children's behavior during interactions with the interviewers, their parents, and play materials. These observations were recorded in clinical notes, and were used in talking with the parents during the second interview.

The second interview, approximately 2 weeks after the first, was with the parent(s) only. They were asked open-ended questions about the family's experiences of war and persecution in the home country, using a method developed by Hjern and Angel (Hjern, 1990). This involved structured questions about the child's psychosocial problems, using a method developed by Cederblad and Höök (1984) in which the interviewer scores each item according to predefined categories on the basis of the open-ended questions. A short version (approximately 30 to 45 minutes) of the method (Hjern et al., 1998), adapted for use by interpreters, was employed because it offered possibilities of comparison with other recent Swedish studies of mental health in children (Cederblad & Höök, 1986; Hjern & Höök, 1990; Ljungberg-Miklos, 1989), and because it allowed the interviewers natural use their observations from the first meeting. Structured questions were also asked about symptoms related to PTSD according to *DSM-III-R* (American Psychiatric Association, 1987), and about parents' attitudes towards talking with their children about the war events they had experienced. Scores on items relating to psychological problems were determined by the interviewer on the basis of observations made during the first visit and of information obtained from the parents at the second. Three or four levels of symptom severity could be coded, depending on the item.

Finally, the interviewer made an overall clinical evaluation of the extent to which both children and parents needed (further) psychiatric treatment. Those judged to be in need of treatment were put in touch with the psychiatric and child psychiatric clinics in the hospital.

ANALYSES

Children's Stress

A "total war stresses" scale was made by summing the standardized scores on the items listed in Figure 18.1. The resulting 15-item scale had an alpha of .80 and was approximately normally distributed. The item "father was soldier" was dropped because of its low item-total correlation. Further analysis showed that this variable had complex associations; children whose father was a soldier ran more risk of threat to the family, difficulty escaping, and need to take shelter, yet members of the family were less likely to be put in a concentration camp.

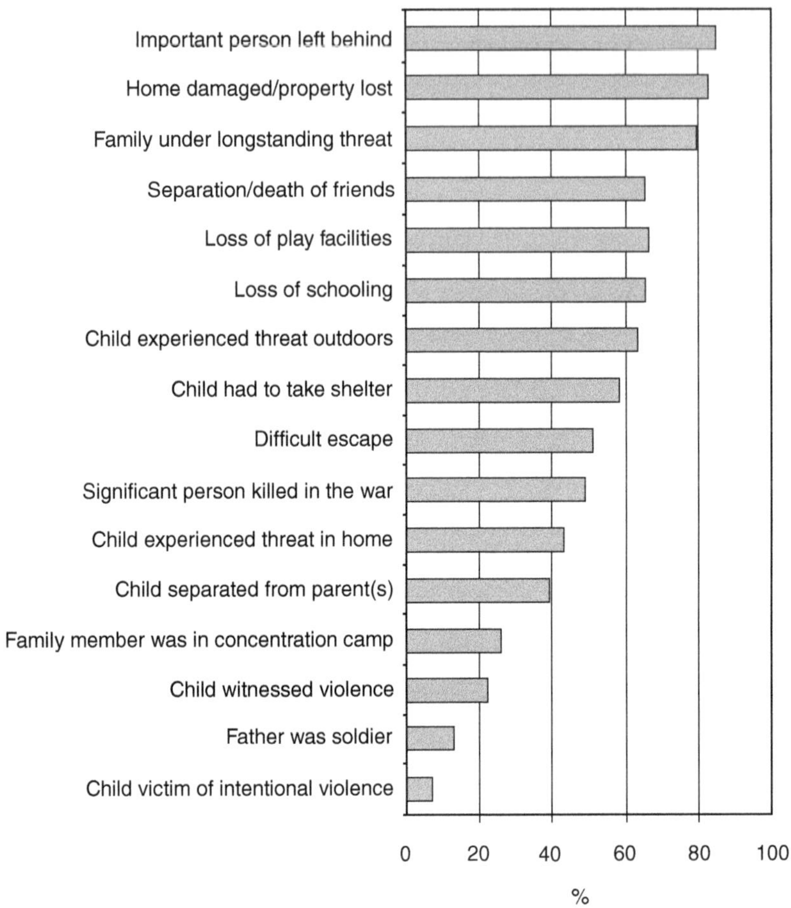

Figure 18.1. War-related stressors and losses experienced by Bosnian children ($N = 99$).

To gain insight into the varieties of stress endured by the children, the total war stresses scale was broken down into subscales that were later used to determine the specific effects of different types of stress on children's problems. Looking for associations at the level of individual items would have generated a matrix of more than 150 correlations, most of them based on rarely occurring items, in which patterns would be hard to find.

Factor analysis (principal components extraction with varimax rotation) was used to determine the structure of the data. For these purposes, the item "father was soldier" was reinserted into the analysis. Five factors, which together explained 64% of the total variance, were extracted. On the basis of these factors, five stress or subscales were constructed by adding up standardized item scores.

These five stressor subscales, each named according to its most important element, were as follows (factor loadings parenthesized): (*a*) violence (α = .68): child witnessed violence (.80), had family member in concentration camp (.66), was victim of intentional violence (.62), lost play facilities (.55), had significant person killed in the war (.44); (*b*) resistance (α = .66): had soldier-father (.78), had difficult escape (.67), had to take shelter (.67), lost play facilities (.51); (*c*) disruption (α = .68): child separated from important friends, possibly by death (.88), lost schooling (.80), had home damaged or lost property (.52). (*d*) threat (α = .63): child threatened in home (.72), family under longstanding threat (.70), child threatened outdoors (.57). and (*e*) loss (α = .61): child separated from parent(s) (.79), left behind important member of extended family (.78), had family member or friend killed (.48).

All these subscales showed a significant degree of correlation with each other, ranging from $r(98) = .26$ to $r(98) = .46$.

Children's Psychological Problems

For statistical reasons, only problems with an incidence of 5% or more were included in the data analysis, thus excluding encopresis, speech problems, headaches, tics, consolation eating, thumb-sucking, and defiance. A scale of "total problems" was made by summing standardized scores on the 16 items (listed in Figures 18.2 and 18.3) that satisfied this criterion, including also parents' assessment of changes in the child as a result of the war. Two PTSD items ("child plays war games" and "child has flashbacks") were omit-

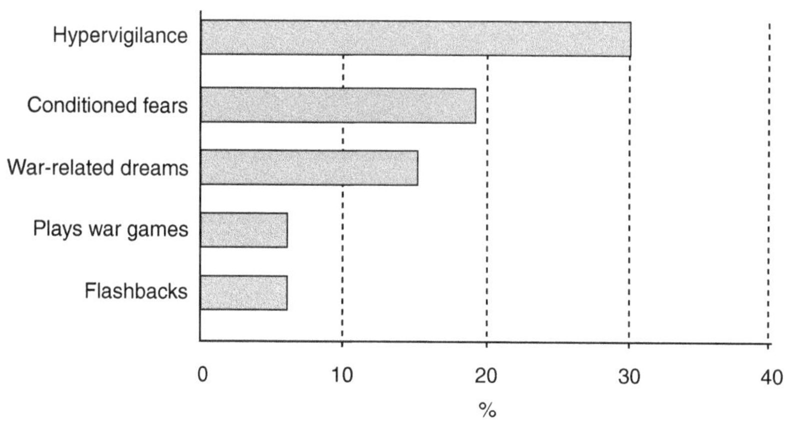

Figure 18.2. PTSD-related symptoms in Bosnian children ($N = 99$).

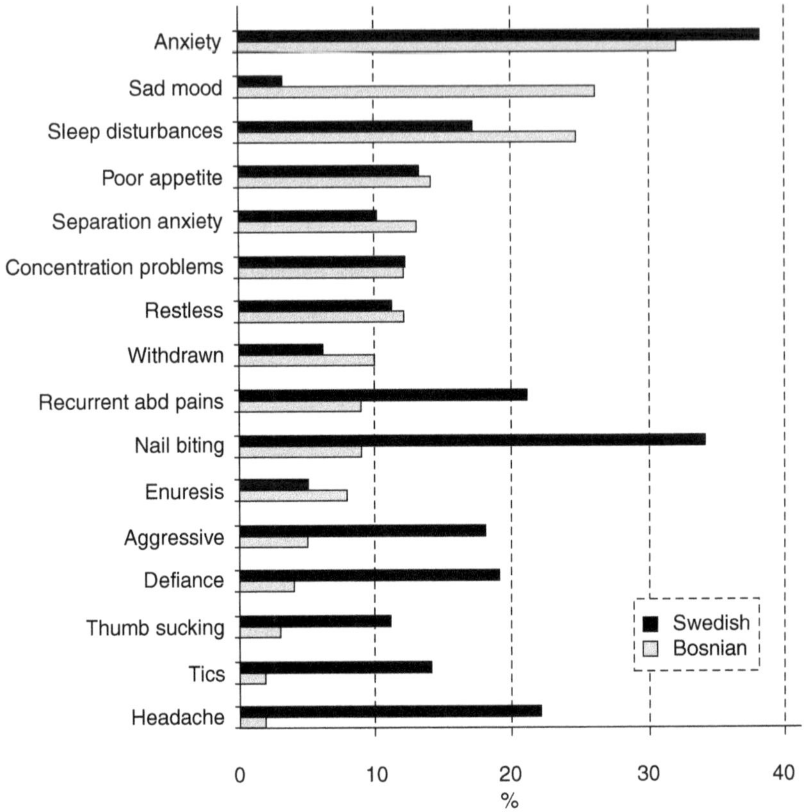

Figure 18.3. Items on Cederblad Symptom Scale: Bosnian 6 to 16-year-olds and Swedish 6 to 15-year-olds.

ted because of their low item-total correlations, as was the item referring to enuresis. The resulting 15-item scale had an alpha of .78. Given its heavily skewed distribution, a square-root transformation was applied.

Using the same procedure as for stressors, problem subscales were constructed on the basis of this list of items (the three items not included in the total problems scale because of low item-total correlations were reinserted into this analysis). Four factors were extracted, which together explained 50% of the total variance.

On the basis of these factors, the following problem subscales were constructed (a square-root transformation was also applied to them): (*a*) behavior problems (α = .71): aggression (.84), restlessness (.79), withdrawal (.62), nail-biting (.53); (*b*) generalized anxiety (α = .72): sleep disturbances (.77), anxiety (.74), separation anxiety (.69), changed by war (.53), concentration problems (.44), war-related dreams (.39); (*c*) phobic and depressive symptoms ($\alpha = .61$): conditioned fears (.74), hypervigilance/startle reactions (.72), sad mood (.51), poor appetite (.45); and (*d*) war preoccupation ($\alpha = .54$): plays war games (.84), flashbacks (.67).

While the first three subscales showed a positive intercorrelation of around .3, the fourth was unrelated to any of them. This suggests that it should not be regarded as an indicator of pathology. Playing war games seems to have been a normal activity among some children, while the question regarding flashbacks may have been misinterpreted as a question about ordinary reminiscences.

The item "child changed by war" was loaded on the factor labeled generalized anxiety. Although the question to parents also referred to sadness, analysis of the item's relationship to other symptom scores showed the strongest association with the items "anxious" and "sleep disturbances," a weak link with "concentration problems" and "separation anxiety," but no significant correlation with "sad mood." It seems that parents were largely guided in their assessment by signs of anxiety in the child.

RESULTS

Stressors

Information about organized violence in the home country was obtained during the second interview with the parent(s) alone.

The organized violence experienced by the refugee families reflected events that took place in their particular home area. To clarify the meaning of the categories listed in Figure 18.1; a more concrete description of the events follows.

Before Escape

Ethnic cleansing. Most families came from areas controlled by Serbian militias and had been victims of the "ethnic cleansing" carried out in these areas. Families from Banja Luka, for example, told of organized repression and discrimination against the Muslim minority. Parents lost their jobs and were subjected to threats and violence from neighbors and paramilitary forces. Those who did not flee at the outbreak of war described having to perform forced labor (e.g., digging trenches or cleaning up after shellings and fires). Violent raids on and thefts from their homes were common, and certain families were repeatedly attacked at night. Muslims were rounded up indiscriminately and sent off to concentration camps. Some parents had to stay away from home for months because of fear of arrest, communicating with their children only through mail or telephone. With no income, the families gradually became impoverished and undernourished.

For the children, the threat from violent soldiers and paramilitaries meant that they had to spend most of the time indoors. All Muslim school teachers were replaced by Serbs, and the teaching of the Christian Orthodox religion was made compulsory. One family described the use of special emblems on the children's clothes to single out those not attending Orthodox classes. Muslim children were excluded from certain activities and given lower grades. The children reported acts of aggression by their Serbian classmates.

Particularly severe acts of oppression and violence were reported by families from the city of Prijedor and its surrounding villages in northern Bosnia. They experienced brutal killings in the city itself and in the camps of Omarska and Keraterm, where most of the fathers and some of the children and mothers had spent at least some days. Two fathers were killed and one disappeared in the camps. The extent of the genocide in this region is illustrated by the fact that most parents reported 10 to 20 relatives and friends killed during the ethnic cleansing campaign. Children in families of which at least one member had been in a concentration camp were particularly heavily affected in terms of traumatic events, losses, and separations.

Combat stress. Some families, such as those from Jace, in central Bosnia, had lived under siege with intense shelling for months on end. The children had not been able to go to school or to play at all for long periods, and had suffered greatly from food shortages. When the city fell, its inhabitants had to run for their lives into the woods. All the fathers in these families had been soldiers at the front for extended periods, and some had been wounded in battle. Most of the families from Sarajevo had also lived under siege for a long time. Some, however, escaped during the early days of the war, and were thus spared the intense shelling, constant fear of sniper fire, and chronic shortage of food, electricity, and water described by others.

Separation and loss. Parents had been forced to hide or were sent to the front as soldiers. Other families were split up when children or other members were sent abroad for safety. Many children had missed schooling because of the war, and most had lost touch with important figures such as friends or grandparents. Almost half the children had had a relative or friend killed in the war. A very high proportion had lost their homes and belongings.

During and After Escape

A difficult or dangerous escape was reported by 53% of the families. A few told of extreme hardships—flight into the woods and walking for months through the mountains into Croatia, or being sent through Bosnia like cattle in locked trains. Many escaped through Croatia, where they stayed in transition for a while before finding their way to Sweden. Many of these families told of dramatic escapes in cars or lorries through areas with heavy fighting.

An "easy" escape meant getting on a bus through Serbia with very little time for preparation or packing. Almost all families coming from Serb-controlled areas reported being allowed to leave only on condition they handed over their homes and belongings.

Transition and uprooting did not end at the Swedish border. The families passed through a mean of 2.3 refugee camps in Sweden; on average, the children changed homes six times (range 2 to 13 times) in the 24 months before the interview.

Stress and Family and Child Characteristics

Some interesting relationships emerged between the stress scales and other characteristics of children and families. Older children scored higher on disruption, as well as loss. Length of time in Sweden was associated with lower scores on total stress, violence, and threat. (This could mean either that the earlier arrivals had experienced fewer of these stressors, or that there was a tendency to report fewer of them as time went by.) Children whose parents talked with them about the war had slightly higher total stress scores, most markedly on resistance [$t(97) = 3.03$, $p = .003$].

Fewer associations than expected were found between the family's place of origin and the sorts of stressors experienced. Children from cities other than Banja Luka had experienced more loss [$t(97) = 3.83$, $p = .0005$], particularly in separations from their parents, since those in cities under siege or close to the front line were often evacuated and sent abroad to stay with relatives. Children in Banja Luka itself scored lower on resistance [$t(97) = 4.02$, $p = .0005$]; for example, none of the fathers from this city were soldiers, since it was involved in military action only during the very last months of the war. Lower scores on resistance were also significantly associated with higher SES [$r(98) = -25$, $p = .02$], but multiple regression analysis showed that location was the more important factor here; having lived in Banja Luka explained the effect of SES, rather than vice-versa. No other associations between SES and the stress scales were noted, suggesting that war stressors had affected all classes somewhat impartially.

PSYCHOLOGICAL PROBLEMS

Children

The incidence of PTSD-related symptoms is shown in Figure 18.2. It is noteworthy that 36% of the children were reported as suffering from hypervigilance/startle reactions or from conditioned fears. Many children were afraid of men in uniform or with a beard, since they associated them with Serbian nationalists. Others were afraid of vans (which had been used to round up Muslim prisoners), and a few absolutely refused to enter forests. In addition, 40% of the children were judged by their parents to have become more nervous or sad since the war. However, 3% were judged to be calmer or happier than before the war.

Comparisons with other groups. Figure 18.3 shows data on items from the Cederblad symptom scale. Those with an incidence of less than 5% are not shown. When norms derived from research with Swedish children were applied to these scores, 11.1% of the Bosnian children were classified as having poor mental health, a rate much lower than the 20% prevalence rate found among Swedish children.

In the clinical evaluation made by the interviewers, which also took indicators of PTSD into account, 8% of the children were judged to be in need of psychiatric treatment.

No significant association was found between any of the symptom scales and the sex or age of the child. A slight negative association was found between the length of time the child had spent in Sweden and scores on total problems [$r(98) = -.23$, $p = .03$], generalized anxiety [$r(98) = -.20$, $p = .05$] and phobic and depressive symptoms [$r(98) = -.24$, $p = .02$]. This association could be entirely accounted for by the negative association reported above between length of stay in Sweden and total stressors. Nevertheless, a tendency for problems to improve with time seems possible; the finding that people who have been in Sweden longer report fewer war stressors could be explained as the result of forgetting or denial. However, even if the negative correlation between children's symptoms and time spent in Sweden is taken at face value, the effect is a weak one.

The only relation between the family's place of origin and the problem subscales was that children from cities other than Sarajevo scored higher on behavior problems [$t(97) = 2.17$, $p = .04$] and war preoccupation [$t(97) = 2.38$, $p = .02$].

Parents

Many of the parents in the sample had suffered greatly in the home country. In 13 families, one or both had been imprisoned in a concentration camp, and another three reported having been tortured during short detentions. Eight of the fathers had fought in the war as soldiers.

Only one parent, a chronic schizophrenic, had been a psychiatric patient in the home country. In 33% of the families, one or both parents had asked in the refugee camp for help with mental or psychosomatic problems, and another 24% had been treated for a somatic illness. During the interview, 22 parents (19%) from 17 families were judged to be in need of further psychiatric intervention.

These 22 parents had higher scores on all the stress subscales except disruption. A particularly strong association with having a family member who had been in a concentration camp emerged: 58% of those who had experienced this stress were judged to need treatment, compared to 14% of those with no such experience.

The 20 children with one or both parents diagnosed as being in need of psychiatric treatment scored higher on total problems [$r(98) = .27$, $p = .006$] and generalized anxiety [$r(98) = .36$, $p = .0005$]. However, multiple regression analysis showed that this association was explained by stressors shared by parent and child, suggesting that concern about the negative influence on the child of the parent's psychopathology may sometimes be exaggerated.

Children's Problems and War-Related Stressors

First, examination of the correlation between the scales of total stress and total problems indicated a clear relationship between war stressors and children's problems, [$r(98) = .34$, ($p = .0005$)]. Second, to obtain more detailed insight into the relationship between stress and problems, the subscales were used as dependent variables in forward stepwise multiple (linear) regression analyses (see Table 18.1). Behavior problems showed no significant relation to war stressors; generalized anxiety was predicted by threat [$t(97) = 3.50$, $p = .0007$]; phobic and depressive symptoms were predicted by

TABLE 18.1
Multiple Regression Analyses Predicting Scores on Symptom Subclases ($N = 99$)

	Standardized Regression Coefficients (β)			
STRESS	BP[a]	GA	P&D	WP
Violence	–0.12	0.18	0.38***	–0.10
Resistance	0.17	0.17	–0.04	0.21*
Disruption	–0.13	0.04	0.05	0.13
Threat	–0.03	0.33**	0.08	0.04
Loss	0.09	–0.03	0.09	0.07
Final adj. R^2	0.00	0.10	0.13	0.03
Final F	0.89	12.18**	16.16***	4.52*
(df)	(5, 93)	(1, 97)	(1, 97)	(1, 97)

Note: BP = behavior problems, GA = generalized anxiety, P&D = phobic and depressive symptoms, WP = war preoccupation.
[a]All variables inserted into the equation.
*$p < .05$; **$p < .001$; ***$p < .0001$.

violence [$t(97) = 4.02$, $p < .0001$]; and war preoccupations were predicted by resistance [$t(97) = 2.12$, $p = .04$].

The subscales of loss and disruption made no significant contribution to the models. These results can be compared with those from two studies of Palestinian children during the Intifada (Baker, 1990, 1991), which noted that the rate of depression, as well as PTSD-related symptoms, increased consistently. The effect on antisocial behavior seemed to depend on the social context in which the children lived, being weaker in communities with a strong religious commitment.

Third, to identify the components of the most salient scales, correlations were examined at the level of the individual items making up a scale. The components of threat that were most strongly related to generalized anxiety were "child experienced threat outdoors" and "child experienced threat in home," thus marking them as the most disturbing stressors for the children. Looking at the associations in the reverse direction, the component of generalized anxiety most sensitive to threat was parents' assessment of whether the child had become more nervous or sad as a result of the war; this appears, therefore, to have been quite a reliable assessment.

Similar analyses showed that phobic and depressive symptoms were associated with all items in the violence scale; the strongest association was with the item "child victim of intentional violence." Conversely, all items on the phobic and depressive symptoms scale showed significant associations with violence, particularly the item "poor appetite."

The variable most strongly associated with war preoccupations was whether the child's father had been a soldier. Both symptoms in this scale (plays war games and flashbacks) were equally associated with the score on resistance. Considering that these supposed symptoms were not associated with any other indications of psychopathology, it is possible that the findings had more to do with growing up in a military family than with trauma or stress, as such.

Mediators of Stress and Problems

The possible role of mediating variables as buffers or amplifiers of the effects of stress was examined by inserting an interaction term into the equation describing the regression of stress on problems. The variables of time in Sweden, age of child, SES, sex of child, and parents' need for psychological treatment showed no significant mediating effects. Whether or not the parents talked with their children about the war did, however, have a significant interaction effect, though not in the expected direction.

The majority (70%) of parents tried not to talk with their children about the war, most commonly because they thought their children were better off without reminders of their suffering in the home country. As reported above, the more severely disrupted children were more likely to have parents who talked with them about the war. It is also interesting to note that all four single mothers thought it was good for their children to talk about past suffering.

The attitude of the majority of parents was thus at loggerheads with the received wisdom among many Western professionals that working through traumatic experiences is important to mental health. A multiple regression analysis examined the interaction between talking about war and the effects of stress (see Table 18.2).

According to the working-through hypothesis, this interaction should be negative; i.e., talking should buffer the effects of stress. However, the interaction was found to be positive [$t(97) = 2.26$, $p = .03$]. There was also a slight main effect of talking, which was associated with lower total problem scores [$t(97) = -2.07$, $p < .05$]. Examination of scatter plots showed that talking about war experiences was associated with fewer problems when the stressors were relatively minor, but at high levels of stress the problems are actually exacerbated. It is ironic that parents tended to adopt this policy toward precisely those children for whom it seems contraindicated, namely those who had experienced more stress.

Need for Treatment

Stepwise multiple regression was also used to examine the predictors of the health professionals' judgment that a child was in need of psychiatric treatment. Variables included the stress subscales, problem subscales, and assessment of one or both parents as being in need of psychiatric treatment. The only significant predictors that emerged were the child's score on the subscales of generalized anxiety [$t(97) = 2.85$, $p = .005$] and phobic and depressive symptoms [$t(97) = 2.59$, $p < .01$]. It appears that mental health professionals pay attention to the symptoms identified here as the major consequences of war stress.

TABLE 18.2
Regression Analysis Predicting Squareroot Transformed Total Symptom Scores

Variable	β
Total stress score	0.24*
Child talks about the war in family	–0.63*
Interaction talking × total stress	0.71*
Final adjusted R^2	0.14
Final *F*	6.20**
df	(3, 95)

*$p < .05$; **$p < .001$.

Children's Social Network

Intercorrelations among the five items relating to children's social networks were weak, and it was not possible to construct scales with any degree of confidence. However, there was a good case for summing the items "sees other children in own home or their home" and "plays outdoors with other children" [$r(98) = .43$], reflecting the amount of contact with other children.

The amount of contact with other children was, as expected, related to the assessment of the child as "withdrawn" [$r(98) = -.30$, $p = .003$]). It also showed a significant positive correlation with the length of time the family had been in Sweden [$r(98) = .36$, $p = .0005$], reflecting the gradual building up of social networks, and with SES [$r(98) = .25$, $p = .02$]. Children who scored low on contact with other children had higher scores for total problems [$r(98) = .26$, $p < .01$]. On the subscales, a significant association was found only with the phobic and depressive symptoms scale [$r(98) = -.22$, $p = .03$]. There were no significant correlations with the stress scales. However, examining associations with individual stress items showed the item "child victim of intentional violence" to have a strikingly high negative correlation with the amount of contact with other children [$r(98) = -.35$, $p = .0005$]. Of the seven children suffering this stress, only one played ("seldom") with other children in his house or theirs, and only three played outside with other children. This suggests a fairly severe disabling effect of trauma, still noticeable after one year. The fact that these children had often been treated violently by other children suggests a possible mechanism for this effect.

Nevertheless, the effects of this particular trauma do not fully explain the negative correlation between contact with other children and total symptoms, for this correlation is also significant in the 92 children who had not themselves been victims of violence [$r(91) = -.23$, $p = .03$]. Since there are no other relationships with war stress, it seems that healthier children play more with other children; the data give no indication of the direction of causality.

Though these findings are inconclusive, they are not necessarily in conflict with those reported by Westermayer (1987), who clearly demonstrated that recreating social networks for Laotians in exile had protective effects. The families in the present study lived in a fairly uniform social situation that would tend to minimize within-group differences in the formation of social contacts.

DISCUSSION

Analysis of the war stressors to which the children and families in the sample had been subjected showed that they could be grouped into clusters that were both statistically homogeneous and psychologically meaningful. Subscales based on these clusters had specific relationships with different sorts of child symptoms.

Effects of Stressors on Symptoms

Symptoms consistent with PTSD were fairly widespread in the sample and could be related, along with symptoms of depression, in the experience of violent events (in particular, these suffered by the children themselves). However, two PTSD symptoms—playing was games and experiencing flashbacks—turned out to have no clinical significance.

An important link was evident between the experience of living under threat and generalized anxiety. It seemed that even when a child was not exposed to violent events, growing up in a family subject to (ethnic) persecution and oppression could drastically undermine development of a sense of security. Recent research in this area has generally been dominated by the concept of trauma. Several researchers, such as Kleber (1995), have emphasized that war traumas are seldom the acute single events presupposed by the category PTSD; rather, they involve plural, multiple, or sequential traumatization. However, such a stretching of the concept risks undermining its utility. Traumatization, as defined by the *DSM*, is undoubtedly a crucial phenomenon in war and organized violence; although threats, hardships, losses, deprivations and uncertainties are also stressors that may have deleterious effects.

Although the two links found between violence and threat and children's symptoms were significant at $p < .001$, the magnitude of the correlations involved (.39 and .33) was not great. Even allowing for a certain amount of measurement error, the relationship between stressors and symptoms is not statistically strong. It should also be borne in mind that the data on experiences of war and children's psychosocial symptoms were collected during the same interview, and that some respondents were expecting referral for psychiatric treatment. These combined factors may have led parents with troubled children to share memories of war events more readily.

The three other stress subscales of resistance, disruption, and loss showed no direct association with symptoms. This does not, of course, mean that they have no long-lasting effects, since the study covered only the aspects of development reflected by psychiatric and psychosocial problem scales; it did not, for example, examine effects on cognitive or moral development.

A somewhat surprising finding was the few effects of age, sex, or parental pathology, which neither buffered nor exacerbated the effects of war stressors. Nor was any direct relationship found between war stressors and the subscale behavior problems.

Comparisons with Other Children

No comparative data were available on the prevalence of the PTSD symptoms examined here in children growing up in peacetime, but figures were available for the items from the Cederblad symptom scale. In comparison with Swedish children of similar age (Cederblad & Höök, 1986), the Bosnian children showed more signs of emotional disturbances, yet markedly fewer psychosomatic and behavior problems. Like the Southeast Asian children studied in Australia by Krupinski and Burrows (1986), the Bosnian refugees scored lower on many problems than did children native to the host country.

The task of interpreting these differences is complicated by the fact that they reflect not only the effects of war stress, but also the influence of cultural and social factors. Concerning the latter, it should be borne in mind that no validation of the method used here has been made outside the Swedish majority population; norms for Bosnian children who have not experienced the stresses of war and resettlement are not available, and there are likely to be culture-based differences between Bosnian and Swedish children in the prevalence of problems. Studies of other refugee children have shown that antisocial behavior and acting-out tend to be lower among Bosnian children (Almqvist & Brandell-Forsberg, 1995; Hjern et al., 1998; Ljungberg-Miklos, 1989). That antisocial behavior is strongly influenced by sociocultural context has been demonstrated in comparisons of teacher-reported child behavior in different social groups in the same society and between different countries (Hjern, 1990). Studies (Weisz, Suwanlert, Chaiyasit, & Weiss, 1993; Weisz, McCarty, Eastman, & Chaiyasit, 1997) of ratings by parents, teachers, and observers in Thailand and the U.S. have demonstrated cross-cultural variations in both the prevalence of problem behavior and the criteria by which it is judged. The higher ratio of internalizing to externalizing problems seen in the Bosnian children than in the Swedish children, may thus reflect cross-cultural differences.

Furthermore, refugee and nonrefugee parents may perceive and report their children's problems differently. Several studies, including a Croatian study of displaced refugees (Zivcic, 1993), have demonstrated that parents in stressful conditions are poor raters of depressive symptomatology and posttraumatic reactions in their children. Children have been shown to shield their most difficult emotions from their parents under stress "so as not to upset the adults" (Yule & Williams, 1990). In view of the strong tendency among the Bosnian parents in the present study to avoid talking about the war with their children, it seems probable that such protective behavior was common among the children, so that (unlike parents in populations where disclosure is encouraged) these parents underestimated some of their children's symptoms.

Given the possibility that parents' perceptions of their children's disorders may have been influenced by their cultural background and war experiences, this study's reliance on these perceptions may seem misguided. However, experienced professionals also played an important part in determining the final ratings. Notes based on 90 minutes of observation of the children with their parents were used in arriving at these ratings, and the interviewer, not the parent, decided the appropriate code for severity of symptoms. While the possibility of bias introduced by the parents cannot be eliminated, short of placing the child under secret surveillance, the problem seems to some extent unavoidable. After all, parents are a privileged source of information about such events as nightmares, bed-wetting, eating problems, and expression of highly personal thoughts and feelings.

The low rates of mental health problems found on the Cederblad scale may also reflect an improvement during the 18 months or so between the children's arrival in Sweden and the study interviews. In a study (Ekblad, 1993) of ex-Yugoslavian refugee children in a refugee camp in Sweden, the frequency of individual child psychiatric symptoms was generally higher than in the present study. However, while the present data on the question of improvement are ambiguous, the children's conditions of life were in many ways favorable; their social environment was better than that of other groups of refugee children studied in Scandinavia (Almqvist & Brandell-Forsberg, 1995; Hjern et al., 1998; Montgomery, 1998). The divorce rate was low, and most of these families had already started recreating social support systems with fellow Bosnians, among them various professionals with child-oriented academic education. Both parents and children were going to school or day-care centers that helped them structure their existence in the host society and find meaning in their daily activities.

Thus, the differences between the Bosnian and Swedish samples might be due to many factors besides the effects of war and organized violence. The most reliable evidence about these effects, therefore, is probably to be obtained from analysis of within-group differences, i.e., the symptom patterns of children in the same sample exposed to various degrees of stress.

Despite the difficulty of interpreting the comparative data, the impression remains that the children in the current sample showed a remarkable degree of resilience. This may have to do with the relatively secure containing environment offered by their families, who shared a strong common culture that enabled them to make sense of suffering in religious and historical terms, as well as to cope with it, as in Summerfield's (1998) concept of "social memory." However, a different research design would be necessary to investigate the influence of such factors empirically, because within-group variance in the present sample was slight.

Likewise, all children in the study shared the stress of being uprooted from a familiar environment and of acculturation to life in Sweden. It is likely that such experiences would affect their mental health, but the present research design did not permit determination of their influence. Further qualitative studies are under way to shed light on the families' successes and difficulties in coping with the after-effects of war stressors.

From the results of the study, it is evident that no simple one-to-one relationship exists between war stressors and the development of symptoms. The same event can have widely differing effects on children and adults. A simple deterministic model of the effects of war stressors is obviously inadequate; many factors at the levels of child, family, and the wider community and culture must be taken into account alongside the stressors experienced.

A simple calculation illustrates the practical consequences. If the stress scales of violence and threat are combined with the symptom scales of generalized anxiety, and phobic and depressive symptoms, the resulting correlation between stressors and symptoms reaches $r(98) = .45$. Selection of the 20 children scoring highest on stressors and the 20 scoring highest on symptoms reveals that only seven children belong to both groups. This demonstrates how difficult it is to estimate children's need for treatment simply on the basis of their traumatic experiences. It is a point increasingly emphasized in the literature but one that is still not taken seriously enough by policymakers, who tend to promote standardized programs for groups "at risk."

Working Through

Most parents in this study evidently did not share the assumption common among Western mental health professionals, that it is good for refugee children to talk about war memories. Present study results, indeed, cast some doubt on the beneficial effects of working through distressing experiences in this particular context. Pennebaker and colleagues (1997), with a sample of middle-aged Americans that included Holocaust survivors, demonstrated beneficial effects on both mental and physical health of sharing distress with others. Yule (1992) has suggested a similar protective effect in school children who survived a ferry disaster. It is possible that these effects differ from present study findings because of cultural context. The traditional value attached in Western cultures to confession and sharing distress can be traced back to early Christendom, where it was described as early as 300 A.D. (Pennebaker, 1997). Though many non-Western cultures have a similar belief, others discourage disclosure (Wellenkamp, 1997). A study of refugee children from the Dinka tribe of southern Sudan (Jeppsson & Hjern, 2001) describes how boys raised as shepherds from an early age are taught to repress fear and distress. Mozambiquans, likewise, talk about forgetting as their normative means of coping. Ethiopians call this "active forgetting" (Summerfield, 1999). Thus, it seems likely that disclosure will have different consequences in different cultural settings. In contexts where disclosure is encouraged, it is likely to increase support and emotional involvement for the victim; in those where it is discouraged, it may evoke contempt and hostility. It is important, therefore, that mental health interventions using a working-through approach be adapted to the context in which they are to be implemented.

In a follow-up study in 22 families from the present study population, data have been collected from child and parent interviews regarding mental health and how the war experiences have been dealt with in the family sphere during the first five years of exile in Sweden. This new data will, we hope, permit new insights into the processing of war memories, and into ways in which talking about the war might be associated with a short-term negative mental health outcome.

REFERENCES

Almqvist, K., & Brandell-Forsberg, M. (1995). Iranian refugee children in Sweden: Effects of organized violence and forced migration on preschool children. *American Journal of Orthopsychiatry, 65,* 225–237.

Almqvist, K., & Brandell-Forsberg, M. (1997). Refugee children in Sweden: Post-traumatic stress disorder in Iranian preschool children exposed to organized violence. *Child Abuse & Neglect, 4,* 351–366.

American Psychiatric Association. (1987). *Diagnostic and statistical manual of mental disorders* (3rd ed., rev.). Washington, D.C.: American Psychiatric Publishing.

Baker, A. M. (1990). The psychological impact of the Intifada on Palestinian children in the occupied West Bank and Gaza: an exploratory study. *American Journal of Orthopsychiatry, 60,* 496–505.

Baker, A. M. (1991). Psychological response of Palestinian children to environmental stress associated with military occupation. *Journal of Refugee Studies, 4,* 21–38.

Cederblad, M., & Höök, B. (1984). *Rendering ock provning are ett instrument for att mata beteenderabbninger has born* [Revision and trial of an instrument to measure distorted behavior in children] (Stressforskningsupport nr. [Stress research report #] 184). Stockholm: WHO Psychosocial Center.

Cederblad, M., & Höök, B. (1986). Var sjatte born har en psykisk storning [Every sixth child has mental disturbance]. *Laskartidiningen, 83,* 935–939.

Ekblad, S. (1993). Psychosocial adaption of children while housed in Swedish refugee camp: aftermath of the collapse of Yugoslavia. *Stress Medicine, 9,* 154–166.

Gantzel, K. J., & Schwinghammer, T. (1995). *Die Kriege nach dem Zweiten Weltkrieg, 1945 bis 1992: Daten und Tendenzen* [Wars since World War II, 1945 to 1992: Figures and trends]. Munster, Germany: Lit Verlag.

Hjern, A. (1990). *The health of newly resettled refugee children from Chile and the Middle East.* Unpublished doctoral dissertation, Huddinge University Hospital, Karolinska Institute, Stockholm.

Hjern, A., Angel, B., & Jeppsson, O. (1998). Political violence, family stress and mental health of refugee children in exile. *Scandinavian Journal of Social Medicine, 26,* 18–25.

Jeppsson, O., & Hjern, A. (2001). *Traumatic stress in cultural context: a study of unaccompanied refugee children from Southern Sudan.* Unpublished manuscript.

Kleber, R. J. (1995). Epilogue. In R. J. Kleber, C. R. Figley, & B. P. R. Gersons (Eds.), *Beyond trauma: cultural and social dynamics* (pp. 299–305). New York: Plenum Press.

Krupinski, J., & Burrows, G. (1986). Psychiatric disorders in adolescents and young adults. In J. Krupinski (Ed.), *The price of freedom* (pp. 123–135). New York: Pergamon Press.

Ljungberg-Miklos, J. (1989). Flyktingbarns psykiska halsa [The mental health of refugee children]. *Socialmedicinsk Tidskrift, 66*, 18–24.

Montgomery, E. (1998). Refugee children from the Middle East. *Scandinavian Journal of Social Medicine* (Suppl. 54), 1–152.

Pennebaker, J. (1997). Confession and inhibition: the beginnings of an approach. In J. Pennebaker (Ed.), *Opening up: the healing power of expressing emotions* (pp. 5–18). New York: Guilford Press.

Pfeffenbaum, B. (1997). Post-traumatic stress disorder in children. *Journal of the American Academy of Child and Adolescent Psychiatry, 36*, 1503–1511.

Stubbs, P., & Soroya, B. (1996). War trauma, psychosocial projects and social development in Croatia. *Medicine, Conflict and Survival, 12*, 303–314.

Summerfield, D. (1998). The social experience of war and some issues for the humanitarian field. In P. J. Bracken & C. Petty (Eds.), *Rethinking the trauma of war* (pp. 9–37) London: Free Association Books.

Summerfield, D. (1999). A critique of seven assumptions behind psychological trauma programmes in war affected areas. *Social Science and Medicine, 48*, 1449–1462.

Svedin, C. G., Back, K., & Wadsby, M. (1994). Mental health among immigrant and refugee children of divorced parents. *Scandinavian Journal of Social Medicine, 22*, 178–186.

Weisz, J. R., McCarty, C.A., Eastman, K. L., & Chaiyasit, W. (1997). Developmental psychopathology and culture: ten lessons from Thailand. In S. S. Luthar & J. A. Burack (Eds.), *Developmental psychopathology: perspectives on adjustment, risk, and disorder* (pp. 568–592). Cambridge, England: Cambridge University Press.

Weisz, J. R., Suwanlert, S., Chaiyasit, W., & Weiss, B. (1993). Behavioral and emotional problems among Thai and American adolescents: parent reports for ages 12–26. *Journal of Abnormal Psychology, 10*, 395–403.

Wellenkamp, J. (1997). Cultural similarities and differences regarding emotional disclosure: some examples from Indonesia and the Pacific. In J. Pennebaker (Ed.), *Opening up: the healing power of expressing emotions* (pp. 293–311). New York: Guilford Press.

Westermayer, J. (1987). Prevention of mental disorder among Hmong refugees in the U.S.: lessons from the period 1976–1986. *Social Science and Medicine, 25*, 941–947.

Yule, W. (1992). Post-traumatic stress disorder in child survivors of shipping disasters: the sinking of the "Jupiter." *Psychotherapy and Psychosomatics, 57*, 200–205.

Yule, W., & Williams, W. (1990). Post-traumatic stress reactions in children. *Journal of Traumatic Stress, 3*, 279–285.

Zivcic, I. (1993). Emotional reactions of children to war stress in Croatia. *Journal of American Academy of Child and Adolescent Psychiatry, 32*, 709–713.

19

Multiethnic Comparison of Adolescent Major Depression Based on the *DSM-IV* Criteria in a U.S.–Japan Study

Yuriko Doi, Robert E. Roberts, Kazuo Takeuchi, and Shousuke Suzuki

Objectives: *To compare the prevalence rates of major depression based on the* DSM-IV *criteria with data from a multiethnic sample of adolescents drawn from the same U.S.–Japan study and to investigate the relation of adolescent major depression to ethnicity.* ***Method:*** *Adolescents aged 12 to 15 years (N = 2,046; 539 Anglo-American, 636 African American, 409 Mexican American, and 462 Japanese adolescents) were studied in 1994 (response rates: 85.3% for U.S. students and 95.5% for Japanese students). The DSM Scale for Depression, a self-administered checklist developed from the Diagnostic Interview Schedule for Children questions on major depression, was used to estimate the prevalence of* DSM-IV *major depression.* ***Results:*** *The overall prevalence rates of major depression without/with impairment were 9.6% and 4.3% for Anglo-American, 13.4% and 6.1% for African American, 16.9% and 9.0% for Mexican American, and 5.6% and 1.3% for Japanese adolescents. The significant association between adolescent major depression and ethnicity disappeared after sociodemographic adjustments. Only fathers' educational attainment and family financial status remained significant (odds ratios: 3.28 to 5.30 for grade school for fathers and 2.62 to 2.78 for being worse off economically).* ***Conclusion:*** *These findings imply ethnicity does not have a significant impact on the risk of adolescent major depression after sociodemographic adjustments.*

Most epidemiological research on child and adolescent psychopathology, including major depression, has been conducted in Western countries (Angold, 1988; Bird, 1996; Fleming and Offord, 1990). Methodological problems have been reduced in criterion and information variance, particularly since the early 1980s when standardized diagnostic criteria and structured diagnostic interview schedules came into wide use (Hodges, 1993; Roberts et al., 1998). In the United States, the National Institute of Mental Health (NIMH) Methods for the Epidemiology of Child and Adolescent Mental Disorders (MECA) Study addressed methodological issues to develop feasible, reliable, and valid methods for the assessment of mental disorders, risk factors, and service use in youths aged 9 through 17 years in a large-scale, population-based survey (Lahey et al., 1996). The NIMH Diagnostic Interview Schedule for Children Version 2.3 (DISC-2.3) used in the MECA study was examined for its acceptability, reliability, and validity (Lahey et al., 1996; Schwab-Stone et al., 1996; Shaffer et al., 1996). For major depressive disorder, concurrent validity was good and higher in youth informants (0.73 and greater) than parent informants (0.55 to 0.60). In contrast, test–retest agreements were moderate in the latter (0.54 to 0.62) and marginal to poor in the former (0.34 to 0.45) (Schwab-Stone et al., 1996). In the MECA study, the prevalence of major depression was 4.8%.

In Japan, there have been only a few epidemiological studies of child and adolescent psychopathology using community or school-based samples. By the use of broad-band case ascertainment of the Rutter Questionnaire, Matsuura et al. (1989) studied 1,860 subjects aged 6 to 12 years and estimated a 3.0% current prevalence of children with emotional and behavioral problems from information obtained from their teachers. They also examined 2,638 subjects aged 6 to 12 years and reported prevalence rates of 12.0% and 3.9% from information obtained from their parents and teachers, respectively (Matsuura et al., 1993). Morita et al. (1993), using combined data from 1,992 junior high school students, their parents, and teachers, who completed the Rutter Questionnaire and Rutter Child Interview, estimated that 15.0% of adolescents have emotional and behavioral problems. Morita et al. identified quite a few students who were adequately referred to appropriate mental health services. Using the narrow-band case ascertainment of the Children's Depression Inventory, Murata et al. (1989) calculated a prevalence rate of 5.9% for depression in junior high school students. A recent study conducted by Sugiwara et al. (1999) used the Child Assessment Schedule and reported a prevalence of *DSM-III-R* major depression of 2.7% in 114 children aged 8 years.

According to the Management and Coordination Agency of Japan (1997), school refusals and school violence have reached record highs and adolescent suicide, caused by bullying and bullying-related crimes are serious problems in Japan. However, as mentioned above, no systematic epidemiological research on child and adolescent psychopathology has been conducted. Such research is an essential component of a sound policy for the provision of mental health services. Four reasons why such this has not been carried out in

Japan are suggested: (1) school boards and teachers are hesitant to permit researchers or interviewers to enter schools to contact their students directly, (2) community-based research on children and adolescents that uses either interviews or questionnaires has not been traditionally done in Japan, (3) diagnostic instruments in Japanese are not widely available in Japan, and (4) some Japanese psychiatrists and psychiatric pediatricians doubt whether standardized diagnostic criteria originally developed in Euro-American society are fully applicable for use with Japanese children and adolescents. Accordingly, the purposes of this study are (1) to apply a paper-and-pencil Japanese version of the DISC-2.3 module on major depression and *DSM-IV* criteria, (2) to estimate the prevalence of adolescent major depression in a nonreferred sample, and (3) to compare such major depression among Japanese adolescents with that of their counterparts in the United States within the same study to examine whether or not there are ethnic differences in major depression.

METHOD

Subjects

In the Teen Life Changes Survey conducted in 1994, questionnaires were obtained from 5,496 students in grades 6 to 8 in a school district in the Houston, Texas, a metropolitan area in the United States, and 504 students in grades 7 to 9 in a public junior high school in Maebashi, the capital city of Gunma Prefecture, Japan. The participation rates were 85.3% for U.S. students and 95.5% for Japanese students. Nonparticipants were students who were absent from school on the day of the survey, students whose parents declined for them to participate, students who themselves declined to participate, and students who had a lot of missing data.

A sample of 2,046 students 12 to 15 years of age (539 Anglo-Americans, 636 African Americans, 409 Mexican Americans, and 462 Japanese) remained for further analyses after exclusion of students who did not respond to any item on gender, age, or the *DSM* Scale for Depression and who belonged to other ethnic minority groups. Ethnic status was self-designated in this study, using the following categories in the U.S. survey: African American, Anglo-American, Cambodian American, Central American, Chinese American, Cuban American, Indian American, Korean American, Mexican American, Native American, Pacific Islander, Pakistan American, Vietnamese American, Puerto Rican, and others. Ethnic status such as Korean ancestry within the Japanese sample in this study was not considered. There were very few such students in the sample.

Procedures

In the U.S. survey, questionnaires were administered in a classroom setting during the regular school day, monitored by project field staff. Passive parental and active student consent procedures were used, after the permission of the school board was obtained. In the Japanese survey, questionnaires were administered in a classroom setting during the regular school day, monitored by each classroom teacher, after the permission of the school board was obtained. When the questionnaires were distributed, students were told they could skip any question or stop at any time if they felt uncomfortable answering the questions. Surveys were administered only in English in the United States and in Japanese in Japan.

Measures

Depression was measured by the *DSM* Scale for Depression (DSD) (Roberts et al., 1997), a self-administered questionnaire developed from the NIMH DISC-2.3 questions on major depression. The original DSD consists of 31 items and asks respondents to choose one response from four answers on a Likert scale: almost every day, often, sometimes, and hardly ever or never. The time frame was the preceding 2 weeks. More details about the DSD are reported elsewhere (Roberts et al., 1997). Four of six items regarding suicide in the original English version were eliminated from the Japanese version at the request of the local school board in Japan. Two retained items were, "Did you wish you were dead?" and "Have you thought about suicide or killing yourself?" Excluded items were, "Have you ever made a plan to kill yourself?" "Have you made a plan to kill yourself in the past two weeks?" "Have you ever tried to kill yourself?" and "Have you tried to kill yourself in the past two weeks?" Therefore, 27 items of the DSD were used for analyses in both the U.S. and Japanese surveys. Cronbach α values (Cronbach and Meehl, 1955) for the 27-item DSD in the current study were .94, .93, .94, and .92 for Anglo-American, African American, Mexican American, and Japanese adolescents, respectively.

Other scales for loneliness, self-esteem, and social support were used to examine the construct validity of the DSD (Nunnally and Bernstein, 1994): the Roberts Loneliness Scale (Roberts et al., 1993), Rosenberg's six-item version for self-esteem (Hops et al., 1990; Rosenberg, 1965), and the Multidimensional Scale of Perceived Social Support (Zimet et al., 1988). In this study, the respective values for the correlation coefficients of the DSD with loneliness, self-esteem, and social support were 0.58, 0.69, and 0.38 for Anglo-American; 0.59, 0.63, and 0.30 for African American; 0.53, 0.56, and 0.27 for Mexican American; and 0.50, 0.48, and 0.24 for Japanese adolescents. All the correlation coefficients were significant beyond the .001 level.

Cronbach α values for the scales of loneliness, self-esteem, and social support ranged from .70 to .94 across these ethnic groups, which were satisfied with criteria of .70 or greater (Nunnally and Bernstein, 1994).

The Japanese version of the questionnaire including the above scales was developed through the process of three translation stages proposed by Brislin (1986); first, the original version was translated from English into Japanese by a bilingual familiar with both languages; then the translated Japanese version was back-translated by another bilingual; finally, both versions in English and in Japanese were examined by other bilinguals. The preliminary Japanese version was pretested regarding words, meanings, and content on each item among Japanese junior high school students who were not involved in the study. After being reviewed by the authors, the final Japanese version for use in this study was created.

In addition, adolescents were asked to provide general sociodemographic information including gender, age, family structure, parental education, and perceived family financial status. Because it was difficult to obtain accurate data on family income from adolescents, they were asked to subjectively report their feeling or impression about the financial situation of their family: "Compared to other students at your school, would you say that your family is financially worse off or better off than other families?" The answers were as follows: much worse off, somewhat worse off, about the same, better off, much better, and don't live at home.

Case Ascertainment

To estimate the prevalence of major depression, we applied a diagnostic algorithm for caseness using the DSD based on *DSM-IV* criteria (American Psychiatric Association, 1994). Adolescents were designated as cases if they reported that they experienced five or more criterion symptoms almost every day, including the core symptoms of depressed (or irritated) mood and/or anhedonia, in the preceding 2 weeks. Shaffer et al. (1996) recommended that caseness be determined by the presence of both diagnostic and severity criteria. Therefore, cases who reported difficulties in their role-functioning at home, at school, or with peers were considered more impaired than other cases. Those who met criteria for major depression and had experienced many problems at home, at school, or with peers were categorized as cases of major depression with impairment.

Statistical Analyses

Chi-square analyses were performed to detect differences in background characteristics among subjects by ethnicity. Two point-prevalence rates for cases without and with impairment were calculated by ethnicity and gender. A χ^2 test (two-tailed) was used to compare the prevalence rates among ethnic groups. To investigate the relation of major depression without/with impairment to ethnicity, logistic regression analysis (Kleinbaum, 1994) was used to determine the odds ratios (ORs) and 95% confidence intervals (95% CIs), adjusting for differences in gender, age, guardian status, parental educational attainment, and perceived family financial status. Main modification effects were tested by inclusion of the interaction terms for sociodemographic variables. The data were analyzed using SPSS, Japanese version 9.0 (SPSS, 1999).

RESULTS

Subjects

The sociodemographic characteristics of adolescents analyzed for this study are shown in Table 19.1. Significant differences in age, guardian status, parental education, and family financial status by ethnicity were found ($p < .001$).

Prevalence Rates of Adolescent Major Depression without/with Impairment by Ethnicity

Two prevalence estimates of cases of major depression without and with impairment are presented for each ethnic group (Table 19.2). All prevalence rates were highest for Mexican American, second highest for African American, third highest for Anglo-American, and lowest for Japanese adolescents. Multiethnic differences in the prevalence rates of adolescent major depression were statistically significant, except for those cases with impairment in male adolescents. Adjusting for impairment in case ascertainment for major depression showed the prevalence rates greatly decreased.

Multiethnic Comparison of Adolescent Major Depression without/with Impairment by Univariate and Multivariate Analyses

Table 19.3 shows the associations of adolescent major depression with ethnicity and other sociodemographic variables such as gender, age, guardian status, parental education, and family financial status using univariate and multivariate analyses. Anglo-American male adolescents aged 12 years living with their biological mother and father, with parents who were high school graduates and about the same family financial status, were used as reference.

TABLE 19.1
Sociodemographic Characteristics of the Study Subjects (N = 2,046)

	Anglo American (n = 539)		African American (n = 636)		Mexican American (n = 409)		Japanese (n = 462)		
	n	%	n	%	n	%	n	%	χ^2
Gender									
Male	249	46.2	298	46.9	190	46.5	228	49.4	1.20
Female	290	53.8	338	53.1	219	53.5	234	50.6	
Age									
12 years	154	28.6	170	26.7	110	26.9	67	14.5	100.90**
13 years	211	39.1	228	35.8	155	37.9	154	33.3	
14 years	146	27.1	185	29.1	107	26.2	141	30.5	
15 years	88	5.2	53	8.3	37	9.0	100	21.6	
Guardian's status									
Mother									
Living with natural mother	491	91.1	575	90.4	375	91.7	460	99.6	37.75**
Living without natural mother	42	7.8	43	6.8	19	4.6	1	0.2	
Not ascertained	6	1.1	18	2.8	15	3.7	1	0.2	
Father									
Living with natural father	350	64.9	259	40.7	259	63.3	439	95.0	302.32**
Living without natural father	168	31.2	319	50.2	118	28.9	20	4.3	
Not ascertained	21	3.9	58	9.1	32	7.8	3	0.7	
Educational attainment									
Mother's education									
> High school	24	4.4	27	4.2	93	22.7	0	0.0	276.52**
High school	115	21.3	86	13.5	76	18.6	103	22.3	
< High school	294	54.5	311	48.9	95	23.2	270	58.4	
Not ascertained	106	19.7	212	33.3	145	35.5	89	19.3	
Father's education									
> High school	20	3.7	24	3.8	77	18.8	2	0.4	260.28**
High school	66	12.2	72	11.3	59	14.4	56	12.1	
< High school	293	54.4	247	38.8	79	19.4	318	68.9	
Not ascertained	160	29.7	293	46.1	194	47.4	86	18.6	
Family financial status									
Same	233	43.2	324	50.9	220	53.8	267	57.8	51.32**
Worse off/much worse off	47	8.7	37	5.8	40	9.8	50	10.8	
Better off/much better off	246	45.6	225	35.4	120	29.3	119	25.8	
Not ascertained	13	2.4	50	7.9	29	7.1	26	5.6	

**$p < .001$.

TABLE 19.2
Prevalence (%) of Adolescent Major Depression without and with Impairment by Ethnicity and Gender

	Anglo-American (n = 539)	African American (n = 636)	Mexican American (n = 409)	Japanese (n = 462)	χ^2
Without impairment					
Overall	9.6	13.4	16.9	5.6	31.57**
Male	8.8	12.8	13.7	5.7	10.12**
Female	10.3	13.9	19.6	5.6	22.62**
With impairment					
Overall	4.3	6.1	9.0	1.3	28.95**
Male	4.0	5.7	6.3	1.8	6.66
Female	4.5	6.5	11.4	0.9	24.60**

Note: Impairment means many problems at school, at home, or with peers.
*$p < .05$; **$p < .001$.

For adolescents with major depression without impairment, univariate analyses revealed significant associations with ethnicity (OR = 1.45, 95% CI 1.00–2.08 for African American; OR = 1.90, 95% CI 1.29–2.80 for Mexican American; OR = 0.56, 95% CI 0.34–0.91 for Japanese adolescents), guardian status (OR = 1.69, 95% CI 1.27–2.26 for living without his or her natural father), parental educational attainment (OR = 2.14, 95% CI 1.27–3.62 for grade school for mothers; OR = 3.48, 95% CI 1.97–6.17 for grade school for fathers), and family financial status (OR = 2.31, 95% CI 1.52–3.51 for being worse off/much worse off). Using multivariate analyses after sociodemographic adjustments, the significant association between adolescent major depression and ethnicity disappeared. Only fathers' educational attainment and family financial status remained significant (OR = 3.28, 95% CI 1.56–6.89 for grade school for fathers; OR = 2.62, 95% CI 1.46–4.72 for being worse off/much worse off). Guardian status of a natural father was not included in the multivariate analysis because an interaction effect with family financial status was identified.

Findings were similar for adolescent major depression with impairment. Univariate analyses demonstrated significant associations with ethnicity (OR = 2.23, 95% CI 1.30–3.82 for MexicanAmerican adolescents; OR = 0.30, 95% CI 0.12–0.73 for Japanese adolescents), guardian status (OR = 2.00, 95% CI 1.33–3.01 for living without his or her natural father), parental educational attainment (OR = 2.60, 95% CI 1.35–4.99 for grade school for mothers; OR = 6.24, 95% CI 2.79–13.95 for grade school for fathers), and family financial status (OR = 2.15, 95% CI 1.21–3.83 for being worse off/much worse off). Not ethnicity but fathers' educational attainment and family financial status were still substantially related to adolescent major depression with

TABLE 19.3
Associations of Adolescent Major Depression with Ethnicity

		Without impairment		With Impairment	
	n	Crude OR (95% CI)	Adjusted OR (95% CI)	Crude OR (95% CI)	Adjusted OR (95% CI)
Ethnicity					
African American	636	1.45 (1.00–2.08)	NS	1.47 (0.86–2.49)	NS
Mexican American	409	1.90 (1.29–2.80)	NS	2.23 (1.30–3.82)	NS
Japanese	462	0.56 (0.34–0.91)	NS	0.30 (0.12–0.73)	NS
Gender					
Female	1,081	1.23 (0.93–1.62)	NS	1.31 (0.88–1.94)	NS
Age					
13 years	748	1.29 (0.89–1.87)	NS	1.36 (0.77–2.38)	NS
14 years	579	1.36 (0.92–2.00)	NS	1.68 (0.95–2.97)	NS
15 years	218	1.01 (0.59–1.73)	NS	1.48 (0.70–3.10)	NS
Guardian status					
Living without natural mother	105	1.36 (0.78–2.40)	NS	1.60 (0.76–3.40)	NS
Living without natural father	625	1.69 (1.27–2.26)	—[a]	2.00 (1.33–3.01)	—[a]
Educational attainment					
Mother's education					
<High school	144	2.14 (1.27–3.62)	NS	2.60 (1.35–4.99)	NS
>High school	970	0.88 (0.59–1.30)	NS	0.74 (0.43–1.26)	NS
Father's education					
<High school	123	3.48 (1.97–6.17)	3.28 (1.56–6.89)	6.24 (2.79–13.95)	5.30 (1.97–14.27)
>High school	937	0.74 (0.46–1.19)	NS	0.84 (0.39–1.79)	NS

TABLE 19.3
(Continued)

		Without impairment		With Impairment	
	n	Crude OR (95% CI)	Adjusted OR (95% CI)	Crude OR (95% CI)	Adjusted OR (95% CI)
Family financial status					
Worse off/much worse off	174	2.31 (1.52–3.51)	2.62 (1.46–4.72)	2.15 (1.21–3.83)	2.78 (1.23–6.26)
Better off/much better off	710	1.03 (0.75–1.41)	NS	0.94 (0.60–1.48)	NS

Note: Impairment means many problems at school, at home, or with peers. References are Anglo-American ($n = 539$), male ($n = 965$), age of 12 ($n = 501$), living with a natural mother ($n = 1,901$), living with a natural father ($n = 1,307$), high school graduate ($n = 380$ in mothers, $n = 253$ in fathers), same in family financial status ($n = 1,044$). NS = not significant.
[a]Guardian status of natural father is not included in the multiple regression analysis because of its interaction effect with family financial status.

impairment in the multivariate analysis (OR = 5.30, 95% CI 1.97–14.27 for grade school for fathers; OR = 2.78, 95% CI 1.23–6.26 for being worse off/much worse off).

DISCUSSION

This is the first published report of a multiethnic comparison of adolescent major depression using the *DSM-IV* criteria in a school-based U.S.–Japan study. The uniqueness of this study was that the samples were directly compared within the same study, the same measures were used for ethnic comparative groups to assess the target disorder based on standardized diagnostic criteria along with severity criteria, and statistical tests were used to examine multiethnic differences or similarities across two nations (Hodges, 1993; Roberts et al., 1998; Weisz and Eastman, 1995). Our findings demonstrate that overall prevalence rates of adolescent major depression ranged from 5.6% to 16.9% by ethnicity (the highest for Mexican American adolescents and the lowest for Japanese adolescents) and were reduced by approximately half to three fourths across the groups by the introduction of severity criteria. After sociodemographic adjustments, ethnicity was not significantly associated with adolescent major depression, although father's educational attainment and family financial status demonstrated a significant statistical association.

The number of epidemiological studies on adolescent depression has progressively increased (Angold, 1988; Bird, 1996; Fleming and Offord, 1990). As these authors pointed out, however, the evidence is less informative than expected because of several problems including sampling, case ascertainment, case definition, and data analyses and presentation. Recent studies have used more sophisticated strategies to minimize the impact of sampling and non-sampling errors, to reduce criterion variance by the use of standardized diagnostic criteria, to reduce information variance by the use of structured diagnostic interview schedules, and to enhance comparability across studies by the use of analytical techniques such as relative risks (Garrison et al., 1992; Lewinsohn et al., 1993; Shaffer et al., 1996).

For example, the MECA study used a probability sample of 1,285 youths aged 9 to 17 years in four geographic areas of the United States (females 47%, non-Hispanic white 51%, African American 15%, Hispanic 28%, other 6%; household income <$10,000 [15%], $10,000–24,999 [18%], $25,000–64,999 [42%], $65,000–99,999 [17%], >$100,000 [8%]) to assess psychiatric disorders using the DISC-2.3 based on *DSM-III-R* criteria; they estimated a current prevalence rate of 4.8% for major depression (Lahey et al., 1996; Shaffer et al., 1996). In the Oregon Adolescent Depression Project, 1,710 randomly selected high school students in grades 9 through 12 (females, 52.9%; non-whites, 8.9%; not living with biological parents, 14.9%; parental education less than high school, 16.5%) were evaluated with the Schedule for Affective Disorders and Schizophrenia for School-Age Children (K-SADS) and Axis V Global Assessment of Functioning based on DSM-III-R criteria (Lewinsohn et al., 1993), in which the point-prevalence rate of major depression was 3.1%. Their findings were very similar to the present observations for Anglo-American adolescents, an overall prevalence rate of 4.3%. Garrison et al. (1992) conducted a two-stage epidemiological study on major depression in a representative sample of 3,283 adolescents aged 12 to 14 in the southeastern United States to examine the prevalence and the relation between major depression and the potential correlates of gender, age, race, family constellation, family functioning, socioeconomic status (SES), and negative life events. The 20-item Center for Epidemiologic Studies-Depression Scale (CES-D) was administered to adolescents for screening in stage 1. In stage 2, the K-SADS and the Children's Global Assessment Scale were used to assess 488 screened adolescents (white males 34.2%, white females 42.2%, black males 10.7%, black females 12.9%; not living with biological parents 9.8%; father's education less than high school 11.3%) with *DSM-III* criteria. The prevalence rates of major depression were 9.0% and 8.9% for males and females, respectively. Although the prevalence rates in their study were slightly higher than the present findings of 4.3% for Anglo-Americans and 6.1% for African Americans, their results were strikingly consistent with the present study in that ethnic difference in major depression was not significant after adjustment for sociodemographic and other variables.

However, other than the present study, there are no cross-cultural studies. Therefore, it is too early to conclude that there are no ethnic differences in adolescent major depression between the United States and Japan. Further cross-cultural epidemiological research is needed to accumulate evidence on how ethnicity or culture impacts the frequency of adolescent major depression and the role of ethnic culture as a risk or protective factor for adolescent major depression.

As Weisz and Eastman (1995) mentioned, multiethnic comparisons of child and adolescent psychopathology across cultures require an etic orientation. An etic orientation refers to a validity of psychological concepts and methodologies across cultures. By contrast, an emic orientation refers to an idiographic viewpoint, such that psychological concepts and methodologies are valid only in their own cultural settings. They also emphasize that researchers should avoid simple-minded comparisons that ignore the distinctiveness of the individual cultures being compared. This fundamental etic/emic issue is both old and new in the cross-cultural applicability of concepts. In the past, Marsella et al. (1973) examined 508 college students (309 Japanese, 87 Chinese, and 112 white) enrolled at the University of Hawaii using the Zung Self-Rating Depression Scale and factor analysis. They speculated that somatic and interpersonal complaints might be more symptomatic among the Asian groups. More recently, Iwata and Roberts (1996) used the CES-D and factor analysis to study 2,016 employees aged 19 to 63 years; they reported that the interpersonal plus negative affect appeared unique for Japanese subjects, indicating the association of interpersonal relations with depressive mood in Japanese subjects. Mezzich et al. (1999) have agreed that more culturally informed research is required to ensure that future diagnostic systems incorporate a genuinely comprehensive framework. Alarcón et al. (1999) also described the important intersections of culture and psychopathology from an emic point of view. The content validity of diagnostic procedures and systems of adolescent major depression across cultures is, however, beyond the scope of the present study. Further investigation is necessary.

The role of SES in adolescent depression should be addressed. In an attempt to measure SES, three indicators have been used most often, mainly for adults: occupation, education, and income. Multiple indicators, at least two of them, are currently recommended to incorporate into the measurement rather than composite indices (Liberatos et al., 1988). As Liberatos et al. pointed out, however, little consensus exists about how to appropriately evaluate SES for children and adolescents. The National Longitudinal Study of Adolescent Health (Add Health) recently examined the association between SES and adolescent health (Goodman, 1999). It used parental reports of household income and a level of the most highly educated parent of adolescent subjects, and adolescent reports of their resident parental occupation to measure SES. An 18-item CES-D was used for assessing depression. Parental education and income remained independent correlates of depression, which is consistent with the findings of our study. Although a mechanism for the correlation of parental education and income with adolescent depression is not clear at present, its negative effects on their psychosocial resources such as self-esteem may exist over time to cause their affective change. Level of education and absolute or relative income are not sufficient for us to understand a mechanism of its effect on adolescent depression, particularly because the data were cross-sectional, thereby precluding examination of temporal ordering.

Limitations

There are general methodological limitations pertaining to this study. First, the present samples from the United States and Japan were not representative because they lived in geographically limited areas and were not randomly selected. Second, four of six items on suicide in the DSD used for this study were excluded from the original DSD; thus comparison with other reports using the latter may not be possible without establishing the equality of these two measures. Third, the test–retest reliability of the DSD was not examined, although its internal consistency showed high reliability. The construct validity of the DSD was demonstrated by significant correlations with external scales. But, strictly speaking, case ascertainment by the DSD was not compared with case ascertainment using structured interviews or clinical diagnosis. However, Boyle et al. (1997) demonstrated that the differences in reliability and validity were small between interviews and checklists for use in cross-sectional prevalence studies of childhood psychiatric disorders. Further investigations on this issue should be carried out.

Clinical Implications

Adolescent major depression tends to be underidentified by parents and teachers because of its internalizing nature (Angold et al., 1987; Edelbrock et al., 1986). Therefore, community-based epidemiological studies of adolescents themselves who are not institutionalized provide more accurate information on prevalence and distribution in the general population than those from the data obtained from surrogate informants or from clinical sources. The findings of this school-based study on adolescent major depression indicate that adolescent major depression was prevalent across ethnicity between two nations. In addition, the results studied within an etic framework suggest no significant ethnic differences in adolescent major depression between two Western and non-Western nations and may facilitate cultural psychiatrists or psychiatric epidemiologists to focus on etic/emic issues in mental disorders.

AFFILIATIONS

From the Department of Epidemiology, National Institute of Public Health, Tokyo, Japan (Y.D.); Behavioral Sciences, School of Public Health, University of Texas, Houston (R.E.R.); Takasaki University of Health and Welfare, Takasaki, Japan (K.T.); and Department of Public Health, Gunma University School of Medicine, Maebashi, Japan (S.S.).

ACKNOWLEDGMENTS

This study was supported by research grant H51867 from the NIMH, U.S.A., and by grants-in-aid 07857027 and 07670423 from the Ministry of Education, Science and Culture, Japan.

REFERENCES

Alarcón RD, Westermeyer J, Foulks EF, Ruiz P (1999). Clinical relevance of contemporary cultural psychiatry. *J Nerv Ment Dis* 187: 465–471.

American Psychiatric Association (1994). *Diagnostic and Statistical Manual of Mental Disorders, 4th edition (DSM-IV).* Washington, D.C.: American Psychiatric Association.

Angold A (1988). Childhood and adolescent depression, I: epidemiological and aetiological aspects. *Br J Psychiatry* 152: 601–617.

Angold A, Weissman MM, John K et al. (1987). Parent and child reports of depressive symptoms in children at low and high risk of depression. *J Child Psychol Psychiatry* 28: 901–915.

Bird HR (1996). Epidemiology of childhood disorders in a cross-cultural context. *J Child Psychol Psychiatry* 37: 35–49.

Boyle MH, Offord DR, Racine YA, Szatmari P, Sanford M, Fleming JE (1997). Adequacy of interviews vs checklists for classifying childhood psychiatric disorder based on parent reports. *Arch Gen Psychiatry* 54: 793–799.

Brislin R (1986). The wording and translation of research instruments. In: *Field Methods in Cross-Cultural Research,* Lonner W, Berry L, eds. Beverly Hills, CA: Sage, pp. 137–164.

Cronbach LJ, Meehl PE (1955). Construct validity in psychological tests. *Psychol Bull* 52: 281–302.

Edelbrock C, Costello AJ, Dulcan MK, Conover MC, Kala R (1986). Parent-child agreement on child psychiatric symptoms assessed via structured interview. *J Child Psychol Psychiatry* 27: 181–190.
Fleming JE, Offord DR (1990). Epidemiology of childhood depressive disorders: a critical review. *J Am Acad Child Adolesc Psychiatry* 29: 571–580.
Garrison CZ, Addy CL, Jackson KL, McKeown RE, Waller JL (1992). Major depressive disorder and dysthymia in young adolescents. *Am J Epidemiol* 135: 792–802.
Goodman E (1999). The role of socioeconomic status gradients in explaining differences in US adolescents' health. *Am J Public Health* 89: 1522–1528.
Hodges K (1993), Structured interviews for assessing children. *J Child Psychol Psychiatry* 34: 49–68.
Hops H, Lewinsohn PM, Andrews JA, Roberts RE (1990). Psychological correlations of depressive symptomatology among high school students. *J Clin Child Psychol* 19: 211–220.
Iwata N, Roberts RE (1996). Age differences among Japanese on the Center for Epidemiologic Studies Depression Scale: an ethnocultural perspective on somatization. *Soc Sci Med* 43: 967–974.
Kleinbaum DG (1994). *Logistic Regression: A Self-Learning Text.* New York: Springer.
Lahey BB, Flagg EW, Bird HR et al. (1996). The NIMH Methods for the Epidemiology of Child and Adolescent Mental Disorders (MECA) Study: background and methodology. *J Am Acad Child Adolesc Psychiatry* 35: 855–864.
Lewinsohn PM, Hops H, Roberts RE, Seeley JR, Andrew J (1993). Adolescent psychopathology, I: prevalence and incidence of depression and other *DSM-III-R* disorders in high school students. *J Abnorm Psychol* 102: 133–144.
Liberatos P, Link BG, Kelsey J (1988). The measurement of social class in epidemiology. *Epidemiol Rev* 10: 87–121.
Management and Coordination Agency Government of Japan (1997). Conduct and behavior problems. In: *White Paper on Adolescents in 1997.* Tokyo: Management and Coordination Agency Government of Japan.
Marsella AJ, Kinzie D, Gordon P (1973). Ethnic variations in the expression of depression. *J Cross Cult Psychol* 4: 435–458.
Matsuura M, Okubo Y, Kato M et al. (1989). An epidemiological investigation of emotional and behavioral problems in primary school children in Japan. *Soc Psychiatry Psychiatr Epidemiol* 24: 17–22.
Matsuura M, Okubo Y, Kojima T et al. (1993). A cross-national prevalence study of children with emotional and behavioral problems: a WHO collaborative study in the Western Pacific Region. *J Child Psychol Psychiatry* 34: 307–315.
Mezzich JE, Kirmayer LJ, Kleinman A et al. (1999). The place of culture in *DSM-IV. J Nerv Ment Dis* 187: 457–464.
Morita H, Suzuki M, Suzuki S, Kamoshita S (1993). Psychiatric disorders in Japanese secondary school children. *J Child Psychol Psychiatry* 34: 317–332.
Murata T, Sarata Y, Tsutsumi R, Shinpo T, Nakaniwa Y, Kobayashi R (1989). A clinical study of depression in childhood and adolescence. In: *Study of Risk Factors and Treatment for Mental Disorders in Childhood and Adolescence.* Shirahashi K, ed. Tokyo: Ministry of Health and Welfare.

Nunnally JC, Bernstein IR (1994). *Psychometric Theory,* 3rd ed, Nunnally JC, Bernstein IR, eds. New York: McGraw-Hill.

Roberts RE, Attkisson CC, Rosenblatt A (1998). Prevalence of psychopathology among children and adolescents. *Am J Psychiatry* 155: 715–725.

Roberts RE, Lewinsohn PM, Seeley JR (1993). A brief measure of loneliness suitable for use with adolescents. *Psychol Rep* 72: 1379–1391.

Roberts RE, Roberts CR, Chen YR (1997). Ethnocultural differences in prevalence of adolescent depression. *Am J Community Psychol* 25: 95–110.

Rosenberg M (1965). *Society and the Adolescent Self-Image.* Princeton, NJ: Princeton University Press.

Schwab-Stone ME, Shaffer D, Dulcan MK et al. (1996). Criterion validity of the NIMH Diagnostic Interview Schedule for Children Version 2.3 (DISC-2.3). *J Am Acad Child Adolesc Psychiatry* 35: 878–888.

Shaffer D, Fisher P, Dulcan MK et al. (1996). The NIMH Diagnostic Interview Schedule for Children Version 2.3 (DISC-2.3): description, acceptability, prevalence rates, and performance in the MECA study. *J Am Acad Child Adolesc Psychiatry* 35: 865–877.

SPSS (1999). *SPSS,* Japanese version 9.0. Tokyo: SPSS Inc.

Sugiwara M, Mukai T, Kitamura T et al. (1999). Psychiatric disorders among Japanese children. *J Am Acad Child Adolesc Psychiatry* 38: 444–452.

Weisz JR, Eastman KL (1995). Cross-national research on child and adolescent psychopathology. In: *The Epidemiology of Child and Adolescent Psychopathology,* Verhulst FC, Koot HM, eds. London: Oxford Medical Publications, pp. 42–65.

Zimet C, Dahlem N. Zimet S, Farley G (1988). The multidimensional scale of perceived social support. *J Pers Assess* 52: 30–41.

20

Psychological Model for Judicial Decision Making in Emergency or Temporary Child Placement

Mary Ballou, James Barry, Kerry Billingham, Beverly Weinger Boorstein, Chris Butler, Rick Gershberg, Julie Heim, Dorcas Lirianio, Sheila McGovern, Susan Nicastro, Jo Romaniello, Kim Vazquez-Nuttall, and Chris White

In emergencies, family court judges must often make rapid decisions, without benefit of thorough information, that have significant impact on people's lives. Action-oriented research was used to develop a model that would bring psychosocial factors to the legal system for the purpose of enhancing the judicial decision-making process in emergency and temporary child placement cases.

Almost three million reports of child maltreatment were made in 1999 in the United States (U.S. Department of Health and Human Services, 2001), and the importance of collaboration between the legal and mental health systems to address the issue of child maltreatment is widely appreciated. Psychologists, mental health counselors, and social workers, both in and out of the court system, are asked to make assessments, evaluations, and recommendations to assist the court in critical decision making. Forensic evaluations may be conducted for competency to stand trial, civil commitment, criminal responsibility, probation, parole, and juvenile delinquency issues.

One of the most significant areas of collaboration is in probate and family court regarding decisions for care, protection, custody, and emergency placement of children. Judges are crucial in the process of ensuring safety for these children. As Hennessey (1989), in an opinion piece for psychologists, wrote:

> Over three million children are at risk of exposure to parental violence each year. Judges are in the best position to ensure due process of the law and to use their authority to coordinate the efforts of the myriad agencies involved in these cases to prevent

> unnecessary delay and to keep the focus on the child, his habitation or his protection. (pp. 1223–1224)

The action-oriented research used in the present study sought to develop a triage model of psychosocial information to assist probate and family court judges in making emergency and temporary placement decisions when lengthy and thorough evaluations are not possible; it did not seek to arrive at any universal truths about judicial decision making but to provide a tool that judges could use in such situations. This tool, termed the psychological model (PM) uses psychosocial research and data to illuminate critical factors relevant to these judicial decisions.

The study reported here employed a qualitative action-oriented research design (Bogdan & Biklen, 1992; Denzin & Lincoln, 1994; Robson, 1993). Action-oriented research is often motivated by a particular need, may involve integration of both qualitative and quantitative research methods, seeks an efficient plan of action to resolve the identified problem, and holds promise for providing useful, practical, "real world" inquiries. Typical action-oriented research studies seek to develop and evaluate tools, programs, and interventions. Current debates about conventional research methodology within post-modern, critical analyses and feminist perspectives have also guided the method of this study's action-oriented research.

REVIEW OF THE LITERATURE

Over the years, judges and clinicians have used several conceptual models to guide them in their opinions regarding child custody disputes. The "tender years" concept, based on the importance of the mother–infant relationship, held that young children need to be with their mothers (Herman et al., 1997; Kelly, 1994); it survived well into the last century so that, except in extreme cases of maternal unfitness, courts generally awarded custody of young children to the mother (Herman et al., 1997). Today, the prevailing legal test in all states is the "best interests of the child" (Finlay v. Finlay, 1925) meaning that judges must determine which arrangement best fulfills the needs of the specific children involved. The benefit of this model is its focus on the child, but the concept remains ambiguous, since in practice it refers to whatever fosters children's normative development (Herman et al., 1997). Goldstein, Solnit, and Freud (1973) argued that the use of the word "best" implies the existence of a good solution for the courts to find. They developed an alternative judicial presumption, the "least detrimental alternative," which implies that all children involved in custody disputes are harmed to some degree, and the best solution is the one that harms them the least.

Children may need to be removed from their homes and placed in temporary custody for many reasons. They may be at risk for harm or neglect when there is adequate evidence of violence—experienced or witnessed—in the home; sexual abuse; marital conflict; custody battles; abandonment; or caretaker removal due to criminal, mental health, battering, or substance abuse issues (Briere, Berliner, Bulkley, Jenny, & Reid, 1996). Unlike custody evaluations, which should involve numerous sources of data, careful consideration of the child's environment and potential caregivers, and time for thorough review by a judge (Sattler, 1998), emergency placements must be decided quickly, with the child's safety as the main consideration. However sudden the incident or quick the order, it is best to use as many sources of information as possible, including schools and state social services, as well as community, friends, family, and neighbors. In most cases, it is still preferable to place the child with a stable member of the family rather than in foster care or with outside agencies. Judges may also consider the fact that placement can be used by parents and attorneys as a "bargaining chip" with which to manipulate terms of ultimate custody.

Several salient themes and areas in need of attention are evident in the literature on child custody. While research, opinions, and evaluation guides are plentiful, little attention seems to have been paid to the issues around emergency temporary placement.

Custody evaluation decisions have frequently been based on attachment theory; in the early attachment literature, while it was acknowledged that multiple attachments could occur, the mother was usually viewed as the primary attachment figure (Ainsworth, Blehar, Waters, & Wall, 1978; Bowlby, 1969). In more recent models (Field, 1996), attachment has been viewed as a relationship that develops between two or more people as they become attuned to each other, each providing meaningful stimulation and arousal modulation for the other. This model provides for multiple meaningful attachments. In addition, research suggests that attachments made to violent caretakers are harmful to the child despite their closeness (Downs, 1997). Such research challenges the traditional bias toward maintenance of the mother–child relationship that is embedded in the psychological and legal systems, and hence offers expanded possibilities for attachment relationships.

As is clear from the literature, multiple sources of data (Sattler, 1998) and general agreement about important factors are both desirable in custody evaluations. However, among guidelines for custody evaluations, there is little standardization, validity and reliability research, or clear analysis of underlying theoretical assumptions. Most cases use an expert opinion as their main source of information, even though the use of multiple sources has shown greater validity; for example, long-term predictions of violence by expert witnesses have had rather low accuracy (Poythress, 1992). It should also be noted that the various guidelines and custody evaluation protocols are not consistent with legal standards (Jameson, Ehrenberg, & Hunter, 1991).

For temporary removal of children by way of an adjudication of dependency, a preponderance of evidence is required. The higher "clear and convincing" standard, established in Santosky v. Kramer (1982), must be reached, to terminate parental rights and make the child available for adoption (Ash & Derdeyn, 1997). Entry to state care is much easier than is exit through the adoption route, a fact that contributes to the large number of children in long-term foster care (Fein, Maluccio, & Kluger, 1990). Separating 6 to 36-month-old children from their primary caregiver is usually considered especially harmful, since this is a period when the motional scaffolding of the personality is being formed (Halfon, Mendonca, & Berkowitz, 1995). Emergency out-of-home placements or custody decisions are intended to be temporary; however, they often affect decisions for permanent placement. While multiple placements may be necessary, children can experience each as a rejection and this may interfere with their later capacity to form intimate relationships (Rosenfeld et al., 1997). Foster care is considered a temporary intervention that may be used in crisis situations until the child's home is safer or more stable. However, research shows that stays in such temporary care can average five years (Widom, 1991).

The literature suggests that judicial decisions may be inconsistent or based on arbitrary factors or issues unrelated to the most important considerations of a case. Miller et al. (1982) compared the action taken in 288 child abuse/neglect cases referred initially to juvenile court, child welfare agencies, or the police. Emergency placement decisions were found to be closely related to which agency received the initial report, but were not explained by factors such as differences in severity of abuse/neglect, family characteristics, or other attributes of case processing. (An additional issue that arose from the research itself was the inadequate resources in many localities and states for the placement of children in emergency situations. Without such facilities, judges are less likely to order placement outside the home.)

STUDY BACKGROUND

Probate and family court judges are frequently called on to make quick decisions for temporary placement of children in cases of suspected child abuse, battering, and neglect by the caregiver. Kunin, Ebbesen, and Konecni (1992), reviewing court records of 282 disputed child custody cases, found that only two factors directly affected judges in their decisions: the child's preference and the recommendations of the forensic evaluator. The evaluator, a clinician, reports to the court or the attorney involved rather than to the parties being evaluated, and the goal of the evaluation is not to treat the child, but to provide objective information and informed opinions to help the court render a custody decision (Herman et al., 1997).

Because these decisions must often be made quickly, there is not always time for the lengthy process of evaluation by and inclusion of court psychologists, outside consultants, background information, or knowledge of pertinent emotional and behavioral histories. As a result, judges in these cases lack the relevant psychological and historical information necessary to assess the significant psychosocial factors when making emergency placement decisions that will be in the best interest of the child.

The goal of the PM is to provide brief but clinically sensitive information for the process of judicial decision making in such situations. As action research, the model brings two important concepts—utility and psychosocial inclusion—to legal decision making; these are particularly important as trends shift to decisions based on the best interests of the child. Briere et al. (1996) noted that until very recently, decisions in such cases had been weighted toward family preservation as a primary means of serving these interests. These two doctrines are clearly just different points on the same continuum, but the best interests of the child are now considered separately from family preservation, although in many cases family preservation remains in the child's best interests. Utility involves a decrease in the jargon and equivocation that are not uncommon in the social sciences; psychosocial standpoints must be rendered clear and useful. The action research project reported here sought to integrate psychological theory and research results around child-caretaker relationships, on the one hand, with legal requirement, on the other, in order to enhance the decision-making process.

The study enlisted a number of exports to provide information and perspectives on the questions being investigated. Many of the participating judges expressed a need for readily available psychological perspectives in child placement situations. Children have an ambiguous status in the courts because, while their best interests are a guiding force, they have no legal status as citizens. Further, they are often unable to advocate for themselves, yet their caretakers may not be their best advocates. Thus, children become vulnerable to adults, some of whom may be more intent on meeting their own needs than on maintaining those of the children. In addition, the shift from family preservation to recognition of the harm that may result from remaining in violent or otherwise unstable families has led many judges to intervene on the child's behalf (Ackerman, 1995: Briere et al., 1996; Grisso, 1987; Jameson, Ehrenberg, & Hunter, 1991).

METHOD

The study was conducted in two phases that involved several methods of inquiry. During phase 1, the triage model that eventually became the PM was developed by triangulating information from various sources. In phase 2, it was evaluated and revised in successive stages by experts in the field.

The design was based on an interdisciplinary approach that involved the input of several expert stake holders, including family and probate court judges, attorneys, social service workers, child psychologists, psychiatrists, guardians *ad litem,* and court advocates. The overarching goal was to develop a triage model that would be credible and useful and would not neglect any of the multiple factors and stances involved in emergency and temporary child placement decisions. Considerable effort was made to use an ecological approach in identifying pertinent factors so as to align the model more closely to real-life situations.

Phase I

Phase I consisted of an initial needs assessment, followed by a literature review, discussions with practitioners in the community, and observations of courtroom proceedings. From the information thus gathered, a draft of the PM was developed.

Needs Assessment

Two family and probate judges in a family court located in Cambridge, Massachusetts, participated in the needs assessment. Both were senior women jurists with a combined service of 35 years in the court. Prior to their appointments to the bench, both had practiced family law. Initial meetings of researchers and judges established the judges' interest in and collaborative commitment to identifying general problems. During the subsequent 2-hour needs assessment discussion, the judges identified several areas that would benefit from psychological input. Among these was judicial decision making in cases of emergency child placement (another was continuance of restraining orders, and this became the focus of a parallel study not reported here). The judges expressed the need for a set of guidelines for quick evaluation of the factors involved, explaining that time demands in emergency situations often compel decision making without the benefit of adequate information, since thorough evaluations are not possible. Resources and caseload were additional factors reinforcing the need for such guidelines.

Literature Review

Once the specific need was identified and clarified, a critical literature review (summarized in the literature review section, above) was performed. Each study was assessed for embedded assumptions, adequacy of design (including sample, measurement, and statistical appropriateness), and inclusion of complex contextual factors. Questionable studies were excluded from further consideration.

Interviews with Professionals

Discussions were held with a variety of community practitioners from state and local services who viewed the issues at hand from varying disciplinary perspectives.

Contact was first made with representatives of child welfare workers in the division of social services, and with legal aid and school psychologists known to the research team. These participants were asked for additional referrals to experts who would represent differing standpoints of position or belief. Interviews were then conducted with individuals working as guardians *ad litem*, child rights advocates, and child psychiatrists, as well as with a child forensic psychologist/lawyer. The several areas of ambiguity and controversy that were identified during these discussions with professionals informed the development of the PM.

Court Observations

Over a period of 1 month, a member of the research team observed (taking detailed notes) proceedings of the Cambridge Family and Probate court, where petitions were being decided in the courtrooms of five sitting judges in *ex parte* sessions. Three of the five judges were female, two were male, and their experience as sitting judges ranged from 2 to 35 years.

The observations provided an understanding of the organization and functioning of the court, as well as some comprehension of the difficulties faced in decisions about emergency placement of children. Procedures, judgments, and other issues were discussed with the judges. Procedural steps were viewed across the entire process, beginning with the petition and the interview by court personnel, followed by the recommendation to the judge and, finally, by the court hearing and judicial ruling. This material helped to add a practical perspective to the information used in developing the PM. For example, the court observations illustrated the need for a model that provided concise and accessible information compatible with the fast-paced nature of courtroom procedure.

PM Development

Information gleaned from the judges' needs assessments, literature review, interviews with involved professionals, and court observations went into the development of the PM. A number of critical psychosocial factors important to decision making were identified, along with questions that could be used to clarify and elicit information for each factor. The factors and questions were couched, so far as possible, in direct language.

In keeping with the action research method, evaluative feedback on the PM was sought by arranging a meeting with interdisciplinary mental health staff of a court clinic. The court clinic functioned in a variety of capacities: treatment, training, research, and evaluation. Most importantly, it dealt with both scheduled and emergency custody, parenting, and placement evaluations for the judges. The court clinic staff consisted of a psychiatrist, three psychologists, and three social workers. Their ages ranged from late 20s through 50s, and their length of experience with evaluations and clinical work with the family courts varied from 4 to 28 years. The feedback from this group included sharing current and in-press research, clarifying the limits of the PM's use, and affirming the utility of such a tool. Among the PM revisions resulting from this feedback were emphasis on use of the PM only when a more thorough evaluation could not be made, and suggestions for its additional utility as an evaluator in judging the adequacy and thoroughness of reports from outside mental health and social service workers.

A revised draft of the PM was submitted to a court social worker in the Probation and Family Service department of Middlesex County Court (Cambridge), an experienced teacher-counselor-court social worker, whose job was to interview petitioners and make recommendations to the court at the request of the judges. She was well acquainted with judicial needs, processes, and specific requirements. Her feedback helped clarify which information should be readily assessable from court records and from the petition itself. She also advised caution in using psychological language and assumptions; for example, she found the term "empathic response" to be specific psychological language. Her input prompted several further revisions to the PM draft.

Finally, an experienced forensic child clinical psychologist with multicultural competence was consulted about the PM in general terms and terms of ethnic, race, and class sensitivities. His evaluation confirmed the study's critical analysis of the predictive use of correlational research, which can lead to the use of risk factors for profiling—a process that often has discriminatory effects on nondominant and nonmainstream groups. Among the revisions prompted by his evaluation was a focus on adaptive coping skills rather than on material measures of class status, since he pointed out that the use of socioeconomic class has potential for bias.

Phase II

For the second phase of the research project, a focus group was formed for additional evaluation and validation of the credibility and usefulness of the PM and its critical factors. Group participants were experts from a variety of disciplines in the field of child services. Members' feedback also proved helpful in further refining the model and identifying its more subtle implications.

Focus Group

Participants. Focus group members had worked in their respective child service fields for periods ranging from 5 to 30 years. They were chosen to reflect the spectrum of professionals involved with children's justice, welfare, education, and health. Among the final group were a child psychologist, a child psychiatrist, a school psychologist who also served as a guardian *ad litem,* a lawyer, a court advocate for child witnesses to violence, a second guardian *ad litem,* and a Department of Social Services (DSS) worker. Of the 12 focus group participants, nine were white, two Hispanic, and one black; ten were female and two male.

Discussion format. The group session was 2 hours long and had two facilitators. Open-ended questions were used to generate and guide discussion of the PM and its relationship to actual issues in the field, as experienced by group members. Each session was videotaped for later thematic analysis. As a warm-up to each session, participants aired their ideas on the topic and suggested questions to be considered. Next, they were asked to evaluate each of the PM factors. Then they were asked whether any factors were missing from the PM factor presentation, whether any factor should be reconsidered, and in what order of priority factors should be listed.

Discussion content. At the initial focus group discussion, group members gave their impressions and experiences of judicial decision making in emergency and temporary child placement, and identified critical factors that should be considered. During later discussions, they evaluated the relevance of each PM factor presented and ranked the items in order of importance. They also considered any foreseeable impact the model might have on children and families.

Data analysis. Specific recommendations and opinions about factors to be included, priorities, adequacy of concepts, and wording and placement of factors were recorded via both verbal discussion and written questionnaires. These data were later analyzed, along with the research team's videotapes and notes. A thematic content analysis was then performed as follows: (a) two members of the research team reviewed tapes and notes, analyzed content related to focus group questions in each factor area, and noted emerging themes; (b) these were coded in accordance with salient themes evolving from preselected categories drawn from the focus group questions and the PM's critical factors; (c) a third member of the research team cross-checked the thematic assessment for reliability. Thus, the PM and its critical factors were evaluated by confirming the extant critical factors and validating the responsibility and utility of the model.

RESULTS AND DISCUSSION

Phase I

In the first phase, areas of controversy and ambiguity were identified with respect to attachment and custody in general, and child custody placement cases in particular. A recurring theme from all sources was that rational, rule-based decisions, even when tempered with compassion, do not always mix well with the multiple and complex factors behind human behavior. While extreme cases are often easy to decide, less extreme ones are frequently unclear and complex, presenting numerous relevant and conflicting factors. For this reason, the best predictions appeared to be based on information of multiple origins, including those consulted in this first phase of the PM evolution.

Another theme arising from this phase was that mandates to consider the best interests of the children were not simple or one-dimensional. While physical safety was a primary consideration, it was not the only issue; children's physical, psychological, educational, and cultural security must coexist with social and emotional relationships, as well as with financial and educational resources.

Development of Critical Factors

Six areas were initially identified as critical in determining whether children should be placed outside the immediate family in emergency placement cases: (1) caretaker's history of behavior with the child or children in question; (2) caretaker's history of violence, including criminal record; (3) presence of substance abuse; (4) presence of mental illness; (5) caretaker's coping skills and parenting ability; (6) such other concerns as the child's consistency in school and child's and caretaker's expressed wishes. These six areas formed the basis for the PM's catalogue of critical factors, and to each was appended a list of specific questions, the answers to which would provide the information required by judges, either during situations of quick decision making, or as a tool with which to assess results of independent evaluations by court personnel. (The list of factors that constituted the final version of the PM can be seen in Table 20.1.)

Phase II

The second phase validated and confirmed the critical factors identified in the first phase. The content of the videotapes and notes of the focus group

TABLE 20.1
Psychological Model: Significant Factors in Considering Emergency/Temporary Child Placement

Factor	Source	Area of Inquiry
Caretaker's history of behavior/ relationship with child		a. Does caretaker meet the child's physical and maintenance needs (shelter, clothing, supervision, health, education, etc.)? b. Can caretaker understand and appreciate child's world changes over time? Does caretaker demonstrate empathy and compassion? c. Does caretaker make reasonable age-appropriate demands on child? d. Can caretaker put child's needs ahead of own?
Caretaker's history of violent behavior	Information from police, court, school, & social system records; DYS, DSS, employment, military, neighborhood, friends, family, former partners, children, etc.	a. Are there credible reports/claims of violent behavior by caretaker? b. Has child witnessed this violence? c. Does caretaker blame others for own aggravation? d. Does caretaker minimize own behavior (violence, drug use, harshness)?
Caretaker's substance abuse		a. What is current and recent substance-using behavior? b. What is caretaker's attitude about past/ present substance abuse? c. Have all self-reports been verified? d. Have all potential sources of information been consulted (present/ past partners, family, neighbors, community members)? e. Is there a safe, nonusing caretaker?
Caretaker's major mental illness	Confirmed diagnosis of psychosis, bi-polar depression, or personality disorder	a. Is the illness controlled at this time? b. Are there careful and consistent professional evaluations of the condition and treatment? c. How do general behavior and care-taking ability change during exacerbation of the illness? d. Are claims by spouse or family credible and externally documented?

(*Continued*)

TABLE 20.1
(Continued)

Factor	Source	Area of Inquiry
Caretaker's adaptive coping skills		a. How does the caretaker respond to stressors? b. Does the caretaker display persistent blaming and refusal to take responsibility for actions? c. Does child's behavior reflect problems (truancy, overly attached to one parent, poor school performance, acting younger than his/her age)?
Other considerations		a. What are the relative benefits of maintaining consistency for the child in school, neighborhood, community, peers, siblings, and kin? b. Note that child's presentation and expressed wishes may or may not be reality based or in his/her best interests. c. Note that caretaker's presentation and expressed wishes may or may not be reality based or in the best interests of child. d. Would this placement be appropriate for a longer-term arrangement? e. Have legal orders been followed (visitation, child support, etc.)? f. Are there members of extended family who would be appropriate caretakers for the child?

discussions were analyzed by members of the research team, using categorical thematic analysis. Organized into categories, the discussions provided several themes relevant to the phase 1 draft of the PM. After analysis of the focus group material, the draft was modified accordingly.

The analyzed content of the focus group discussions provided useful information for model validation and revision. The discussions in response to questions took place at three levels. At the first level was a general discussion of what currently influenced judges in making emergency child placement decisions; at the second level were thorough and lengthy considerations about ideal custody evaluations; the third level specifically evaluated the draft PM.

The first general question to the group of experts asked them to identify which considerations were important for judges when deciding on placement issues. Those named matched the ones already covered in the draft PM.

For instance, the focus group participants identified the needs of the child in terms of both health and safety, and included both physical and emotional dimensions. The focus group also identified the level of emergency, legal situation, family history, and possible caretakers as important considerations. The concurrence of these general points with information already required in court documents or in the PM provided validation of the model.

The second level of discussion, that of factors in ideal evaluations for custody, identified a wide range of considerations: (1) a thorough assessment of the child (e g., needs, level of functioning, attachment, and risk or danger); (2) historical and caretaker elements, such as empathy, knowledge of development, substance abuse, home environment and interactions: (3) the consequences of failure to act, the presence of other options than removal, and the advisability of imposing as few changes as possible: (4) matching the child's needs and caretaker's abilities in identifying the best caretakers for the child; (5) the use by judges of information from other professionals involved with the children (e.g., school staff, psychological services, social services) in specifying orders within the custody judgments; (6) adequate follow-up on placements.

Discussions supported thorough evaluations and perhaps even legislation and guideline revision. For example, the replacement of the underlying philosophy that children are parents' property with considerations of the child's best interests would call for systemic change, whilst evaluations needed for some of the more complex recommendations would involve experienced professionals. Indeed, these issues of policy change, judicial training, collaboration with other professionals, and valid and reliable custody evaluation guidelines are currently areas in which considerable advocacy and work is being done (Briere et al., 1996). This general discussion was included so as not to lose sight of the big picture, even though the focus of the PM was primarily on emergency placements that lacked the luxury of thorough information-gathering and evaluation.

The third level of discussion addressed this use of the PM in emergency judicial decisions and content analysis offered several themes relevant to the model. These themes were used both to validate the existing draft model and to guide revision.

In considering what could be dropped from the PM, the focus group agreed that without regard to current status and functioning, certain aspects of parents' past history were irrelevant and should be removed. Current or recent violence, substance abuse, criminal behavior, or uncontrolled major mental illness were seen as relevant because they might affect the child and could have a substantial impact on the caretaker's abilities; other elements of past history were seen as unnecessarily complicating and perhaps prejudicial. Herman et al. (1997) suggested that the issue should not be the diagnosis per se, but rather the effect of any psychiatric impairment on the parent–child relationship and whether it was dangerous for the child. They also pointed to the prognosis, the parent's insight into the disorder, and level of compliance with treatment regimens as important.

The PM's factors dealing with major mental illness and substance abuse were accordingly revised to reflect likely prognosis or length of sobriety. However, historical considerations within the factor of violent behavior were not revised, since the triangulated information from the first phase indicated that past history of violent behavior was germane and probably predictive of future behavior. The focus group members did not agree on this point, as they did about substance abuse and other sorts of criminal behavior and mental illnesses: some considered past (though not current) history prejudicial, while others thought of violence as an enduring form of behavior that is often still present even if not reported.

Several themes emerged in response to the question of what new considerations should be included in the PM. Among these were the agenda of the party presenting the petition, recent events, the child's age/developmental stage and wishes, earlier considerations of placements, family history with courts and social services, and resources available. The several important areas of consideration thus revealed were consistent with the custody literature but did not fit well with the factors developed in the model for assisting judges in emergency decision making. Rather, they involved information better gathered by court personnel and presented to the judge with the petition, since they require information-gathering (e.g. police reports, court and school records, and evidence from other family members) and social science judgments (e.g., child's development stage and petitioners' agenda) not readily available to judges through observation and questioning from the bench. In consequence, the description of the PM's use was expanded to include overt suggestions for collection and organization of such information by court personnel prior to the emergency petition, if at all possible.

Once the findings from phase 2 had been incorporated into the draft PM, the utility of the revised version was reviewed by two judges who had not been participants in the study. Both judges worked in the Plymouth County (Massachusetts) family and probate court and were often involved in such cases. Over the course of a 2.5-hour meeting, both reported the PM to be a helpful tool that they intended to start using in their own practices.

CONCLUSION

In general, the content, form, and intent of the PM were judged positively by the experienced professionals who formed the focus group (indeed, they gave enthusiastic support to the notion of such a model). They found it relevant to matters of emergency placements, and endorsed it as a necessary and potentially useful aid to judicial decision making in such placements. In highlighting several areas and identifying additional information important for evaluation and consideration, the group was helpful in further revisions to the PM, including the development of introductory recommendations.

Thus, it seems that action research holds promise for interventions and evaluations in existing situations and with socially useful issues. The PM reported here was created through such research in response to a judicial need: as an aid to judicial decision making it has merit and promise. The wedding of psychosocial factors to legal considerations may not yet exist in legal training, but some justices see an acute need for it, and it may eventually emerge as a result of interdisciplinary collaboration. Such collaboration is certainly in keeping with the philosophy of the best interests of the child, which is becoming more prominent than the philosophy of family preservation that has ruled decision making in the recent past. Moreover, the PM promises utility for judicial decisions by providing perspectives that free judges from unintended consequences of harmful families, adult conflicts, and general social policy that deeply affect the future of children.

Interdisciplinary projects in research and in action are intriguing, and their results can be both useful and distinct from results obtained from the perspective of a single discipline. In this study, research and development of the PM brought together several disciplines, with the result that the model represents both social science and legal studies. Construction and use of the PM could not have been achieved from the perspective of either profession alone.

This project also raised questions and possibilities concerning the training of judges and changes in the focus of mental health and social services. As well as law and the rules of evidence, training of judges in the use of the PM and in the psychosocial thinking behind it seems indicated. So too, psychological evaluations need to incorporate knowledge of legal strictures and real-life needs and time frames. Judges who use the PM in their courtrooms will need to understand that it is appropriate only for emergency child placement decisions, since more thorough and lengthy evaluations and recommendations are preferable when time allows. They will also need to appreciate that other orders besides those of placement and follow-up are necessary to secure the best interests of the child. Other court personnel should also be educated in these respects.

Further development of and research on the PM are desirable. Judicial training, outcome evaluations, and comparative studies of use and nonuse are certainly warranted. Development and evaluation of the model as a potential guide for judges in assessing the adequacy of reports by other professionals is a promising direction of investigation. The perspectives of multiple cultural groups should be explored and addressed. Finally, the model is one that lends itself to adaptation to other areas in which judges must make quick decisions that affect the welfare of vulnerable people; indeed, a companion study to the project reported here included a PM for continuation of restraining orders. This is a particularly likely direction for expansion of the PM, given the present cultural trend of turning to the courts to settle interpersonal disputes. If courts (or courts with the assistance of the social sciences) continue to be used as sites for redress of family dysfunction and discord, then interdisciplinary collaboration is an especially desirable strategy for ensuring the safety and protection of our society's most vulnerable members.

REFERENCES

Ackerman, M. J. (1995). A clinician's guide to child custody evaluations. New York: John Wiley.

Ainsworth, M. D. S., Blehar, M., Waters, E., & Wall, S. (1978). Patterns of attachment. Hillsdale, NJ: Lawrence Erlbaum.

Ash, P., & Derdeyn, A. P. (1997). Forensic child and adolescent psychiatry: a review of the past 10 years. *Journal of the American Academy of Child and Adolescent Psychiatry, 36,* 1493–1503.

Bogdan, R., & Biklen, S. (1992). Qualitative research for education. Boston: Allyn & Bacon.

Bowlby, J. (1969). Attachment and loss: Attachment (Vol. 1). New York: Basic Books.

Briere, J., Berliner, L., Bulkley, J., Jenny, C., & Reid, T. (Eds.). (1996). The APSAC handbook on child maltreatment. Thousand Oaks. CA: Sage Publications.

Denzin, N., & Lincoln, Y. (Eds.). (1994). Handbook of qualitative research. Thousand Oaks, CA: Sage Publications.

Downs, R. K. (1997). A new paradigm for the representation of the children: the kindercentric model. *Divorce Litigation, 9,* 221–234.

Fein, E., Maluccio, A. N., & Kluger, M. (1990). No more partings: an examination of long-term foster family care. Washington, D.C.: Child Welfare League of America.

Field, T. (1996). Attachment and separation in young children. *Annual Review of Psychology, 47,* 541–562.

Finley v. Finlay, 240 NY. 429,148 N.E. 624 (1925).

Goldstein, J., Solnit, A. J., & Freud, A. (1973). Beyond the best interests of the child. New York: Free Press.

Grisso, T. (1987). The economic and scientific future of forensic psychological assessment. *American Psychologist, 42,* 831–839.

Halfon, N. G., Mendonca, A., & Berkowitz G. (1995). Health status of children in foster care. *Archives of Pediatric & Adolescent Medicine, 139,* 386–392.

Hennessey, E. (1989). The family, the courts, and mental health professionals. *American Psychologist, 44,*1223–1224.

Herman, S. P., Dunne. J. E., Ayres, W., Arnold, V., Benedek, E., Benson, R. S., Bernet, W., Bernstein, G. A., Bryant, E., Bukstein, O., Gross, R. L., King, R., Kinlan, J., Leonard, H., Licamele, W., McClellan, J., & Shaw, K. (1997). Practice parameters for child custody evaluation. *Journal of the American Academy of Child & Adolescent Psychiatry, 36,* 57S–69S.

Jameson, B., Ehrenberg, M., & Hunter, M. (1991). Psychologists' rating scales of the best-interest-of-the-child custody and access criterion: a family systems assessment model. *Professional Psychology, 28,* 253–262.
Kelly, J. B. (1994). The determination of child custody. *Future Child, 4,* 121–142.
Kemp, A. (1998). Abuse in the family: an introduction. Pacific Grove, CA: Brooks/Cole.
Kunin, C. C., Ebbesen, E. B., & Konecni, V. J. (1992). An archival study of decision-making in child custody disputes. *Journal of Clinical Psychology, 48,* 564–573.
Miller, B., Shireman, J., Burke, P., & Brown, H. F. (1982). System responses to initial reports of child abuse and neglect cases. *Journal of Social Service Research, 5,* 95–111.
Poythress, N. G. (1992). Expert testimony on violence and dangerousness: roles for mental health professionals. *Forensic Reports, 5,* 135–150.
Robson, C. (1993). Real world research: a resource for social scientists and practitioner-researchers. Oxford, UK: Blackwell.
Rosenfeld. A. A., Pilowsky, D. J., Fine, P., Thorpe, M., Fein, F., Simms, M. D., Halfon, N., Irwin, M., Alfaro, J., Saletskey, R., & Nickman, S. (1997). Foster care: an update. *Journal of the American Academy of Child & Adolescent Psychiatry, 36,* 448–457.
Santosky v. Kramer, 455 U.S. 745 (1982).
Sattler, J. (1998). Clinical and forensic interviewing of children and their families. San Diego, CA: Jerome Sattler.
U.S. Department of Health and Human Services. (2001). Child maltreatment 1999. Washington, D.C.: Government Publishing Office.
Widom, C. S. (1991). The role of placement experiences in mediating the criminal consequences of early childhood victimization. *American Journal of Orthopsychiatry, 61,* 195–209.

Permissions

DEVELOPMENTAL TOPICS

1. Attachment for infants in foster care: the role of caregiver state of mind. Dozier, M., Stovall, K.C., Albus, K., & Bates, B. *Child Development,* 2001, 72, 1467–1477. Reprinted with permission of the Society for Research in Child Development.
2. Child–parent attachment and children's peer relations: a quantitative review. Schneider, B., Atkinson, L., & Tardif, C. *Developmental Psychology,* 2001, 37, 86–100. Copyright 2001 by the American Psychological Association. Reprinted with permission.
3. Separation anxiety in parents of adolescents: theoretical significance and scale development. Hock, E., Eberly, M., Bartle-Haring, S., Ellwanger, P., and Widaman, K. *Child Development,* 2001, 72, 284–298. Reprinted with permission of the Society for Research in Child Development.
4. "I got some swords and you're dead!": Violent fantasy, antisocial behavior, friendship, and moral sensibility in young children. Dunn, J., & Hughes, C. *Child Development,* 2001, 72, 491–505. Reprinted with permission of the Society for Research in Child Development.
5. Ordinary magic: resilience processes in development. Masten, A. *American Psychologist,* 2001, 56, 227–238. Copyright 2001 by the American Psychological Association. Reprinted with permission.

BIOLOGY AND BEHAVIOR

6. Behavior phenotypes for genetic syndromes: a reference guide for psychiatrists. Moldavsky, M., Lev, D., & Lerman-Sagie, T. *Journal of the American Academy of Child and Adolescent Psychiatry,* 2001, 40, 749–761. Copyright 2001 by Lippincott, Williams and Wilkins. Reprinted with permission.
7. Approaches to gene mapping in complex disorders and their application in child psychiatry and psychology. Asherson, P., & Curran, S. *British Journal of Psychiatry,* 2001, 122–128. Reprinted with permission.
8. Functional neuroanatomy of visuospatial working memory in fragile X syndrome: relation to behavioral and molecular measures. Kwon, H., Menon, V., Eliez, S., Warsofsky, I., White, C., Dyer-Friedman, J., Taylor, A., Glover, G., & Reiss, A. *American Journal of Psychiatry,* 2001, 158, 1040–1051. Reprinted with permission.

9. Memory: an overview, with emphasis on developmental, interpersonal, and neurobiological aspects. Siegel, D. *Journal of the American Academy of Child and Adolescent Psychiatry,* 2001, 40, 997, 1011. Copyright 2001 by Lippincott, Williams and Wilkins. Reprinted with permission.
10. Infant temperament and the brainstem auditory evoked response in later childhood. Woodward, S., et al., *Developmental Psychology,* 2001, 37, 533–538. Copyright 2001 by the American Psychological Association. Reprinted with permission.
11. Temperamental contributions to social behavior: the moderating roles of frontal EEG asymmetry and gender. Henderson, H., Fox, N., & Rubin, K. *Journal of the American Academy of Child and Adolescent Psychiatry,* 2001, 40, 68–174. Copyright 2001 by Lippincott, Williams and Wilkins. Reprinted with permission.

CLINICAL ISSUES

12. Pervasive developmental disorders in preschool children. Chakrabarti, S., & Fombonne, E. *JAMA*, 2001, 285, 3093–3099. Reprinted with permission.
13. Open trial of risperidone in 24 young children with pervasive developmental disorders. Masi, G., Cosenza, A., Mucci, M., & Brovedani, P. *Journal of the American Academy of Child and Adolescent Psychiatry,* 2001, 40, 1206–1214. Copyright 2001 by Lippincott, Williams and Wilkins. Reprinted with permission.
14. Two-year prediction of children's firesetting in clinically referred and nonreferred samples. Kolk, D., Day, B., Bridge, J., & Kazdin, A. *Journal of Child Psychology and Psychiatry,* 2001, 42, 371–380. Reprinted with permission.
15. Predictors of later schizophrenia and affective psychosis among attendees at a child psychiatry department. Cannon, M., Walsh, E., Hollis, C., Kargin, M., Taylor, E., Murray, R., & Jones, P. *British Journal of Psychiatry,* 2001, 178, 420–426. Reprinted with permission.
16. A further look at the prognostic power of young children's reports of depressed mood and feelings. Ialongo, N. Edelsohn, G., & Kellam, S. *Child Development,* 2001, 72, 736–747. Reprinted with permission of the Society for Research in Child Development.

CULTURE AND SOCIETY

17. Mother's functioning and children's symptoms 5 years after a SCUD missile attack. Laor, N., Wolmer, L., & Cohen, D. *American Journal of Psychiatry,* 2001, 158, 1020–1026. Reprinted with permission.
18. Effects of war and organized violence on children: A study of Bosnian refugees in Sweden. Angel, B., Hjern, A., & Ingleby, D. *American Journal of Orthopsychiatry,* 2001, 71, 4–15. Reprinted with permission.
19. Multiethnic comparison of adolescent major depression based on the DSM-IV Criteria in a U.S.-Japan study. Doi, Y., Roberts, R., Takeuchi, K., & Suzuki, S. *Journal of American Academy of Child and Adolescent Psychiatry,* 2001, 40, 1308–1315. Copyright 2001 by Lippincott, Williams and Wilkins. Reprinted with permission.
20. Psychological model for judicial decision making in emergency or temporary child placement. Ballou, M., Barry, J., Billingham, K., Boorstein, B., Butler, C., et al., *American Journal of Orthopsychiatry,* 2001, 71, 416–425. Reprinted with permission.

For Product Safety Concerns and Information please contact our EU
representative GPSR@taylorandfrancis.com
Taylor & Francis Verlag GmbH, Kaufingerstraße 24, 80331 München, Germany

www.ingramcontent.com/pod-product-compliance
Ingram Content Group UK Ltd.
Pitfield, Milton Keynes, MK11 3LW, UK
UKHW021719240926
475702UK00029BA/1426

* 9 7 8 0 4 1 5 6 4 5 8 7 4 *